WORKING WITH YOUR DOCTOR

Getting the Healthcare You Deserve

WORKING WITH YOUR DOCTOR

Getting the Healthcare You Deserve

Nancy Keene

O'REILLY™

Cambridge · Köln · Paris · Sebastopol · Tokyo

Working with Your Doctor: Getting the Healthcare You Deserve
by Nancy Keene

Copyright © 1998 O'Reilly & Associates, Inc. All rights reserved.
Printed in the United States of America.

Published by O'Reilly & Associates, Inc., 101 Morris Street, Sebastopol, CA 95472.

Editor: Linda Lamb

Production Editor: Claire Cloutier LeBlanc

Printing History:

> July 1998:   First Edition

Permissions for quotations appear on next page.

ISBN: 1-56592-273-5

To my parents
Bill and Doris Keene
for teaching me to ask questions and search for answers

Contents

Preface

THE ESSENCE OF MEDICINE is the relationship between two humans—you and your doctor. This central relationship—based on trust—evolves with time and experience with one another. Sensitivity to emotional needs and time to listen are essential ingredients in developing a satisfying patient-doctor relationship. However, over-reliance on technology and changes in the economics of medicine threaten this partnership.

How you receive medical care is fundamentally shifting. A narrow focus on the biology of disease and use of cutting-edge technology have developed at the expense of the human dimension of medicine. Large health care organizations are replacing private practices, changing the type of medicine doctors have traditionally offered. Malpractice premiums have forced some doctors to practice defensive medicine—prescribing drugs or tests not because they are needed, but simply to protect themselves. In other cases, managed care organizations reward physicians for restricting care, and sometimes doctors aren't even allowed to tell you about options that are considered too expensive. The fear of malpractice litigation has spawned a climate of distrust and suspicion between doctors and patients. The distinction between life and death has blurred due to a boom in technological wonders, creating complex ethical dilemmas.

In addition, much criticism has been leveled at doctors: that they are arrogant, over-reliant on machines, uncaring. Many people dread going to the hospital because they feel powerless and diminished. Modern medicine can perform technological marvels, but compassion seems to be increasingly rare. Although treatment options abound, informed decision-making is not universal. People are flocking to alternative health care providers in large numbers.

These massive changes in health care delivery may leave you wondering whom you can depend on and who has your best interest at heart. You may be confused about how to be heard or how to thread through a bureaucratic practice or managed care plan. Many patients are learning that they can't assume someone else will take care of things. You can't trust that you can keep the same doctor or that he is unaffected by changes in your insurance plan. You can't rely on your primary physician to always be up to date on the latest treatments of all conditions.

In this changing environment, the passive patients of the past are becoming increasingly rare. But to fully share decision-making with your doctor, you need to know what your health needs are, the best way to meet those needs, and how to get information. You also need to know your own rights and responsibilities, as well as your doctor's. This book will help you create a partnership with your doctor based on trust, respect, and good communication.

Why I wrote this book

My experiences with doctors over the last twenty years have dramatically changed the way I interact with them. When I was hit by a school bus while riding my bicycle to classes in college, I was feisty enough to convince the doctor (he turned out to be the chief orthopedic resident) to try to set and cast my numerous fractures rather than operate and pin the bones back together. But I didn't know enough to have family and friends check out his credentials or make sure I was getting antibiotics (I wasn't, and I developed a serious infection) or even adequate pain relief. I endured months of rehabilitation after the bicycle accident crushed my lower leg and severely injured my arm.

Since those days, I've been hospitalized for many problems ranging from almost silly—surgical excision of a Tanzanian bug which had burrowed into my neck during a trip to Africa—to very serious—major emergency surgery for a ruptured ovarian cyst. One of my babies was born at a teaching hospital which housed laboring mothers in dingy rooms and encouraged anesthesia, while the second was born at a community hospital with comfortable birthing rooms and warm staff. I spent two and a half years advocating for and supporting my young daughter through horrifying but successful treatment for childhood leukemia. In these many encounters with medical professionals, I have enjoyed occasional superb care for which I will be forever grateful, some dreadful care when I was least able to defend myself, and much in the mediocre middle.

I've also seen medicine from the other side. While obtaining a degree in biology in the 1970s, I supported myself with jobs in a large regional medical center affiliated with a medical school. I worked in the blood bank, the coronary care unit, a medical laboratory, and as a member of the IV team. For many years, I volunteered for a busy rescue squad, and moved through the levels of training from emergency medical technician (EMT), to shock trauma technician (ST), to paramedic. I taught both EMTs and STs for several years at a local community college and in the emergency room. I grew to know, and respect, the hospital staff.

What I discovered—often the hard way—is that the two most powerful weapons in dealing with doctors are information and an assertive but friendly attitude. I learned how to access information quickly, use the information to develop questions for my physicians to help me understand my illness and treatment options, and communicate my concerns and decisions. I have forged close, satisfying relationships with my current physicians, and you can, too.

In order to become an empowered patient, you won't need to go through the same kinds of experience and learn from the same mistakes. Nor do you need to depend on superhuman vigilance, in-depth medical knowledge, excellent insurance, or the luck of the draw. You can learn the specific, practical skills you need to get good medical care and to have healing encounters with your doctor.

This book will tell you how I, and dozens of others, made changes in our approach to medical care, with excellent results. More importantly, it will give you the tools you need to make the same kind of changes in your own care.

What this book offers

This book provides the guidance you need to confidently and effectively take on a more active role in maintaining health and seeking out the best medical help when needed. Taking charge requires educating yourself about your condition and learning communication skills to enable you to describe your symptoms to your doctor, ask questions, and negotiate treatment options. Practical steps to improve your relationships with medical caregivers and develop a method of constructive medical decision-making are presented.

This book will help you become an assertive, but understanding, medical care consumer. It will help you comprehend some of the stresses affecting your doctor and provide some strategies for working around the problems. You will learn about your responsibilities as well as your doctor's.

But most of all, the information in this book will help you shed old patterns of submission or aggression toward your doctor. You are hiring a person with specialized knowledge, which you may desperately need, but you are the ultimate decision-maker. You will learn how to form a relationship rather than an uneasy and temporary alliance. The combination of assertive information gathering, questioning, and negotiating described here will help you forge a close partnership with your doctor.

The quotes

The stories in this book are from both patients and doctors. Most are from interviews or unsolicited writings from patients active in online support groups. Many of the stories concern serious conditions or diseases. Why this preponderance of serious stories? Where are the cases of mild psoriasis or stomach flu or inoculations? I intentionally spoke to heavy users of the medical system because they are most likely to encounter problems. If your life or health depends on your interactions with your specialist, problems of communication must get resolved quickly. If the way a radiation technician treats you can result in a fracture of your already weakened and patched-together bones, that interaction deserves some scrutiny. In contrast, if you see a doctor infrequently for routine, minor complaints, you won't have as much invested in the relationship, might not notice as much, and may not feel as compelled to work on a better relationship.

We can learn much from these medical "frequent fliers." They are familiar with the territory, navigate the system frequently, and have much at stake. Their stories are disproportionally presented in order for us to learn from their experiences. They share their own strategies for everything from getting test results quickly to how to forgive a mistake.

Doctors, as well, eloquently describe the joys and frustrations of their relationships with their patients. They labor in the trenches every day, and their words illuminate some of the pressures on the other side of the stethoscope.

All of the stories are absolutely true, although some names have been changed to protect privacy. Every word was spoken or written by a patient, a patient's loved one, a doctor, or a nurse. There are no composites or editorializing—just the actual words of people who wanted to share with others what they have learned in their medical journeys.

How this book is organized

In these chapters, you will learn strategies for each phase of your relationship with your doctor. Chapter 1 looks at why it is in your best interest to become actively involved in your own care. Then you will learn effective methods to evaluate your needs and choose a doctor who will be a good match (Chapter 2). If you are insured by a managed care organization, you will have to take special precautions to ensure a good, working relationship with your doctor (Chapter 3). Once you have found a doctor, clear communication will start the relationship out on the right foot (Chapter 4). In a patient-doctor relationship, many times problems arise because expectations of one side or the other are not realistic or are not being met. Chapters 5 and 6, on physician responsibilities and patient responsibilities, respectively, clarify the roles in this partnership.

In any relationship, friction is inevitable. Chapter 7 gives tips on how to solve problems before they become insurmountable. Chapter 8 explains when it is in your best interest to get a second opinion, and how to find the best doctor for the job. If it is necessary to consider changing doctors, Chapter 9 discusses your options.

Next we look at topics you'll encounter in treatment. Occasionally, all patients are prescribed drugs, tests, or surgery, but close questioning is necessary to determine whether the risks outweigh the benefits (Chapter 10). Next comes a basic guide to taking action if you have been wronged (Chapter 11). Chapter 12 illuminates a subject that is often misunderstood: clinical trials. And Chapter 13 describes in detail how to research your medical condition and share your findings and questions with your doctor.

I have also included five appendices for reference materials: patients' bills of rights, names and addresses of medical specialty boards, sources of information on specific medical conditions, sources of information on general medical topics, and names and addresses of professional medical search organizations. There is a list of additional reading materials if you wish to delve into a topic in greater depth.

Since patients come in two sexes, I did not adopt the common convention of using only masculine personal pronouns. Because I do not like using he/she, I have alternated personal pronouns within chapters. This may seem awkward as you read, but it prevents half of the readers from feeling excluded.

What you will find in this book is a wealth of practical, personal advice to help demystify medicine and enrich your relationship with your doctor. This book will help you return to the historical roots of medicine: a human relationship based on understanding and compassion, not service agreements and high-tech machines.

Acknowledgments

THIS BOOK IS A PRODUCT of twenty years of being a patient, taking care of patients, reading the biomedical and popular literature on medical topics, and communicating with hundreds, perhaps thousands, of medical professionals, patients, parents of patients, and siblings of patients. We have talked in the hospital, on the telephone, in person, in writing, and over the Internet. I am deeply grateful for the insights of every person who has helped me in my many medical journeys, as well as contributed to the development of the ideas and words in this book.

I especially appreciate the many women and men, doctors and patients, who shared their stories in these pages. Their words illuminate the multifaceted patient-doctor relationship. Thank you: Kirsten, Mike, Jan Aguirre, Judith M. Amory, Carol M. Anderson, Dan Aranoff, LaDonna Breidfjord Backmeyer, Kathleen A. Barry, Eve Beattie, Bonnie Bodie, Laurie Borgman, Jeff Bowen, June Brazil, Barbara Brenner, Marianne Brosseau, Victoria E. Brown, Caren Lieberman Buffum, Stephanie Carey, Robert M. Crisp, Ph.D., Claire Diamond, Caroline Diepenbrock, Wendy Dowhower, Steve Dunn, Nancy Dyson, Pam Elliott, Patty Feist, Tracy Flinders, Kate Forgach, Nicholas French, A. Gifford, Roxie Glaze, Deborah Gominiak, Carol M. Goshorn, Karen M. Gray, Ph.D., Kathryn G. Havemann, Wick Hunt, M.D., F.A.C.E.P., Sue Hunter, Laura J. Hutchins, Frank James, M.D., Angela Jensen (for Kirsty), Renee Kaplan, Bill Keene, Doris Springer Keene, Mary Ellen Keene, Mary Kelley, Kathleen Kenny, Madeline Holmes LaBonte, Barbara B. Lackritz (alias Grannybarb), Lauren Dieguez Langford, Nichole Libbey, Guy Litalien, Nancy M. Lucci, Joyce Maltz, Nick Marciano, M.D., Pat Mauceri, Pamela McAllister, Trish Miller, Ruth Natanson, cancer survivor and social worker, Ann Newman, Mark Newman, Robin Aspman-O'Callaghan, M.Ed., Leah Paley, Robert T. Palladino, Bob Panoff, Sandra Pilant, Lynne A. Rief, Steve Sapovits, Judith M. Schumann, Mark W. Schumann, Connie Scott, Brenna Scoville, Kirsten Skeehan, Rosanne Skopp, Cathi Smith, Theresa Smith, M.A., Anne Spurgeon, Doreen Stakor, Mark W. Steinberg, N.D., Nan

Suhadolc, Andrea J. Thomas, R.N., David Turetsky, Ralene Walls, Carol Weimer, Pam Went, Kimbra Suzanne Wilder, Patti Wiley, Mary Lee Stout Zapor, Lynn Zimmerman, and those who wish to remain anonymous.

Many people from diverse disciplines provided valuable comments and suggestions on various parts of the manuscript. Thank you, Steve Dunn, Patty Feist, Wendy Harpham, M.D., Kathryn Havemann, J.D., Honna Janes-Hodder, Doris Keene, Bill Keene, Linda Peeno, M.D., and Ralene Walls, and many others who carved time from busy schedules to review and improve the book.

Special thanks to editor Linda Lamb for gentle suggestions, vast knowledge, and inspiration; to editorial assistant Carol Wenmoth, for her attention to detail and unfailing good cheer; and to Tim O'Reilly, publisher and friend, for his belief in and support of the patient-centered guides.

Any errors, omissions, misstatements, or flaws in the book are entirely my own.

CHAPTER 1

Taking Charge of Your Health Care

Education is a powerful weapon. In medicine, it can save your life.

—Robert Arnot, M.D.
The Best Medicine

THE PATIENT-PHYSICIAN RELATIONSHIP—grounded in mutual trust and compassion—is the center of medicine. Yet, often patients spend more time finding a car mechanic than they do a competent doctor. When they do go to a doctor, many find themselves passively following the doctor's advice and sometimes resenting it, or worrying whether they are getting the best available treatment. Very few ever question the doctor or request second opinions. Even fewer double-check dosages or read up on prescribed drugs.

You need to be involved to get the best medical care. A crucial first step is to invest the time to find a doctor who is smart, caring, and up to date. You're also more likely to trust a doctor who really knows you—one who knows your medical history, understands your needs, and talks to you about your likes and dislikes. Research has shown that patients who work as partners with their physicians feel more in control, tolerate treatments well, and take more responsibility for their health. Moreover, if you have a close relationship with your doctor, you are more likely to be diagnosed accurately and recover quickly.

When doctors know their patients well, they tend to spend more time with them and devote more resources to their problems. They are also less likely to make mistakes and more likely to research options. Forming a partnership with your physician will benefit you in numerous ways.

But how can you be sure that you are getting good health care? Medical care in the United States ranges from superior to abysmal. We have the finest research and technology in the world, yet one of the highest infant mortality rates of all the industrialized nations. Life expectancies range from the 40s to the 80s, depending on where you live, your genetic background, and how you live your life. In addition, the health care system in the U.S. is undergoing rapid and fundamental change, which may profoundly affect the level of care you receive.

Despite the very effective technologies available that have greatly increased life spans and pushed previous scourges such as diphtheria and polio to near extinction, more and more people are becoming disillusioned with modern medicine. Some describe feeling like nonpersons, mere collections of body parts and assortments of physical processes that various specialists focus on. They feel that the person in the body—and the life experiences, thoughts, and values that make up that person—are ignored by the great medical machine. They feel diminished.

Historical views of physicians

Today, patients have access to sophisticated medical information from books, health newsletters, online information, and home kits that test everything from blood pressure to ovulation. Many illnesses can now be effectively treated, and advances in technology—from gene therapies to in-utero surgery—proliferate.

Why then, with longevity increasing and cures available for a multitude of diseases, are patients abandoning the medical profession in droves? As Eric Cassell, M.D., says in *The Healer's Art*:

> *The tools are magnificent; the drugs are fantastically effective; the electronic technology is a wonder to behold. And yet in the midst of this justified hyperbole we find it necessary to see what has gone wrong.*[1]

Indeed, many things have gone wrong or stayed wrong. In distancing themselves from patients and withdrawing into rational discussion of disease processes, doctors began to lose a vital therapeutic tool: the bond of physical touch. For centuries, touch was employed by physicians to comfort and diagnose, although today it has been almost completely replaced by machinery. Medicine, in some ways, has become a soulless technology. Lewis Thomas, in *The Youngest Science*, states:

> *Many patients go home [from the hospital] speedily, in good health, cured of their diseases. In my father's day, this happened much less often, and when it did, it was a matter of good luck or a strong constitution. When it happens today, it is more frequently due to technology.*

There are costs to be faced. Not just money, the real and heavy dollar costs. The close-up, reassuring, warm touch of the physician, the comfort and concern, the long, leisurely discussions…are disappearing from the practice of medicine, and this may turn out to be too great a loss for the doctor as well as the patient. This uniquely subtle, personal relationship has roots that go back into the beginnings of medicine's history, and needs preserving. Once lost, even for as short a time as one generation, it may be too difficult a task to bring it back again.[2]

There are numerous books that describe the increased technology, decreased time, and odd lack of humanity in Western medicine. Max Lerner, in his book *Wrestling with the Angel*, sums it up:

There are still authentic doctors, young and old, who retain their healing touch and whose authority shines through, evoking a responsive chord of life-affirming self-belief in the patient. I can bear witness to this in instances of my own experiences with my doctors. I wish it were true of more doctors, in the service of more patients.

Why isn't it? Part of the key may lie in the freezing of the roles of both the doctor and patient, the doctor's in presenting his diagnoses and therapies from on high, the patient's in accepting them passively. Whatever interaction takes place is routine. Nothing touches a spring of affirmation in the other. The entire model tilts toward the rigid.[3]

In addition to the loss of human touch, a second problem is medical education itself. One cannot produce caring, thoughtful individuals by running them through a gauntlet of insults, exhaustion, and depersonalization. Young doctors work thirty-six hour shifts, learn from other student doctors to call less-than-desirable patients "crocks" and "gomers" (an acronym for "get out of my emergency room"), and are encouraged to value high-tech interventions over prevention. Too often, patients are referred to as "the liver in room 201." Many medical students who begin with idealistic goals of helping people and providing a service to humanity end up swallowing the hidden curriculum of treating people as objects. In *Gesundheit!*, Patch Adams, M.D., describes this phenomenon.

The greatest shock I experienced in medical school came during discussions with teachers about the doctor-patient relationship. The overwhelming majority emphasized the importance of professional distance. This meant maintaining a scientist's detachment and dealing with

patients as if they were experiments in a laboratory. The "distance ethic"
was extended to the wards, where doctors described patients as diseases,
lab values, signs, symptoms, or treatments. I was amazed that a group of
doctors "on rounds" could hover around the bed of a human being,
staring at, poking, and even undressing him or her with little more con-
sideration than was given to dogs in the physiology lab.[4]

In addition, most medical students are ill-equipped to deal with health, as they learn little about nutrition, exercise, or other methods to prevent illness. Perri Klass, a pregnant Harvard medical school student, wrote in *A Not Entirely Benign Procedure*:

In our reproductive medicine course, the emphasis was on the abnormal, the pathological. We learned almost nothing about normal pregnancy; the only thing said about nutrition, for example, was said in passing—that nobody knows how much weight a pregnant woman should gain, but "about 24 pounds" is considered good...We learned nothing about any of the problems encountered in a normal pregnancy; the only thing said about morning sickness was that it could be controlled with a drug...We learned nothing about the emotional aspects of pregnancy, nothing about helping women prepare for labor and delivery. In other words, none of my medical school classmates, after the course, would have been capable of answering even the most basic questions about pregnancy asked by the people in my childbirth class.

The professor discussed ectopic pregnancy, spontaneous abortion, and major birth defects. I was eight months pregnant. I sat there rubbing my belly, telling my baby, don't worry, you're okay, you're healthy. I sat there wishing that the course would tell us more about normal pregnancy, that after memorizing all of the possible disasters, we would be allowed to conclude that pregnancy itself is not a state of disease.[5]

A third problem is increasing specialization. The knowledge base is so vast in medicine today that one person simply cannot know it all. The economics of medical education encourages young doctors to enter subspecialties in order to pay off onerous debts incurred during the long years of training. Professors in medical school often denigrate the general practice specialties and encourage young doctors to become specialists. Doctors working in preventative medicine or public health are held in lower esteem than those in surgery or cardiology. The emphasis on "interesting" cases—rare and complex diseases or disorders—predisposes many students to long for the odd, the obscure. The subtle, personal relationships of the past, based on years of care and in-depth conversations, are increasingly rare.

In addition to the many changes wrought by advances in science and technology, another fundamental shift is occurring in medicine that has the potential to dramatically alter not only the care you receive, but also the doctor who provides it. Managed care is on the scene, and all the rules are changing—fast. Many patients are finding that they must change doctors under the rules of their plan, or, even if they keep the same doctor, he is operating under guidelines—based on cost-effectiveness—created by an insurance company. A battle is shaping up between managed care organizations and doctors, many of whom are forming their own provider groups to bypass the insurance companies. Meanwhile, large HMOs continue to buy up smaller, sometimes nonprofit groups.

Where does this leave you, the patient? Probably worried. But you have more power than you think. In these changing times, you can affect the quality of your health care by taking an active role. The people who are the most assertive, who arm themselves with the most information and talk to their doctors, are going to get the best care.

The first step in assessing your current care is understanding how the doctor's agenda may differ from yours.

How doctors' decisions are influenced

Patients often assume that their illness is the doctor's sole concern, and that decisions are based strictly on what is best for them. This is not always the case. Doctors' decisions are based on a host of competing interests and pressures, in addition to being directly affected by human problems such as lack of sleep or family conflicts. There are many agendas that can consciously or unconsciously affect doctors' treatment of patients.

Time and money

Providing high-quality care for patients takes time. Spending more time with each patient, however, means seeing fewer patients and making less money. Practicing state-of-the-art medicine also requires keeping up with new developments in medicine by reading journals or attending conferences, both of which take time away from patients, resulting in lower incomes or less free time.

I get the bum's rush every time I go to my doctor. I wait forever, then I'm whisked into a cubicle, spend ten minutes getting examined, then he's gone without even making eye contact. I feel like I can't even get a word in without ruining his day. I don't like it.

Choices on how to allocate limited time and how the doctor is paid directly affect medical decision-making. Because most fee schedules pay more for tests and procedures than for taking histories, doctors who spend a lot of time with patients doing thorough examinations and learning about the patient's family, eating habits, exercise program, and stresses make less money. Writing prescriptions takes less time than discussing lifestyle changes, but it allows doctors to see more patients daily, thereby increasing incomes. Giving an electrocardiogram generates more income than listening to the heart; doing a coronary bypass is more lucrative than assessing the patient's eating and exercise habits and encouraging healthy changes; removing a wart pays more than reassuring a patient that it will do no harm.

Doctors who get paid by the procedure, especially if they have a financial interest in the equipment or facility, tend to order more tests than doctors on straight salaries. On the other end of the spectrum, HMOs often tie the doctor's salary or bonuses to how well he keeps costs down, sometimes causing inappropriate withholding of tests or procedures. Chapter 3, *Getting What You Need from Managed Care*, explains this potential conflict in detail. Thus, there may be factors other than concern for your health that influence the medical care you get from your doctor.

One doctor sums up the reasons for taking the time to form a partnership with your doctor:

I think what's going on in medicine today is antithetical to what medicine really should be. To me, medicine is a relationship between two people, and that relationship is based on trust and understanding. It fascinates me that in double blind, controlled drug studies, about 30 percent of the people in the placebo group get better. That's a powerful phenomenon. Part of that, I am convinced, is the trust and confidence of the patient in the advice and human relationship with their doctor. What's happening in our society is that in the last twenty years doctors have bought into the idea that what they do is a commodity. Far too often, the doctor-patient relationship is reduced to this technical fix, assembly line medicine. Quite frankly, that's not medicine. Rather, medicine is a healing event that requires the participation of both people and knowledge of one another. The patient has to know and trust me. There is a need for me to reveal some of who I am to a patient—and they reveal who they are—in order for healing to take place. And that takes time.

Philosophy

Doctors differ enormously on their philosophy of practice—that assemblage of beliefs, opinions, and values that color all decisions. A woman with breast cancer could consult a surgeon, an oncologist, and a radiologist, and get three completely different opinions of how to treat her disease. In general, doctors tend to treat as they were taught. Hence, surgeons generally recommend operations, internists give drugs, radiologists have a bias toward X-ray treatment. Not only are there big differences between individual doctors, there are striking regional differences as well. Where you live, your gender, and the color of your skin may dictate the type of medical treatment you receive.

Age, sex, race, and address affect medical care

The Harvard Medical School Department of Health Care Policy studied variations in the use of coronary angiography (X rays of the heart after injection of a radioactive substance) in patients who had suffered a heart attack. They found that the procedure was used most for young, white males. Blacks had less access to the procedure than did whites; women were less likely to receive the procedure than were men. The racial differences were most pronounced in the southeastern states. Also, older patients were less likely to receive the procedure. There were also wide variations among states; for instance, patients in Montana were three times more likely to have the procedure than were patients in Rhode Island.[6]

Most patients mistakenly assume that treatment plans are based solely on scientific fact. Opinion, that thing that everyone has one of, determines treatment more than you might realize. In fact, the doctor's philosophy of practice colors decisions in extremely significant ways.

- **Importance of prevention**. Some doctors emphasize a healthy lifestyle to prevent or control illness. If you see such a physician, he might recommend changes in diet, smoking, alcohol consumption, and exercise to control your coronary artery disease. Other doctors, with a different philosophy regarding prevention, might simply refer you to a surgeon for a coronary artery bypass. Some patients are unwilling to take responsibility for their health and wish for a "magic bullet" in pills or surgery; others desire to try all preventative methods first. Try to pick a doctor whose views on preventative care match yours.

- **Personal value system**. You may be the type of person who needs to research your condition to feel comfortable, while others want to pick a competent doctor and rely on her wisdom. To find a good match, you'll need to discuss your values with your doctor and express clearly what you want from her.

> *My primary care doctor told me something of immense value several years ago when I needed to see a specialist for an acute condition. She said, "We need to pick your doctor carefully because I know you. You are an information seeker. We need to make sure that we find someone philosophically aligned with you or you are going to clash. You know, doctors occupy a continuum of medical philosophies, and you need to find a match. There's also the question of different communication styles—we need to find a good talker. Let's make sure we find the right person." That advice has guided me for years. I put in the time now, and reap the benefits of good medical relationships later, when I really need them.*

Other kinds of mismatched values can also cause problems. If your gynecologist staunchly opposes abortion for any purpose, you might not be referred for genetic testing early in pregnancy or be given the option of amniocentesis. Conversely, if your religious beliefs forbid the use of blood products, your surgeon might refuse to operate without your consent to receive blood if necessary. A mismatch in values between doctor and patient almost guarantees conflict.

- **Level of intervention**. Some doctors—whose motto is "life at all costs"—aggressively treat disease until all options are exhausted. Some patients desire this no-holds-barred approach. Other doctors are more selective in their use of technological intervention and experimental drug therapies. Patients of these doctors would probably be given a range of options, with the risks and benefits of each discussed. A good match in medical aggressiveness helps to create an effective patient-physician partnership.

- **Patient roles**. Patients are sometimes equal partners in their medical relationships. The doctor presents all known facts, gives his opinion and explains its basis, answers the patient's questions, and respects the patient's right to make the ultimate decision. Other doctors give only partial information and restrict or redirect questions. Some doctors make all decisions for their patients and expect submissive compliance. A few doctors expect to be treated as the ultimate medical authority, revered and obeyed. In his book *Doctors and Patients: What We Feel About You*, Peter Berczeller, M.D., states his position:

> Our expectation is that all patients will give us immediate obedience and respect—and 100 percent of the time at that! ...besides, if we have sacrificed so much of our time and energy for the ultimate sake of our patients, should we not at least be rewarded by their keeping quiet and doing what we tell them to do?[7]

Unless you take the time to find out, you won't know whether your doctor's philosophy is autocratic or democratic.

Curiosity

Doctors are often intellectually curious, especially when dealing with rare or perplexing illnesses or when training medical students. In these cases, tests and procedures are often performed to find out more about a disease than to influence treatment. In some settings, a patient may be treated as simply a body; his illness may be viewed as a puzzle to solve rather than something that is impacting his life. Doctors and medical students sometimes forget that tests are expensive and often cause side effects. Moreover, adults need to miss work, plan time to recuperate, make child care arrangements, and endure whatever tests are given. Often these issues are not discussed or even considered prior to orders being written. Sherwin B. Nuland, M.D., in his book *How We Die*, labels this curiosity:

> The quest of every doctor in approaching serious illness is to make the diagnosis and design and carry out the specific cure. This quest, I call The Riddle, and I capitalize it so there will be no mistaking its dominance over every other consideration. The satisfaction of solving The Riddle is its own reward, and the fuel that drives the clinical engines of medicine's most highly trained specialists. It is every doctor's measure of his own abilities; it is the most important ingredient in his professional self-image...Every medical specialist must admit that he has at times convinced patients to undergo diagnostic or therapeutic measures at a point in illness so far beyond reason that The Riddle might better have remained unsolved.[8]

Boredom

Some doctors are bored. After the excitement of training in large medical centers where many rare and complicated cases are thoroughly studied and discussed, opening a practice can be a letdown. Doctors who provide primary care spend day after day explaining why antibiotics won't work for viral infections or how to prevent constipation in children. For a newly pregnant young woman, each visit to the doctor is a chance to discuss every aspect of the exciting pregnancy, but for the obstetrician it may be just another time to recite the litany that he has recited thousands of times before. Many patients notice a difference in treatment when they develop a challenging illness or a rare abnormality.

> I had an OB/GYN who I thought just had a lousy bedside manner
> (and only later found out he had a drinking problem). He was pretty
> darn bored during my first pregnancy. Then I had an inverted uterus
> during delivery (a one-in-a-million complication in women, although
> rather more common in dairy cows). He became very interested in me
> then, as were all his colleagues; I had become an interesting case. All
> during my next pregnancy, he was also very attentive. I couldn't shake
> the feeling that he was hoping that I'd have an inverted uterus again, and
> become an even more rare statistical anomaly.

Teaching

The interests of doctors and patients may sharply diverge when trainee doctors are involved. Many sick patients at training hospitals are familiar with the discomfort associated with having five pairs of hands palpate a tender abdomen or having a student struggle to draw blood from a small vein. In *Patient Beware*, Cynthia Carver, M.D., describes an experience that happened to her in a maternity clinic prior to her entry to medical school:

> Off went my clothes, and on went the little white gown. The nurse
> helped me up onto the examining table and put my feet in stirrups...and
> draped a sheet over me. The sheet prevented me from seeing anyone
> seated between my legs, but left my genitals exposed to the world at
> large...
>
> After ten minutes or so the doctor came in, and to my relief he was
> middle-aged, friendly and non-threatening. He examined me gently but
> thoroughly, and as he finished told me that everything was fine.

I started to withdraw my feet from the stirrups, but the doctor stopped me, saying, "Just stay there for a minute. I'd like another doctor to check you." ... Suddenly there were four young men standing there, all gazing at my bottom as he pointed out the details of my anatomy. He then relinquished his place between my legs to one of the young men and instructed him to repeat the pelvic exam. I was horrified. I started to cry.[9]

Many people do not realize that training of student doctors extends into the operating room, where senior physicians supervise residents as they learn their trade. All students have to practice to become competent, but you can be in charge of when, where, and how by scrutinizing consent forms and discussing all aspects of your care with your primary doctor.

When my husband needed delicate surgery on the nerves in his arm, we traveled over a hundred miles to go to a surgeon with an excellent reputation for hand and arm surgery who operated at a large teaching hospital. When we went in for the pre-op visit, we were seen by two residents, one of whom handed us a two-sided piece of paper covered with small print. Buried on the second side was the section in which patients gave permission for the surgeon "and his colleagues" to perform the surgery. When we told the two young residents that we had traveled a great distance to have Dr. D. perform the surgery, one became quite frosty and told us huffily that he had "two and one-half years experience" and his senior resident had "six years experience." When you are in your seventies and some fresh-faced youngster crows about his two and one-half years of experience, it's not too impressive. He was obviously offended that we would question his credentials, or worse, refuse to let him perform this surgery. Nevertheless, we scratched out "and his colleagues" and had Dr. D. do the surgery.

When you are treated in a teaching hospital, most of the orders for your care are written by doctors-in-training—residents or interns—who are fearful of missing anything that their instructors might point out. Young doctors routinely work more than 100 hours each week, are required to memorize huge volumes of information, and sometimes experience a boot camp mentality in which humiliation and contempt prevail. This training frequently results in exhausted, fearful young men and women who are afraid of making mistakes and do everything in their power to cover all possibilities. Of course, these multiple tests and procedures protect the student from the wrath of his instructor, but may not be in your best interest.

Politics

Political problems of all stripes can affect the treatment a patient receives from a doctor. HMOs sometimes restrict a physician's ability to refer patients for specialized care or may restrict referrals to a specialist within the same plan—who may not be the best person for the job. Hospitals may discourage or even forbid referrals to physicians not on staff.

Office politics sometimes affects patient care. For instance, doctors who are extremely competitive may feel uneasy asking a colleague for an opinion, even if they are unsure of a diagnosis or best treatment. Residents may order unnecessary tests in order to impress their instructor. A physician who also is a researcher may encourage, sometimes even pressure, patients to enroll in a clinical trial to further his own professional goals rather than presenting options and allowing patient choice. For-profit hospitals sometimes put making money above providing good patient care. Political pressures such as these may consciously or unconsciously drive doctors' decision-making.

In *M.D.: Doctors Talk About Themselves*, one physician describes the rapidity of changes wrought by politics at his hospital:

> The children's hospital where I work used to be run by doctors; now it's run by businessmen. We used to advertise our excellence by publishing in journals, by teaching, and by presenting our studies in medical meetings. Now we do marketing. At the same time that the hospital is telling us we've got to make money to keep our departments going, we're told we have to publish or perish to keep our academic appointments. I'm at a point where I can't staff my department as I should. And all of this has happened in the last five years. The speed has been unbelievable.

> We used to work for patients. It was our responsibility to do as well by them as we could. We were their advocates. No doubt we'd sometimes screw up or order too many tests, and some of us were probably lousy doctors, but the bottom line was that we were working for them. Now we're working for the company that owns the hospital.[10]

Defensive medicine

Doctors do not want to be sued. To lower their risk of getting sued, doctors often order unnecessary tests and prescribe unnecessary drugs. They want to be able to show that they did everything possible, they covered all the bases.

Studies show, however, that this type of defensive medicine does not lower the risk of getting sued. What most determines whether a doctor is sued is whether the patient likes the doctor and feels cared for.

Physicians' perceptions on the risk of being sued

A group of scientists at Harvard University studied physicians' perceptions on the risk of being sued and how this perception affected their practice. They found that physicians in the study estimated that 19.5 out of 100 of their colleagues would be sued in a given year, approximately three times the actual risk. In addition, the doctors estimated that 60 percent of problems caused by negligence would result in a suit, which is 30 times higher than the actual risk. Fewer than 2 percent of the patients in New York injured by negligence actually filed malpractice claims. Physicians responded to their fear of malpractice suits by increasing their use of tests and procedures, spending more time discussing the risks of medical care, spending more time on paperwork (e.g., the patient's chart), and reducing the scope of practice.[11]

Unfortunately, defensive medicine has thrown out the concept of "watchful waiting." In the past, doctor and patient would agree to keep an eye on the condition, which would often resolve with time. Not anymore. Now, defensive medicine inflates the cost of medical care and subjects patients to the risks, discomforts, and expense of unnecessary tests and drugs.

Impaired doctors

Impaired doctors are nothing new. However, the stresses of being a doctor are bad and getting worse. The rise of HMOs is dramatically changing health care delivery and making some physicians extremely uncomfortable. Many third-party payers are second-guessing physicians' judgments and often refusing to pay for prescribed treatment. Paperwork requirements increase constantly. Patients are more educated and far more demanding than in the past. In addition to these stresses, doctors with addictive tendencies may be sorely tempted by the availability of drugs at their hospitals.

Most state medical societies have recognized the problem of drug usage by doctors and have responded by implementing special treatment programs for impaired physicians. A recent editorial in the *Journal of the American Medical Association* recommends:

> All [medical] societies should follow the lead of the 25-plus states that now prohibit physicians from prescribing controlled substances for themselves or for their immediate families. Second, the physicians of physicians should be encouraged to seek urine tests for opiates and blood tests for sedatives in any physician patient who presents as a diagnostic enigma. Third, hospitals should have procedures in place to refer addicted physicians for appropriate treatment, including well-supervised and long-term random screening of their urine for drugs. Fourth, I propose that some medical staffs establish trial programs of random urine screening tests for all of their members.[13]

Taking charge will improve your medical care

Active participation improves medical care dramatically. By choosing your doctor carefully, you will be assured of her competence, philosophy, ability to communicate well, and affiliation with an excellent hospital. You will establish a relationship based on shared history and respect and, over time, will feel comfortable with both your doctor and your care. Ideally, your doctor will help you devise a long-range health plan to prevent illness to the extent possible. When you are ill, you will have a doctor who will coordinate all referrals, tests, and medications to ensure that you get the care you need, but no more.

Being an involved partner in your medical care has far-reaching consequences.

Mistake prevention

Mistakes occur because human beings provide medical care. An often-
quoted Harvard study estimates that 80,000 people in the U.S. are killed
annually by medical errors.[14] Being involved helps you catch the inevitable
mistakes.

Mistake causes death of health columnist

When 39-year-old Betsy Lehman, health columnist for the *Boston Globe*
and mother of two small children, died suddenly at the world-renowned
Dana-Farber Cancer Institute, it was not a tragic result of her breast cancer.
Rather, it was due to a horrifying mistake: an overdose of the powerful
anticancer drug cytoxan. A physician at the hospital misinterpreted the
amount of the toxic drug to be given and wrote an order for four times the
correct dose. For four days, Betsy Lehman was given the massive overdose,
unquestioned by the three seasoned pharmacists filling the prescriptions,
the supervising physicians who countersigned the deadly order, or the
nurses giving the drugs. In addition, she was given a fourfold increase of
two other drugs, one to protect her bladder—at the quadrupled dose, the
effects on humans are unknown—and the other to increase the toxicity of
the cytoxan.

Despite horrendous side effects, including vomiting tissue, abnormal blood
results, two electrocardiograms showing damage to the heart, and Lehman's tearful entreaties that something was wrong, no one caught the mistake. She died alone in her hospital bed on December 4, 1994.[15]

In case you are starting to think that hospitals corner the market in errors,
they don't. A recent study showed that prescriptions presented to 100 randomly selected pharmacies resulted in 24 dispensing errors, of which 4 were
clinically significant. In addition, oral and written information given to
patients regarding their prescriptions was found to be woefully inadequate.[16]

Doctors, nurses, and pharmacists all make mistakes. The information contained in Chapter 10, *Questions to Ask About Tests, Drugs, and Surgery*, will help you spot these errors and correct them before they harm you or your loved ones.

Having a competent doctor

The minute you walk into a hospital and state that you have no primary physician, you're playing the medical equivalent of Russian roulette. You may get a top staff physician with excellent skills or a student just out of medical school. Unless you have planned ahead and chosen your doctors carefully, you are at a big disadvantage in obtaining top quality care.

> *I needed emergency surgery for a ruptured ovarian cyst. I was lying in an exam room, while a resident tried to start an IV. Another person in a white coat came in, and immediately bumped into a tray of instruments, sending them flying. He then introduced himself as my anesthesiologist, to which I replied, "No, you're not." I knew it was a training hospital, and the last thing I wanted was an uncoordinated trainee anesthesiologist. He looked shocked and said, "Yes, I am." I told him, the other resident, and the two nurses in the room to leave and send in my husband for five minutes. They said we didn't have time because I was losing blood and needed to get into the operating room. I told them that I wouldn't give permission for the surgery if I didn't have a few minutes with my husband. They really didn't seem to know what to do, so I said kindly, "Please just leave the room," and they left. As soon as my husband came in, I said, "Go page an attending anesthesiologist." Luckily, he knew the head of anesthesia (he had gone to school with his son). He rushed out to page him and, remarkably, ran into him in the hall. He asked him to do my anesthesia, and the doctor kindly said yes.*

An important component of choosing a competent doctor is choosing the right health plan. Often, insurance or network limitations narrow the choices before you even have a chance to consider the possibilities. If you choose a low-cost health plan in order to save money, you usually sacrifice either quality of care or number of doctors from which to choose. Chapter 2, *Finding the Right Doctor*, and Chapter 3, *Getting What You Need from Managed Care*, discuss these issues in detail.

Having a doctor with whom you feel comfortable

Remember when you were home sick as a small child how comforting it was when your mother would give you chicken soup and ginger ale, tuck in your blankets, and smooth your hair back from your hot forehead? Most of us have memories of comfort food and actions that soothed us when we were sick. Without implying that a doctor should act like a parent, having a doctor with whom you feel comfortable provides those same anticipated comforts. You expect to see the same face and hear that familiar voice. Just those expectations can help you feel better.

Contrast those feelings with the worry that accompanies a first visit to an unknown doctor when you are feeling feverish and ill. You wonder if he will realize how really sick you are and react with warmth. You don't know what to expect, and it can leave you feeling bereft in your time of need. What happens if the encounter is less than satisfactory? You may be too ill to defend yourself; you may feel powerless, diminished, and sicker.

Taking the time before you are sick to find a doctor and cultivate a satisfying relationship with him will ensure that you have a competent and comfortable person to turn to when you are ill.

> My daughters and I always look forward to a trip to the pediatrician's office—even though someone usually has to get sick before we go. Dr. M. and his nurse are always cheerful and pleased to see us. They have a gentle way with both children. Whenever there is a problem with insurance or laboratory results, we work together to solve it. When things are tough, they give us a hug before we leave. I trust them and depend on them.

Becoming educated on medical issues

Doctors' responsibilities include educating patients about the causes and treatments of various medical conditions. Unfortunately, patients don't always get the full picture from their doctors for all of the reasons discussed earlier. Being a savvy patient includes researching the best doctors, the best hospitals, and the range of options for specific conditions. Knowing how to obtain this information arms you with the facts you need to help develop a satisfying collaboration with your doctor.

Part of the process of becoming educated about medical matters is learning how to say no to a medical procedure or drug and explaining why. If you know a lot about your condition, but still dutifully obey the doctor whether you agree with his decisions or not, you will not be better off medically. If, on the other hand, you have a generalized distrust of modern medicine and tend to say no to any intervention, you deny yourself the benefits of the many marvelous scientific advances of this century. What is needed is a balance: enough education so you feel equipped to make decisions based on facts, with the understanding that there is much to be gained by selective use of modern medicine's wonders. Learning to say no on occasion may not win you any popularity contests, but it may improve your medical care.

Becoming responsible for a healthy lifestyle

Part of becoming an involved patient includes accepting responsibility for the part you play in your own health. This includes developing a lifestyle that increases the chances of staying healthy. Eating a good diet, exercising, limiting smoking and drinking, and avoiding stress are all under your control, not your doctor's. Many illnesses have some lifestyle components. The doctor is seen only after a certain amount of damage has been done. When you shoulder your part of the burden and encourage the doctor to carry his part, you are well on the way to a satisfying health care partnership.

I trust all my doctors to be entirely human. That is, I trust them to, from time to time: make mistakes, forget, overlook things, mix up facts and memories, be rushed, be distracted, be impatient, be unaware that their biases are biases, etc. I also trust them to care, to want to do a good job, to try to stay on top of things and never make a mistake. And don't forget, as with any profession, there is a spectrum from good to bad, and every doctor lies somewhere along it at any time, and it might vary a lot. Bottom line: they're just people. And that's sufficient reason to watch, check, and question.

CHAPTER 2

Finding the Right Doctor

I consider my patients according to my ability and my judgment
and never do harm to anyone.

—From the oath of Hippocrates, fifth century B.C.

IMAGINE THAT YOU NEED emergency medical care. The following scenarios illustrate two very different possibilities for how that care might be delivered, depending on whether or not you have an ongoing relationship with a doctor you trust.

In the first scenario, you walk into an emergency room, and tell the admitting clerk that your chest hurts and it is hard for you to breathe. You are taken back to a curtain-encircled cubicle, and a young doctor (actually a first-year resident) comes in to examine you. She asks numerous questions about your medical history, takes your blood pressure and pulse, counts your respirations, and does an EKG. In her mind she tries to evaluate how much pain you are in and whether this is a heart attack, pneumonia, a stress-related ailment, or one of the many other possibilities. You are in severe and increasing pain, but don't want to interrupt or seem a complainer. The resident walks out of the room for a moment, carrying the paper from the EKG. You feel a crushing sensation in your chest, and you black out.

In the second scenario, you have been seeing a family practice doctor for years. He knows that you have stable, satisfying family relationships, a job that you enjoy, and an extremely healthy lifestyle. You have told him many times that you eat less than 20 percent fat in your diet, and walk five miles a day because your father and grandfather both died young from heart attacks, and you want to live to see your grandchildren. A few years ago when you developed kidney stones, your doctor saw that you hated to complain and suffered great pain with stoicism. When you called the doctor this morning to tell him of the feeling of severe indigestion and breathlessness, he told you to go to the emergency room immediately and promised to meet you there.

You're worried, but you start to relax when you see your doctor at the door. He greets you with a handshake and introduces a cardiologist. Both doctors look at your EKG while a technician starts an intravenous line. When your doctor goes to put an oxygen mask on you, you say, "Come on, I don't need that, it's just indigestion." He says, "You are going to be fine, but I can tell that you are in pain. You'll feel better with a little oxygen." The cardiologist knows from his examination that you have had a heart attack, so he starts a medication immediately and makes arrangements to admit you to the coronary care unit.

Having a competent doctor who knows you and your medical history usually results in more satisfying medical care. As the above scenarios illustrate, having a trusted doctor to turn to in times of need is not only reassuring, but often medically superior. It is an investment in your future health, and perhaps life, to spend time finding a doctor who is capable of taking care of your medical needs and whose medical philosophy and style matches your own.

The ideal time to select a doctor is when you are well. When healthy, you have the time and energy to research the doctor's credentials, conduct an interview, and get to know her. You are at a distinct disadvantage if you meet a doctor when you are ill. You will be stressed and in pain, which will lessen your ability to communicate effectively. You will not have had time to check the doctor's credentials, so you may worry that this doctor may not be the best available for your situation. In fact, the doctor may be an intern, fresh out of medical school, or a seasoned, compassionate practitioner. The doctor will not have your history available to better help diagnose and treat your illness. You may not like her bedside manner, but will have limited options for immediately changing doctors.

This chapter outlines a step-by-step plan for finding the right doctor for your special circumstances. You will learn how to determine the type of doctor that you need, the type of relationship that you want, how to ferret out the best candidates and learn about their credentials. You'll examine how your medical care is affected by the way a doctor is paid. You'll look at ways to interview a doctor and make a decision. It takes some thought and a bit of time to follow these steps, but it is an investment from which you will reap many benefits in the years to come.

Determine the type of doctor you need

WANTED: Doctor. Must have all-encompassing knowledge of every disease, condition, disorder, whether minor or life-threatening. Must be able to make an accurate diagnosis every time. Must have up-to-the-minute information on all possible treatments, medications, research, including those from non-Western traditions. Must be able to unfailingly prescribe optimal plan for relief, recovery, cure. Must have extraordinary skills in perception of patients' physical/emotional/social/spiritual needs and be able to communicate with patients perfectly. Must be continuously available and ultimately affordable. Must be kind, gentle, wise. Must know top experts with all of above qualities should referral to specialist be necessary. Please reply immediately. Otherwise I'm going to have to go to the bother of getting personally involved in my own health care.

Before you begin searching for a new doctor, you need to define your medical needs. Are you seeking a long-term relationship with a physician to oversee all of your medical care, or a single consultation for a specific problem? Are you looking for an obstetrician to deliver your baby in a manner you find comfortable? A superb diagnostician to try to pull together many elusive but troubling symptoms? A specialist for a second opinion on treatment options for a newly diagnosed cancer? Determining what type of doctor you need is the first step in taking responsibility for your medical care.

The three main types of physicians to choose from are primary care doctors, specialists, and super-specialists. The best doctor for you depends on your age, sex, medical history, and personality. If you're a 25-year-old woman starting a family, for example, you'll need a doctor affiliated with a hospital that has excellent departments of obstetrics, gynecology, and pediatrics. If you are in your fifties and have heart trouble, your doctor should be an internist or cardiologist.

One doctor should oversee all of your medical care. Most healthy people choose from the primary care specialties: internal medicine, family practice, and pediatrics. However, if you have a chronic disease that requires many visits to doctors each year, you might choose a specialist for that disease as your primary physician. For instance, if you have diabetes, your primary doctor might be your endocrinologist. If you have a rare or complex illness, a super-specialist who focuses on just one small slice of medicine may be the best person for you.

Primary care doctors

Primary care doctors are the generalists in medicine. They can handle the majority of problems that you will develop, as well as get to know you as a person, not as a single body part that needs attention. Your primary care doctor will ensure that multiple medications from different physicians don't react unfavorably or cause intolerable side effects. He will make sure that you get the care you need, and no more.

Your primary care doctor should refer you to a specialist if the need arises, and during complicated illnesses will coordinate the services of several professionals. Ideally, he will function as the quarterback for your team—seeing the overall picture and ensuring that the various members of the team work together smoothly.

> Our family doctor took care of all five of my children. The kids went in for yearly physicals and shots. For injuries, he would meet us at the office or hospital for evaluation and stitches. When I needed a series of shots after a surgery, I walked around the block to their house, and his wife (a nurse) gave me the shots in their living room.

> He did untold good deeds for people. For instance, when I was chairman of our parish of Catholic Charities committee, I got a call that a family was living in an animal shed, dirt floor, no water or bathroom. When I went over to see what I could do, I thought the baby had whooping cough. I called our doctor, and he went out and visited the family and coordinated medical care and services for them. He never sent a bill to families with more than eight children. He also made house calls. When we needed a specialist, he would recommend a person, then make the arrangements for us.

The three main types of doctors who provide primary care are internists for adults, pediatricians for children, and family practice doctors for people of all ages. Doctors in these fields have completed four years of medical school, and three or four years of internship and residency. In contrast, general practitioners—depending on the state in which they practice—may have little or no training after completing medical school.

In managed care settings, primary care doctors serve as "gatekeepers," the primary access to more specialized care. As growing pressure is applied to lower costs, these HMO physicians are required to handle more responsibility and are more likely to restrict access to a specialist (see Chapter 3, *Getting What You Need from Managed Care*).

Specialists

Specialists focus on one disease or one part of the body and are trained to treat complex or rare problems that are beyond the expertise of primary care physicians. For instance, if your primary care doctor discovered a mass in your breast, he would send you to a surgeon for an evaluation and a biopsy. If the mass proved to be cancerous, your primary care doctor or surgeon would then refer you to an oncologist for evaluation and treatment. The specialist usually serves as a consultant to examine you, operate on you, or make recommendations for a specific problem, whereas your primary physician serves as ombudsman and interpreter. If you have a serious disease or are getting older, you may be seeing several specialists, but your primary doctor should coordinate all of your medical care.

When your primary doctor refers you to a specialist, she will usually forward all relevant records, and may even make the appointment for you. In return, the specialist will send a report on the results of the examination and/or treatment to your primary care doctor. James E. Payne, M.D., in his book *Me Too: A Doctor Survives Prostate Cancer*, explains how he chose a specialist in radiation oncology:

> Doctor Williams named two radiation oncologists with whom he had developed a positive professional relationship and recommended them for my consideration. I interviewed both.
>
> The first physician was an older man (my age). During my initial appointment he took my medical history and did a physical examination. I thought the physical examination was perfunctory and less than useful. Although he found no anorectal abnormality on examination (and I gave no history of colon problems), he said he wanted me to have a barium enema or colonoscopy (my choice) before beginning the anticipated radiation therapy. I assumed that was standard procedure, so I called a local gastroenterologist and arranged for a colonoscopy.
>
> The second radiation therapist that I visited, Dr. John H. Wilbanks, was frank, candid, positive—a real "can do" person—and up-to-date clinically and academically, by my evaluation. I chose him. He saw no reason for a colon examination, so I canceled the colonoscopy.[1]

Super-specialists

Super-specialists are physicians with a deep knowledge of a very narrow area of medicine. For instance, a pediatric endocrinologist might deal solely with a specific type of growth abnormality in children. Patients often consult these super-specialists for second or third opinions to discover the very newest treatments or technologies available for a specific problem or for a diagnosis of a rare disease. They are also consulted by patients prior to proceeding with an experimental treatment for a serious or life-threatening problem. These physicians—who usually work at university medical centers—are researchers, not generalists.

When I was first diagnosed with multiple myeloma, a relatively uncommon form of cancer, I decided to research the treatment options before I consented to any treatment. One of my oncologists actually told me that I was going to die if I didn't start the chemotherapy right away. Instead, I found out about the International Myeloma Foundation, looked at who was on the scientific advisory committee, then went on the Internet asking for recommendations from others with myeloma.

I received several recommendations to see one of the doctors on the advisory committee of the IMF. I live in New York and he lives in Los Angeles. But I just called him on the phone, and he actually answered it himself. He talked to me for about a half an hour, then asked me to send him my records. He told me that he had treated several people with myeloma who also had lupus (my situation) and that they responded to treatment differently than those with just myeloma. He has made specific suggestions on my treatment and has talked to me many times. He is extremely well known in the field, and has helped me sort out my options several times on the phone. We still have never met.

Consider types of practices

After you decide on the type of doctor that you need, consider the different kinds of practices available. If you are comfortable seeing different doctors, and think that three heads are better than one, a large group might be your best choice. If, on the other hand, you wish to see the same doctor routinely, a solo or small group practice may be more appealing. If you are choosing a doctor for your child, a large, bustling practice may be perfect for an outgoing, exuberant child, but a solo or small practice might be more appropriate if your child tends to be withdrawn around strangers.

The different types of practice are:

- Multi-specialty group: a group containing a range of specialists, for example, internists, surgeons, and radiologists.

- One specialty group: a group of ophthalmologists, for example.

- Office in hospital: an oncology group operating out of a hospital clinic, for example.

- Partnership: two obstetricians working in partnership, for example.

- Solo: a doctor who practices alone.

Define the type of relationship you want

Before shopping for a doctor, it's important to think about what type of relationship you want. Some patients are comfortable with a tough, old-school doctor who will tell them what to do. They just want to find a competent person, let him call the shots, and get in and out of the office quickly. Other patients like to research their conditions, and want and need a doctor who will discuss their findings, so a high priority is finding a doctor who schedules more time with each patient and is willing to answer questions. They desire a partnership in which decisions are made jointly.

Finding a doctor you can really work with means seeking out someone compatible. If you want a lot of information—and all your questions answered—you need a doctor who can't be easily threatened, who takes time with you, and who loves to teach and share his/her reasoning process. Some people actually prefer the old style paternalistic doctor, though, who takes care of you, shields you from information that might be upsetting, etc. Personally, I think that's a bit risky.

Courtesy and respect are essential components in all successful interpersonal relationships. In medical relationships, knowledge and skill are also vital. Depending on the type of service you need, each of these components is more or less important. For instance, if you need a surgeon for an outpatient procedure, his interpersonal skills may not be as important to you as those of your lifelong general practitioner. If you plan to use a pediatrician only for shots and sports physicals, you might search for someone who runs an efficient office. On the other hand, if you like to talk over various child rearing issues in depth with your child's doctor, you need to find someone who is personable and willing to spend time on a consistent basis.

As you can see, a bit of self-analysis is required. Try to think about your temperament and needs as you read the following statements:

- I like my doctor to be authoritative.
- I like my doctor to explain the options and then let me choose.
- I prefer a male doctor.
- I feel more comfortable with a female doctor.
- I want an older, more experienced doctor.
- I like a younger doctor.
- I need a warm, caring doctor.
- I just want my doctor to be competent.
- It makes me uncomfortable if the doctor does not know all the answers.
- I appreciate it when the doctor is honest and says, "I don't know."
- I like to feel that the doctor is in control.
- I think that the doctor is providing a service that I can accept or reject.
- I want my doctor to take care of all my medical needs.
- It's important for me to find a doctor who will ask for a consultation if necessary.
- I like a doctor who will give me a hug or a pat on the arm.
- I expect a doctor to be a professional I consult, not my friend.
- I like to spend a lot of time talking to my doctor about everything that affects my health.
- I just want to get in and out of the office quickly.
- I need someone who is willing to answer my questions thoughtfully.
- I want the doctor to tell me what to do.
- I don't like the doctor to prescribe drugs if I can avoid it.
- I expect the doctor to give me a prescription if I am sick.
- I want the best medicine has to offer—regardless of cost.
- I expect the doctor to talk over less expensive treatments and drugs, if any are available.
- I want the doctor to be accessible; I don't like seeing or talking only to the nurses.
- I like seeing nurse practitioners; I find them to be less intimidating.

- I need a doctor who is open-minded about medical alternatives—acupuncture, nutrition, herbs.

List the characteristics of a medical care provider that are most important to you, such as honesty, competence, warmth, caring, optimism. When you combine the characteristics that are important to you with your desires clarified from the above list, you will have a good idea of what you want and need from your doctor. With this understanding, there is one more important trait to consider: the doctor's philosophy of practice.

Doctors occupy all portions of the aggressive-to-conservative medical spectrum, as do patients. Your job is to find a good match. Some doctors will routinely recommend experimental or risky treatments, while others are more comfortable using the tried and true remedies until the newer treatments have been thoroughly studied. Some doctors disregard quality-of-life issues and will continue to treat as long as there is a treatment available. Continuing life at all costs is their goal. Many patients desire this "do everything that can be done" philosophy in their doctors. Other patients want to assess the risks versus the benefits to their length and quality of life.

Some doctors give antibiotics for every earache, others do not. Some doctors counsel lifestyle changes to control hypertension, others write a prescription. What is your preference? If you choose a doctor with a philosophy at odds with yours, you both might feel uncomfortable as your relationship develops.

After many hospitalizations for a variety of ailments, I have finally learned to tell the doctor up front what I am like and ask if he is comfortable with that. I am a strong dose. I am well versed in medical matters, am an excellent researcher, and ask many questions. They are educated, pertinent questions; I am not wasting time. I just need to know. I tell them in our first meeting that knowledge is my comfort, and I need to share decision making. If they are not happy with that arrangement, we part ways early, before we make each other miserable. But, when I find doctors whose style matches mine, we have wonderful, satisfying relationships.

Locate potential candidates

Your pool of candidates may be severely limited by your insurance plan. Make sure that the potential candidates are part of your plan's network.

There are numerous ways to locate potential candidates, some better than others. Preferred methods are:

- **Recommendations from professionals**. If you are looking for a family doctor, ask a specialist such as your gynecologist or ophthalmologist for a recommendation. If you know any hospital nurses, ask them whom they go to and why. Other professionals' opinions to obtain might be your dentist, mental health professional, or pharmacist. If you need a specialist, ask your family doctor for a referral (see Chapter 8, *Getting a Second Opinion*). If you are new to the area and don't have many personal or professional contacts, walk into your local hospital and ask several nurses for a recommendation. Go to the nurses station on the pediatric floor if you are looking for a pediatrician, and just ask whoever is handy. Walk into an emergency room during business hours on a weekday, ask to speak to a nurse, and explain that you are new to the area and wondered if she would give you a few names of highly respected internists (or whatever type of doctor you require). Most people who choose this method generally find that nurses are helpful, friendly, and willing to share information.

  When I needed to choose a pediatrician for my children, I asked my gynecologist who she took her children to. She told me who she went to, but recommended someone else in the same practice. Then, I asked a couple of emergency room nurses and doctors who they thought was the best pediatrician in town and they all said the same person. We've been going to him for years now and he's wonderful.

- **Recommendations from friends**. Ask several friends whose opinions you respect for their recommendation. Don't settle for an answer like, "He's so nice." Instead, ask questions such as how much time he spends per appointment, how long is the average time spent in the waiting room, how friendly the staff is, and how willing he is to answer questions.

  I was looking for an expert in sports medicine, so I asked a physical therapist friend of mine who ran marathons for a recommendation. She gave me a thumbnail sketch of each doctor in the area, and ended by suggesting one physician and gave her reasons why.

- **Support group**. If you have an illness for which there is a local support group, ask members of the group for recommendations. If there is a national support group (see Appendix C), call or write for their literature, then call several members of the scientific advisory panel, explain your situation briefly, and ask for recommendations.

- **Employer's benefits manager**. If you work for a self-insured company, ask the benefits manager. Often the person in charge of personnel benefits will know most of the physicians in the area and their billing practices. Call to see if she has a recommendation.

- **University medical schools**. If you live near a university, call the head of the clinical residency program, explain your situation briefly, and ask for a recommendation of one or more doctors with excellent clinical skills who practice locally.

Poor methods for choosing a doctor are:

- **Picking one out of the yellow pages**. This is taking medical potluck. You could get an extremely well-qualified physician, or someone who lost privileges in a neighboring state for negligence and has recently relocated to your area.

- **Calling the number seen on a television advertisement**. These referral services are paid for by doctors and are merely advertisements. In addition, most doctors with good reputations fill their practices with referrals from patients or other physicians and do not need to advertise their services.

- **Asking the local hospital for a recommendation**. They will only refer you to physicians with admitting privileges at that institution. The doctor may be excellent or she may just be the newest person hired.

Evaluate credentials

Once you have narrowed down your list to several candidates, try to learn as much as you can about them. No matter how good a doctor's bedside manner is, she can't give you the best available care if she is not up to date in her technical knowledge and skills. On the other hand, stellar credentials do not guarantee an excellent doctor; knowledge and skills are of dubious value if they are not used with good judgment and compassion. Ideally, you want someone with excellent credentials, a personality that complements yours, and a philosophy of practice aligned with your values.

Training

A basic understanding of medical training is necessary to evaluate credentials.

- **Medical degree.** Doctors complete an M.D. degree after four years of college and four years of medical school. To be licensed, some states require only one year of internship—training in a hospital setting—after completion of medical school. Surprisingly, after licensing, doctors can call themselves specialists in any field—pediatrics, dermatology, even surgery.

- **Residency.** Almost all doctors, however, complete three to seven years of rigorous training after medical school. In the first year of clinical training after medical school, the doctor-in-training is called an intern or first-year resident. These medical school graduates are not licensed physicians. In the subsequent years of clinical training in an area of specialty, young doctors are called residents.

- **Clinical fellowship.** After residency, some doctors continue their training in a subspecialty for one to three more years. This additional training is called a fellowship. For instance, a doctor could spend three years in a residency in internal medicine, then several more years studying cardiology. During the years of fellowship training, doctors are called fellows.

  The purpose of a fellowship is to provide advanced training in clinical techniques in a specialized area of medicine. Some fellowships are approved by the appropriate medical specialty board (see next section) and others are not. To check if a fellowship was an approved one, call the hospital where the fellowship took place, or contact the medical board for that specialty.

Board certification

The American Board of Medical Specialties (ABMS) is the premier medical specialty certification board for M.D.s. It certifies physicians in 24 different areas of specialized practice. To earn ABMS board certification, physicians must have three to seven years of post-medical-school specialty training, must meet requirements for experience, and must also pass rigorous written and oral examinations.

Approximately two-thirds of the 600,000 doctors in the U.S. are board certified. Some specialty boards require periodic recertification, while others do
not—for example, family practice doctors need to recertify every six years.
Unless your doctor has recertified within the last decade, board certification
will not guarantee that his skills and knowledge are current. Since medical
knowledge is constantly increasing, if your doctor took the exam in 1976,
he may be twenty years out of date. What board certification does guarantee
is that the doctor met a minimum standard of excellence at the start of his
career. It also ensures that you are not seeing a doctor with a general license
but no additional training who is merely calling himself a specialist.

There are many well qualified—and some eminent—physicians who are not
board certified. Some older physicians, and those who combine clinical
practice with research at large medical centers, may not be board certified.
In general, however, it is best to hire a doctor who has been board certified
in a specialty or subspecialty to ensure the highest level of expertise.

The specialty boards certified by the ABMS are listed in the table, "Specialty
Boards."

Specialty Boards

Specialty Certification	Area of Expertise
Allergy and immunology	Allergies, asthma, problems of the immune system
Anesthesiology	Anesthetics for surgery, pain control
Colon and rectal surgery	Rectal and intestinal surgery
Dermatology	Skin
Emergency medicine	Emergencies
Family practice	General medicine for all ages
Medical genetics	Genes, inherited disorders
Internal medicine	General medicine for adults, many sub-specialties
Neurology	Disorders of the brain, spinal cord, nervous system
Neurological surgery	Brain and spinal cord surgery
Nuclear medicine	Use of radioactive substances for diag-nosis, therapy, research
Ophthalmology	Eyes and eye surgery

Specialty Boards (continued)

Specialty Certification	Area of Expertise
Obstetrics and gynecology	Pregnancy, birth, reproductive system
Orthopedic surgery	Surgery of extremities and spine
Otolaryngology	Ear, nose, throat
Pathology	Microscopic examination of tissue, cells, fluids
Pediatrics	General medicine for children
Preventative medicine	Improving the health of individuals
Physical medicine and rehabilitation	Treatment of impairments of body systems using exercise, prostheses, electricity, heat, light
Psychiatry	Mental, addictive, and emotional disorders
Plastic surgery	Surgical reconstruction and cosmetic surgery
Radiology	X rays and ultrasound
Surgery	General surgery
Thoracic surgery	Surgery of the organs in the chest
Urology	Genitourinary medicine and surgery

The ABMS program is recognized by the American Medical Association (AMA). Beware of "self-designated" specialty boards that are not recognized by the AMA. The boards may have limited experience requirements or may just charge a fee for membership.

A subspecialist is a physician, already board certified, who has obtained further training and certification in one or more of the 83 medical subspecialties certified by the ABMS. For instance, preventative medicine has four subspecialty certifications: aerospace medicine, general preventative medicine, occupational medicine, and public health. Doctors board certified in internal medicine can obtain a subspecialty certification in seventeen different areas, including cardiovascular disease, endocrinology, gerontology, and hematology. Whatever your problem or illness, there are doctors who specialize in diagnosing and treating it.

When asked about qualifications, some doctors say that they are "board eligible." This means that they have completed medical school and residency, but have not yet taken the board examinations, or they have taken them and failed. If the physician you are interviewing has just completed a residency, being board eligible is reasonable. However, some doctors who are not able to pass the examination may use this term indefinitely.

Board-certified physicians are referred to as Diplomates of the Board. Some of the colleges of medical specialties (e.g., the American College of Radiography) have several tiers of additional recognition. For instance, beyond basic board certification, the term "fellowship" is recognition within a specialty group of an individual's outstanding work, study, community service, or contributions to the field. This honorary certificate has nothing to do with the portion of training called fellowship discussed earlier in the chapter. These honors normally indicate that the doctor is well qualified to practice in the specialized field. For example, the initials F.A.A.P. after an M.D. mean not only is she a board-certified pediatrician, but a fellow of the American Academy of Pediatrics as well. Physicians usually prominently display their diplomas, certificates for board certification, and fellowship.

Checking credentials

Many people feel embarrassed to ask doctors about their professional qualifications. If this sounds like you, relax. It is easy to discover a doctor's training and licensing just from a visit to the library or by making a few phone calls. Don't rely on what a doctor calls himself or how he advertises in the yellow pages. One Harvard study found that, on average, 12 percent of the doctors listed as specialists in the yellow pages in Hartford, Connecticut, were not board certified in a specialty. For instance, there were thirty doctors listed as plastic surgeons, but thirteen (43 percent) had no specialty certification in the field. Of eighty-five psychiatrists listed, eleven (14 percent) were not board certified.[2]

Several sources can be checked to verify the credentials of your doctor:

- **Medi-Net**. By far the easiest way to check on your doctor's credentials is to simply call Medi-Net, a new consumer information service that provides health care consumers with a background check on any doctor who is licensed to practice in the United States, including credentials, degrees, training, board certification(s), as well as any disciplinary actions or sanctions taken against the doctor. Each complete Medi-Net physician profile costs $15.00 per doctor. Preliminary information is provided on the telephone, with detailed reports mailed or faxed to callers usually the same day. To order a report, call toll-free 1-888-ASK-MEDI (275-6334) or 1-800-972-MEDI (972-6334). Or see their web page at *http://www.med-i-net.com/welcome.html*.

- **American Medical Association Directory of Physicians in the U.S.** This multi-volume set, published every two years by the AMA, lists every physician in the U.S. In the first volume, there is an index that lists physicians alphabetically. This resource contains the doctor's name, medical school attended, year licensed, primary and secondary specialty, type of practice, board certification, and physician recognition awards. If your local library does not have this directory in their reference section, call your regional library and ask the reference librarian to look up the name of the doctor whose credentials you are checking. You should be able to get this information from the librarian over the phone.

For those with access to the Internet, the AMA has made its Physician Select database available on the Web at *http://www.ama-assn.org*. Click on Doctor Finder. This searchable database contains credential information on all U.S. licensed physicians. There are more than 650,000 M.D.s and Doctors of Osteopathy in this database, which can be searched by physician's name and state, or by medical specialty and state. By clicking on Definition under each specialty, users can find information on the subspecialties included under it.

This database contains office address and phone number, gender, year graduated, residency training, board certification, and whether the doctor is a member of the AMA. In addition, users are informed whether the doctor has received a Physician's Recognition Award, signifying annual documented completion of 50 hours of continuing education.

- **Official ABMS Directory of Board-Certified Medical Specialists**. This multi-volume set of books is published yearly and can be found at most public libraries and on the Web at *http://www.certifieddoctor.org*. The ABMS directory lists board-certified U.S. and Canadian physicians, and includes information on specialty, when certified, medical school and year of degree, place and dates of internship, place and dates of residency, fellowship training, academic and hospital appointments, professional association memberships, type of practice, and current address, telephone, and fax. If a physician is not listed in the directory, he may not have been certified at time of publication or he may have requested to be omitted from the directory.

Smaller libraries may not carry this directory because of cost. If this is the case, call the reference librarian at your regional library or the closest medical school library, and ask her to look up the information and give it to you over the phone. Librarians routinely provide this service. Certification can also be verified by calling the ABMS certification telephone number: 1-800-776-CERT.

- **State medical licensing board**. Your state medical licensing board should be able to tell you the status of your doctor's license, when she was first licensed in the state, and the status of any misconduct charges or disciplinary actions. Professional discipline is unusual, but when it does occur, it becomes a matter of public record. On the Internet, consult Docfinder at *http://www.docboard.org/doc_find/doc_find.htm* to check physician licensing information for Arizona, California, Iowa, Massachusetts, North Carolina, and Texas.

There's a general practice doctor in our town who has been disciplined for sexually abusing several patients and making inappropriate comments to others. In order not to lose his license, he paid an $11,000 fine, must have a chaperone in the examining room at all times, and is required to get continued psychological counseling. I worry that new people in town won't know of his history unless they call the state licensing board to check.

In November 1996, Massachusetts became the first state to open the state Board of Registration in Medicine files to the public. Now patients have access to the following information about doctors licensed in Massachusetts: business address, specialty, board certification, education and training, whether they take new patients or Medicaid patients, where they have hospital privileges, awards received, peer reviewed publication, any hospital discipline, board of medicine discipline, malpractice payments for the last ten years, and criminal convictions. To contact this service, call 1-800-377-0550 or (617) 727-3086. Or see their web site at *http://www.docboard.org/ma/ma_home.htm*.

- **Public Citizen Health Research Group**. This group, founded by Ralph Nader in 1971, publishes a three-volume set of books that lists doctors who have been disciplined by state or federal agencies for incompetence, negligence, substance abuse, patient abuse, or the inappropriate distribution of prescription drugs. The title of the 1996 edition is *13,012 Questionable Doctors*. They also publish state editions of *Questionable Doctors*. Check the reference section of your library for the latest edition or call (202) 588-1000 to order. PCHRC can also be contacted by email at *public_citizen@citizen.org* or through their web site at *http://www.citizen.org*.

- **National Practitioner Data Bank**. Since 1990, the U.S. Department of Health and Human Services has been collecting information on all physicians in the U.S. Any disciplinary actions by state licensing boards or medical societies, malpractice payments, and revocation or limitation of a doctor's license by a hospital or clinic must be reported. One of the purposes of the data bank is to provide health care providers with a method for identifying possibly incompetent practitioners. In the past, doctors could simply cross a state line and continue to practice, with state authorities ignorant about their past problems. Unfortunately, consumers do not have access to this information. If citizens pressured their elected representatives to eliminate the restrictions on access to the data bank, it would be possible to make a more informed choice of medical care providers.

Understand how the doctor is paid

There are basically three ways that doctors in the U.S. are paid for their services:

- Fee-for-service: A fee for each service that they provide.
- Salary: A yearly salary or hourly wage.
- Capitation: A flat fee for each patient.

Each of these payment methods directly affects doctors' compensation and may profoundly influence their medical decision-making. In addition, health care plans and insurance companies devise bonuses and disincentives to shape the type and costs of medical care provided under their plans. What follows is a brief description of each payment type and its potential impacts on your medical care. For additional information on salary and capitation systems, see Chapter 3, *Getting What You Need from Managed Care.*

Fee-for-service

Fee-for-service is the traditional method of paying for medical care in the U.S. In a fee-for-service system, the doctor bills for each service provided, including examinations, laboratory tests, and surgeries. In most fee-for-service systems, some services are more lucrative than others. For instance, insurance companies generally pay little for interviews and examinations. But every time a "procedure"—such as blood tests, X rays, or heart catheterization—is performed, the doctor is handsomely compensated.

This system provides a financial incentive for ordering too many tests and surgeries. Additionally, doctors have a potential conflict of interest because they are ordering tests from which they derive a profit. The potential conflict increases if the physician gets a bigger reward by having the test or X ray performed at a facility that he fully or partially owns. Fee-for-service systems allow doctors to refuse to care for patients who are uninsured or for whom the doctor will receive only partial payment—for instance, Medicaid patients. A major problem with the system is that it encourages technological intervention at the expense of holistic care. A big benefit is that it gives doctors freedom to treat patients without restrictions and allows patients to change doctors without restrictions.

> *Every time my son gets a sinus infection, which is just about every time he gets a cold, the pediatrician wants to do a sinus X ray. I am bothered not only by the radiation, but I have an uneasy feeling because this group of doctors owns the X-ray facility next door. He was required by law to tell me that he has a financial interest, and he did, but it makes me uneasy. He always fills out an X-ray referral sheet, and I always say no.*

Salary

With the number of HMOs and large group practices increasing, more doctors are working for salaries than ever before. Doctors who are paid a straight salary have no financial incentive to order more or fewer tests. However, many salaried physicians work under plans with bonus and penalty provisions that directly link services with compensation. Some types of bonuses and penalties are:

- HMOs that give the doctor a yearly budget for tests. If the doctor exceeds his budget, the difference comes out of his pay. Conversely, if the doctor comes in under budget, he may receive the difference as a bonus.

- Bonuses tied to the overall performance of the group or HMO. The lower the costs across the board, the higher the bonuses for all of the doctors. In other words, the less money the doctor spends on her patients, the more she keeps.

- Withholding salary. Similarly, some plans withhold a percentage of the salary, which is returned at the end of the year if the HMO plan makes a profit. This system encourages peer pressure within the group for all physicians to keep costs down (i.e., order fewer costly tests and surgeries).

Capitation

In some HMOs, doctors are paid a monthly, flat fee for each patient. These "by the head" systems encourage doctors to take on more patients than they can handle, decreasing time per appointment and increasing waits. Because doctors lose money on complex and time-consuming cases, they favor younger and healthier clients. Capitation systems create conflicts for doctors who want to provide comprehensive care for all of their patients, yet lose money by doing so.

One doctor describes his anguish about the capitation system in *M.D.: Doctors Talk About Themselves*:

> I had a patient, a man in his early forties, who called me up one afternoon complaining of chest pain that was radiating out to his left arm—a classic symptom of a heart attack. This guy is about my age, and I had been friends with him. He had become my patient through a capitated HMO that I had signed up with. They are called "capitated" because I got a monthly fee, a per head payment, for each of my patients. My fee ran eight dollars per patient. The idea, of course, is that most patients don't go to the doctor, so it is supposed to average out.
>
> I called the ambulance to pick him up, and I called ahead to the hospital coronary care unit. Then I phoned his wife at work to break the news to her, and I rushed over to the hospital to be there when he arrived. I made all the right moves medically. And at the hospital, I also tried to calm his fears, as well as his wife's. That takes a lot out of a doctor's hide,

trying to help people through the emotional side of this. There's a lot more to taking care of a heart attack patient than just prescribing the right drugs.

But something bothered me about this case, and that was my own realization that when he called to tell me he had chest pains, my first reaction—before anything else crossed my mind—was, "You can't do this to me. I only get paid eight dollars a month to take care of you."[3]

If you are one of the 70 million Americans insured by a managed care plan, get a copy of your plan's preferred provider list. The candidates to interview should come from this list, and it saves time to make sure they are accepting new patients before you spend time checking their credentials.

The first interview

After you have assembled a short list of candidates and evaluated their credentials, it is time to interview. No matter how many recommendations you receive or sterling credentials you have uncovered, until you have a candid conversation with the human behind the stethoscope, you will not know if she is a person with whom you feel comfortable. Many doctors, especially those just opening a practice and those who truly like to get to know their patients, are more than willing to sit and chat for ten to fifteen minutes.

I am a long-term survivor of Hodgkin's disease and I needed a specialist to provide skilled follow-up care. I heard about a doctor from my hematologist and some friends who'd had good experiences with him. I wrote him a letter explaining my situation and saying that if he was accepting new patients, I'd like to set up an appointment.

Well, at my first appointment, I was delighted. He knocked, instead of walking right in, shook hands, introduced himself (without the Dr. in front of his name!), and sat down with me to take the history while I was still in my regular clothes. We went over exactly what things we need to be concerned about at this point and what I need to do in terms of screening, infection prevention, etc., in a very reassuring, non-scary way. The way he individualized everything just felt so comforting.

At this first meeting, your purpose is twofold: describing yourself and your expectations, and finding out about her attitudes, communication style, and office policies. A simple, nonthreatening way to phrase a question is to start by saying, "Tell me about..." Of course, the questions you ask must be tailored to your specific needs, but some suggested questions for the first interview are:

- What types of services does the practice offer? Of these, which do you provide, and which are provided by others, such as nurse practitioners or physician's assistants?
- Are you and your staff skilled in the areas of my special needs?
- How many patients do you see each day? How long does an average visit last?
- In which hospital(s) do you have admitting privileges?
- What is the telephone call policy? Do you offer advice or renew prescriptions over the phone?
- Who covers the practice after office hours and when you are on vacation?
- What is the average cost for an office visit, and other services, including laboratory tests? Does the office bill directly to my insurance company? If the charge exceeds the insurance "reasonable fee," do you waive the excess?
- What is your philosophy of practice? Are you more comfortable with patients who want to be health care partners, or do you prefer patients who readily accept recommendations? Do you mind answering questions? How would you feel if I ever asked for a second opinion?
- How do you feel about discussing treatment options with the patient?
- Are you comfortable discussing complementary or alternative treatments?

If you are interviewing a specialist, such as a surgeon, refer also to Chapter 10, *Questions to Ask About Tests, Drugs, and Surgery.*

When interviewing the doctor, clearly state your interests and expectations. Share your medical needs and goals; for example, if you are diabetic, you might want help managing your chronic illness through diet rather than insulin. Be honest. After all, the doctor has to feel confident that he will be able to work successfully with you, too.

> *When my daughter was diagnosed with a life-threatening illness, her pediatrician botched the diagnosis. I forgave him, simply because I know doctors are human. But I was clear in telling him what I needed from him*

as the difficult and lengthy treatment began. It soon became apparent that he was either too busy or just not interested in working with the specialists at the Children's Hospital. He wasn't keeping track of her lab work or results from procedures. I decided to change doctors. When I interviewed the new doctor, I was brutally honest. I told him that I knew he was busy and had many very ill kids in his practice. I told him that I knew they took a lot of time and a deep emotional toll. But I desperately needed someone who kept track of things, was comfortable with very sick kids, and was competent to manage the case. I was so overwrought that I cried. I told him that I was not a problem parent, but that I did ask many questions and I asked him how he felt about that. We had a very honest exchange of information and feelings. He walked me out to the door, hugged me, and reassured me that we would get through this together. He has been wonderful to us for years. I still ask lots of questions, I take him articles to read, and we occasionally disagree. But I trust him and he respects me and I couldn't ask for more.

If the idea of interviewing doctors makes you uncomfortable, another option is to go in for a first visit with a minor complaint such as a cold, a headache, difficulty sleeping, even a fungus infection on your toe. Tell the clerk when you make the appointment that you would like to schedule some extra time to get acquainted with the doctor since this is your first visit. Pick a problem that will allow you to keep your clothes on. It's impossible to have a balanced, comfortable chat about philosophy, fees, and types of practice when you are lying on a gurney looking up.

When you first meet the doctor, say something open-ended such as, "I'm having a problem with (a cold, constipation, a sore toe) and I'd like to discuss possible approaches for dealing with it." After talking about the problem, ask if he would mind telling you a bit about his background and philosophy of practice. This is the time to ask the types of questions listed above for the interview. Even if the visit is a roaring success, see the other doctors on your list. You might not find another that you like as well as the first, but you will learn a great deal about different methods, styles, and approaches to patients. When you return from each interview, write down your thoughts and feelings, and the doctor's responses to your questions.

If you are interviewing a doctor for your child, bring him along for the initial meeting. Before the appointment, explain to your child what you are doing and why. Share the questions that you intend to ask, and find out if he has any questions to add to the list. During the interview, think about whether this doctor will be a good match. For instance, if your youngster is shy, does the doctor sense this in the interview and respond with a quiet voice and nonthreatening manner? Does she talk to your child or just you? After the appointment, ask your child's opinion on the doctor's personality, warmth, and information-sharing. Examine your own feelings about how your child was treated by the office staff, nurses, and the doctor.

Making a decision

After you complete your interviews of the top two or three candidates, review your notes and assess your feelings. In making a decision, you might consider the following: Were the staff and front office personnel friendly and helpful? Remember that these are the people with whom you will deal most frequently. Did the doctor seem compassionate, genuine, caring, reassuring, optimistic? Did he seem gloomy, intimidating, reserved? How forthright did he seem? Were you comfortable with the amount of information that was shared? Would you feel secure discussing personal or embarrassing problems with this doctor? Did you sense that you could have a good rapport and a strong relationship with this person? Did he treat you as an intelligent partner in the medical decision-making process?

I want information, I want to know what all the options are, I want to know what is going on in my body, I want to know everything. I think active participation makes an ideal patient. If it drives your M.D. crazy (I've seen it happen to some of my medical providers) then it's the wrong M.D. We should never let our doctor's impatience or lack of time intimidate us or prevent us from asking every question we need answered.

I now have an oncologist who not only patiently answers all of my questions (without ever making me feel foolish or annoying for asking), he actually asks me questions like, "Your counts are so good this week— what are you doing?" And then he listens with an open mind when I explain my nutritional plan. I feel like he and I are co-seekers in this search for a healing plan. I also have a gynecologist who tells me everything. She describes in detail what she is doing during the exam, what she sees, what she thinks, and even holds up a mirror if I want to see what she is seeing. She answers my questions even before I ask them. I hope everyone can find doctors like these.

Think about whether this doctor will be a good team player. One of the consequences of our health care changes has been a decentralization of care. Although the physician is still, in essence, the team leader, other persons—nurses, physical therapists, chaplains, social workers—may also be critical to your care. If you have a complex illness that requires the services of many professionals, choose a physician who is a good team player.

> *Traditionally doctors had little respect for nurses, much less respiratory therapists, physical therapists, and other professionals with whom they worked. But the time has come now where we each have a part to play.*

Even doctors sometimes need to choose a medical caregiver, although they often describe themselves as difficult patients. In his book, *Me Too: A Doctor Survives Prostate Cancer*, James E. Payne, M.D., describes his feelings about his first meeting with a surgeon:

> *Dr. Williams had scheduled my next appointment…to meet one of his new urological associates and have him examine me and review my case. Then we three could discuss the findings of my metastatic workup and make concrete plans for my definitive treatment.*

> *Dr. Williams's new partner was undoubtedly a very bright young urologist. It was obvious that he had an impressive grasp of urological knowledge and was very thorough, but his professional persona did not favorably impress this former surgeon. To be specific, his digital rectal examination of my prostate was rough, prolonged, and hurt like hell. In my judgment, he definitely lacked the empathetic personal touch so important in the practice of the healing arts.*

> *During my own clinical years, and as a teacher of surgery, I sometimes felt intellectually inferior to the brightest of my capable and learned staff of young university-trained surgeons. I noted, however, that many of them seemed too mechanical in their approach to patient care, which often offended my sensibilities. During my teaching rounds I had insisted that my students be "gentle doctors" whether performing an examination on an alert patient or doing an operation under anesthesia.*

> *Either I got through to Dr. Williams during his surgical training or he remembered my admonitions and treated me according to my teachings—I like to believe it was the former. His examinations were always*

*deliberate and very gentle. Although his younger associate was obviously
very sharp and knowledgeable, I wouldn't have allowed him to be my
primary surgeon because of his roughness.*[4]

Dr. Payne took charge of his medical care by hiring a physician whom he
trusted to be his medical coordinator, asking him for recommendations,
then interviewing the candidates who would provide services that he
required. By following the steps outlined in this chapter, you too can find a
doctor with excellent credentials, a comforting manner, and a philosophy in
harmony with yours.

*I did a poor job of selecting my own doctors. I chose them because
they were friends. Now, with the wisdom of hindsight, I could make
a better choice. First, I would be concerned with integrity. The
blindest purchase we make in our life is medical care. We have no
basis of comparison. So I want my doctor to have integrity. I want
to make sure that his advice is for my benefit and not his—or hers.*

*Next, I would want to know about the doctor's knowledge. What
school did he graduate from? Where was his residency? Does he
have specialty boards? Has he kept up? What do his colleagues
think of him? What is his track record in treating my illness?*

*Only after these questions are answered would I concern myself
with questions of personality. Is he sympathetic? Does he listen?
Does he communicate? Are we compatible? Sympathy is high on my
list, but what good is sympathy if a doctor doesn't have
knowledge?*[5]

—Edward Rosenbaum
A Taste of My Own Medicine

Getting What You Need from Managed Care

It is an unfortunate fact of life that even previously good doctors can have their medical judgment colored by the psychological and monetary pressures some HMOs impose.

—Alan Steinberg, M.D.
The Insider's Guide to HMOs

MANAGED CARE HAS BEEN AROUND since the 1920s, when doctors first contracted with businesses to provide medical care for their workers for a set fee. In 1973, companies with twenty-five or more workers were required to offer a choice between traditional insurance and health maintenance organizations (HMOs). Enrollment in managed care plans began to soar—from six million in the mid-1970s to over seventy million in 1997. The resulting rise of managed care organizations has forever changed the way in which medicine is practiced.

The huge growth of HMOs makes it likely that now or in the future you will be impacted by this new kind of health care delivery. Even if you keep the same doctor, under managed care she may be working under guidelines you are unaware of, created by the insurance company. Decisions about your care—time to spend on an appointment, what treatments to recommend or not to mention—can be based on guidelines determined by the HMO as to what is cost-effective for a large number of people in the aggregate rather than what is best in your individual case. Your doctor might alter how she practices without your even knowing it.

Health care delivery in the U.S. is in flux. HMOs differ widely on services and programs; independent surveys that provide concrete comparisons and ratings of HMOs are just now emerging. Some consumers are demanding more participation in decisions that affect their care. Doctors and their organizations are examining changes to their profession and deciding on responses.

Health care delivery—who will get care, who decides on what the care is, who will pay, who will be paid, how care will be regulate—is an issue of public policy as well as an issue affecting individuals. Laws are being enacted, at state and federal levels, in response to complaints about health care delivery. For example, recent laws prohibit insurers from mandating discharge twenty-four hours after a normal birth or on the same day as a mastectomy, if patient and doctor agree on the need for a longer hospital stay. Battles over the control of decision-making are ongoing. No one knows what the face of managed care will look like in the next several years, except that it undoubtedly will be different from managed care today.

This chapter will not predict the future. It doesn't say whether a particular HMO is good or bad. And it doesn't take a stand on public policy issues or say that one method of health care delivery is intrinsically the most fair or best use of finite health care dollars.

This chapter does point out some things to be aware of. Since the system has dramatically changed, you need to learn how to get the best coverage for yourself and your family. You also need to understand how insurance through an HMO might impact your relationship with your doctor and how to take steps, if necessary, to form a different partnership. This chapter will define managed care, provide a brief overview of the different types of managed care plans, give tips on how to pick the best plan for your family, and discuss how many patients prevented or coped with problems of managed care.

What is managed care?

Managed care is a catch-all term describing a system that combines coverage of health-care costs and delivery of health care for a prepaid premium. Instead of paying claims submitted by independent doctors or hospitals, managed care companies employ or have contracts with doctors and hospitals that set policies for what they can or can't do. For instance, they use an authorization process to limit access to specialists, cut down on self-defined unnecessary procedures, and reduce money spent on prescription drugs.

In the not-too-distant past, most patients had insurance that simply paid doctors and hospitals for treatment with no strings attached. This type of arrangement is called fee-for-service. You see the doctor of your choice, and he is free to prescribe treatments, drugs, or referrals to specialists without input from the insurance company. Managed care organizations, in contrast, try to keep costs down by controlling services. Managed care firms use a variety of methods to control costs.

- **Preventative services.** Most managed care companies emphasize prevention services (screening tests such as mammograms, counseling to stop smoking, providing childhood immunizations) to control costs. It is often cheaper to prevent future disease with lifestyle changes or minor interventions now, rather than pay for treatments later, so long as the same company will be paying the cost for an individual's health care throughout his life and that company is willing to act now for the financial long term. In practice, studies show a wide variation in such preventative services. Some managed care groups try to enroll only healthy patients (called "cherry picking") and then just hand out brochures on low-fat diets or the need for exercise, while others take an active role in monitoring healthy habits.[1]

- **Using "gatekeepers."** Primary care providers (PCPs) are the cornerstone of managed care. They deliver the majority of health care services needed by their patients. The theory is to coordinate all of the patient's care as well as to send patients to specialists only if it is truly necessary. However, in order to reduce costs, some HMO primary care providers are encouraged to manage conditions that may be beyond the scope of their training rather than refer patients to specialists. Many plans have financial incentives (rewards for keeping referrals to a minimum or punishments for too many referrals) to limit visits to specialists. For example, if you need a colonoscopy (visual examination of the colon using a long tube), your PCP might do the procedure himself rather than send you to a gastroenterologist. You are given a less costly, and potentially more hazardous, procedure without being informed that this procedure is usually performed by a specialist.

- **Limiting choice of doctor.** Patients who sign up with managed care organizations are required to choose a physician from a list of doctors who are employees or who have signed contracts to participate in the plan, follow its rules, and accept plan payments as payments in full for services. If your current doctor is not on the list, you'll have to switch to one who is. If your doctor is a member of the plan but later leaves, you will have to choose another doctor from the list.

The university at which I work organized their own HMO and required all employees to sign up with a PCP on their plan or face a reduction in coverage. I was upset by this forced change and the associated time required to research and choose a new doctor. My options were also limited somewhat because several of the approved PCPs already had full patient loads and not all physicians in the region participated in the plan. So, I asked several friends and acquaintances (including a couple of doctors, my chiropractor, and a few others whose opinions I valued). I made a short list of candidates and spoke with each. I chose a fellow who shares similar sensibilities and, perhaps coincidentally, is close to my own age. I am comfortable with him, have received excellent care, and appreciate the efficiency with which his office functions. I get in and out quickly without feeling rushed.

- **Limiting choice of facilities**. Usually, managed care groups require patients to use specific hospitals and testing facilities. You may have to travel farther to get care from the HMO.

- **Limiting duration of hospital stays**. Laws have been passed regulating minimum stays after childbirth and outlawing "drive-through" mastectomies. But, for most surgeries, managed care organizations encourage doctors to discharge patients quickly to keep costs down. One doctor writes about being pressured to discharge patients from the hospital earlier than he feels is safe:

    Interestingly enough, this system has a lot of "hold harmless" types of clauses. This means that it is always the responsibility of the physicians to keep the best interests of patients in the forefront, even if the insurance company is not! They can make the doctors' and patients' lives miserable with threats of non-payment and throwing the doctor off the provider list, but it is still the doctor's problem if something bad happens after the patient is discharged. Pretty cushy little arrangement, don't you think? They can do whatever they want and it is NEVER their problem. The unfortunate thing is that the doctor and the patient can insist that the patient stay, but a bureaucrat can look at it and deny the payment so the patient is stuck with the bill. Insurance companies are treating medicine as they would any other business, cutting costs to increase profits. Who benefits from these increases? Not the hospitals or doctors, that's for sure. The czars at the top of this food chain get their money off the top and could give a rat's ass what is done with the money left over.

- **Controlling drugs given**. Most managed care organizations have a formulary—a limited list of preferred drugs available at a reduced cost. Medications not on the formulary cost more for the patient, and the plan doctors are strongly discouraged from prescribing them.

- **Using utilization management**. Even though a service is listed as covered in the policy handbook, it may be denied by the group's utilization committee. The managed care firm develops "practice guidelines" and approves or rejects treatment based on these guidelines.

Suicide follows treatment denial

A psychiatry patient in California had the number of inpatient days reduced by a utilization management company. The patient committed suicide and a lawsuit was filed. The court ruled that a complaint could be lodged against both the doctor and utilization management company, since the suit was based on whether the utilization company had sufficient information on which to base a decision. The case has been interpreted to mean that there is a cause of action against managed care companies if their utilization management system is fundamentally flawed or negligently designed.[2]

Changes in how medical costs are reimbursed herald a major shift in health care delivery in the U.S. The focus has veered from the patient's well-being to cost containment. If you join a managed care organization (or have no choice because your employer contracted with one), you need to change your assumptions about your relationships with your health care providers. You may no longer have a doctor who is a partner, interested only in your health. Instead, she may be under pressure to perform specialized services herself, limit referrals, and try to keep her job by keeping all of her patients' costs down—including yours. You can get excellent care from your HMO, but you may have to work hard to get it. Jerome P. Kassirer, M.D., editor-in-chief of the *New England Journal of Medicine*, wrote:

> On the one hand, doctors are expected to provide a wide range of services, recommend the best treatments, and improve patients' quality of life. On the other, to keep expenses to a minimum they must limit services, increase efficiency, shorten the time spent with each patient, and use specialists sparingly...I believe that increasingly the struggle will be more concrete and stark: physicians will be forced to choose between the best interests of their patients and their own economic survival.[3]

Remember, each type of health insurance has biases and weaknesses. Traditional fee-for-service tends to err on the side of doing too much for a patient, while HMOs err on the side of doing too little. HMOs' fixed budget requires that, if one patient is given more, someone else must make do with less. Managers, without a medical degree, may call the shots on your medical care. If you stay alert for these tendencies, ask good questions, and get the facts, you should be able to learn about all of the options and make informed choices.

Types of plans

There are variations on a few main themes in health care delivery. The four main types of programs are fee-for-service, independent practice associations, preferred provider organizations, and health maintenance organizations. They vary by who bears the risk of incurring costs and who decides what treatments are necessary. In places where doctors treat patients with different types of insurance, unsavory practices can develop as described by a doctor in the following story.

> I belong to a group of doctors who have contracted with our hospital to provide services for all emergency patients for a set salary. This has eliminated the big problems that other ERs are experiencing. What happens in some places is that the doctors grab the fee-for-service charts (called the juicy charts) and do everything they can to avoid the personal pay, managed care, Medicare, and Medicaid charts. I've heard many tales about people fighting over charts because the insurance determines how much they get paid for their services. You can see a doctor walking around with five charts under his arm so that he gets the paying patients. Of course, those people then wait forever, but the doctor gets more money.

Fee-for-service (unmanaged care)

The traditional type of insurance coverage most patients in the U.S. are familiar with is fee-for-service private practice, in which the insurer pays the doctor for each visit or service. In this system, insurers are uninvolved third parties in the financial interactions between health care providers and patients. Patients go to the doctor of their choice, and the doctors treat patients as they see fit, without any oversight from the insurance company. Doctors spend as much time with each patient as they want, can order as many tests as they wish, and write prescriptions for the drugs they choose. Patients are free to hire and fire doctors, as well as go to the hospital of their choice. Approximately half of all insured Americans currently use fee-for-service insurance. (Chapter 2, *Finding the Right Doctor*, also discusses fee-for-service medicine, and points out some possible conflicts of interest between doctors and patients in this system, including reliance on high-tech interventions and unnecessary testing and surgery.)

Prior to managed care, there were no incentives to contain costs. Health care costs spiraled up for decades, and the insurance companies passed the cost on to their policy holders by increasing premiums. The number of uninsured persons swelled. Costs of medical care rose dramatically, as did the incomes of doctors.

> *I've had both traditional insurance and an HMO. I liked the old way better. It did cost more money with the deductible and 80/20 coverage, but I knew that my doctors would lay all the options on the table. Then, I could decide how far to go with testing and treatment. It also seemed less rushed. Now, I feel like I cause problems if I ask questions. My doctor doesn't like it much either. He told me once, "This managed care just doesn't give me the time I need to do a thorough examination. Drives me crazy." Even though we have a long history, I feel a bit less trust. He's getting pressured to cut costs and I worry if that will hurt my care.*

Today, most fee-for-service companies include managed care elements like pre-authorization for surgeries, precertification, utilization review, and sometimes formularies (lists of approved drugs).

Independent practice association (IPA)

An IPA is a group of independent, private practice physicians who have banded together in an association that contracts with various HMOs. The physicians agree to accept a set monthly fee per patient (capitation) in exchange for providing all medical care for HMO members. They are not compensated for the actual medical care given.

All of the risk moves from the insurers to the doctors and from a very large pool of people to a much smaller pool of people—those seen by a single practice. For instance, if one patient treated by the group needs a quarter-million-dollar kidney transplant, that could consume all of the profits for the year. In extreme cases (an unlucky year for patients) the doctor could go broke by giving his patients the care they need.

These flat fee systems encourage doctors to take on as many healthy patients as possible because they lose money treating patients with complicated or time-consuming illnesses. Capitation systems create a stark ethical conflict for doctors: treat patients and lose money. The threat of financial risk (or in extreme cases, insolvency) diminishes their ability to be caring and objective physicians.

Late referral ends in death

Thirty-four-year-old Joyce Ching was a member of a California independent practice association. Her two primary care physicians were paid 28 dollars a month per patient, significantly higher than the national average. They also had to pay directly for any test or referral they made. When they signed on with the IPA, the doctors agreed to take on the individual risk for each patient's care; they did not share in a risk pool.

In August 1992, Joyce went to her primary care physician to investigate her rectal bleeding, abdominal pains, and abnormal bowel movements. During the exam, her doctor detected a mass behind her uterus. Joyce's husband asked for a referral to a specialist, but instead, the doctor ordered a pelvic ultrasound and gave her a prescription for pain relievers. The pain continued, and five days later she asked again to see a specialist. Two weeks later she again called, and was told she had to come in to see the primary care physician before she could get a referral. She saw a different doctor in the practice who refused to send her to a specialist and recommended that she change her diet. In great pain, she called seven weeks later asking for a referral and was refused.

In late October, Joyce and her husband went in again to see the doctor, who again refused to refer her to a specialist. Joyce's husband refused to leave the office until he got a referral or a diagnosis. The primary care physician ordered a barium enema X-ray exam which revealed colon cancer. In November, Joyce finally saw a specialist who immediately operated, but to no avail. The cancer had spread and Joyce died several months later, leaving behind her husband and a four-year-old son.[4]

Preferred provider organization (PPO)

A preferred provider organization is a type of health insurance in which a managed care organization contracts with private practice physicians to provide medical care for subscribers. The doctors accept lower fees and agree to controls on their work in exchange for increased patient volume. Thus, patients are steered to doctors with records of low-cost care. Subscribers can use a doctor who is not a preferred provider, but the PPO will pay a lower percentage of the bill.

I work at a medium-sized hospital and always thought that we had wonderful insurance. I belong to a PPO. Most doctor visits are a $20 co-pay (no well visits). All inpatient expense is covered at 100 percent if provided at the hospital at which I work. This always worked great for us. Throughout the years, I had two children, two operations, my son was hospitalized as well as my husband. We never had any inpatient out-of-pocket expenses. But when our daughter needed specialized surgery, our pediatric surgeon would not do it there because we do not have a pediatric intensive care unit. So when Tracy needed to go to another hospital on our PPO plan, I found out that our insurance was not as good as I thought. Even though the other hospital was on the plan, they only pay 60 to 85 percent of services and inpatient costs.

Coverage and services vary considerably among plans. One mother of a child who required extensive medical services for years describes how well her PPO plan worked for her family.

I am a member of a PPO (have been for many years) and find it is wonderful. When my daughter was undergoing treatments five years ago, I had no problems with out-of-town/network coverage (at full rates); my biggest problems were always with getting timely payments, but coverage itself was never an issue. With the new year, we now have a co-pay of $10 per doctor visit (but no other costs for routine preventative or illness visits, which used to be 20 percent) and the prescription costs have also gone up a bit, but I suppose that's a small price to pay.

I have prevented problems by getting full coverage for out-of-network services (both the surgeon and hospital were out-of-network) because there was no similar specialist inside the network.

Health maintenance organization (HMO)

An HMO is a type of heath insurance in which the health care is provided by the insurer for a prepaid monthly premium rather than by independent physicians. These insurers are usually for-profit corporations that try to provide cost-effective health care through preventative medicine and limitations on service. They often hire their own doctors, whose salaries are often adjusted based on how effectively they keep costs down.

HMOs charge a small co-payment for each service provided, for example, ten dollars for each office visit and seven dollars for each prescription. Typically, there is no required deductible (a specific amount of money that is paid before insurance coverage begins).

The two most common types of HMO are staff and group. In staff model HMOs, all care provided to members is given at HMO facilities run by salaried doctors who are employees of the HMO or insurance company. In group model HMOs, service is provided by several groups of doctors who have contracted to care for members for a certain level of payment. These doctors are usually paid under a capitation arrangement.

Computer printouts keep doctors in line

Forbes magazine described how one HMO mails computer printouts to its 3,000 primary care providers outlining costs. One key number is the doctor's monthly average compared to the other HMO doctors' averages. The HMO also has rewards for doctors who do procedures themselves rather than refer to specialists, and penalties for too many referrals. Also computed into the averages are the costs to each PCP from referring specialists. For instance, if the diabetic patients sent to an endocrinologist cost 40 percent more than average, it hurts the PCP's paper performance by running up his costs. The HMO's chief executive, whose previous career was in data management, described one incentive that encourages the plan's doctors to study the numbers on the printouts: "They get to keep their jobs."[5]

Plans vary, and subscribers' feelings about them are varied as well. Two patients who are heavy users of HMO services describe their feelings.

HMOs have some benefits as well as problems. Some of their good points are:

- *The physicians in an HMO have a collegial rather than a competitive relationship, and when specialists are needed they work as a team with the primary care physician and other HMO staff in treating the patient. There is a good amount of communication between the various HMO physicians and often meetings between the various physicians (including the primary care physician) treating a complex case.*

- The HMO hospital is not generally a teaching hospital, thus the hospital care is given only by experienced physicians; there are no physicians in training "practicing" on you as a patient.

- The HMO has established guidelines of care for all of the medical staff to follow in treating routine illnesses. Thus, if you go to the emergency room or a physician other than your regular caregiver, the treatment prescribed is consistent and the medication will be the same. The medical staff has printed instructions of care for several reoccurring conditions our family members have had. This is reassuring to me.

- The HMO is like living in a small town. Everybody knows everybody else. The primary care physician knows the specialist you will see, the pharmacist, the lab technician, the therapist, and they pick up the phone and talk to each other if there are any questions or problems. This also means they can bypass the system when they need immediate results from the lab or X ray or wherever. Also, if there is an urgent medical problem, the primary care physician is able to access the entire HMO system to arrange immediate care. We have had this happen on more than one occasion. We were very grateful to be swept into the system, and doors opened for us when our situation was critical.

- There is absolutely no paperwork or claim forms with the HMO. There may be a small co-payment for some services with some plans, but that's all. There are no complicated hospital bills or forms to complete after an illness. There is also no worry that part of the cost of care will be disallowed by the medical insurance coverage.

· · · · ·

I don't know why they have the audacity to call it a health maintenance organization, when it seems more and more like a TFD: Treatment Filtering Disorganization! It's a health maintenance organization because they want people who will maintain their health (which is why they mainly have people in the working sector). They do not want to deal with people whose health has not been maintained, i.e., who get sick. HMOs are not like traditional hospitals that make money (or used to) when people get sick and so compete for patients. HMOs lose money big time *when people get sick because it's a prepaid plan and they don't get to charge for additional treatments or hospitalizations, etc. The bottom line is, your illness upsets the profit margin.*

How to pick a plan

Most people spend more time shopping for a CD player than for an HMO— even though this is a purchase that could impact your health care and perhaps save your life. Your choice of doctor, hospital, and services is greatly limited under managed care, so you really need to shop around to find the best deal for yourself or your family. All plans are not the same. You'll want to make sure that what you are paying for with your monthly premiums, and the company that you are counting on when you need help, offer the valuable services that you need. You'll also want to ensure that the plan(s) you consider will allow you to continue to see all of your current doctors, to preserve the relationships you have created.

In many cases, however, employees have to accept whatever plan is provided by the employer, and those companies that offer choices don't always offer good ones. Even if you have no choice, asking questions and reading policies will help prepare you to negotiate for services should the need arise.

The following is a list of questions that will tell you more about the company and the plan you are considering. To find out answers to the questions, read the actual contract (not glossy promotional material), ask your benefits manager at work, and also talk to your doctor.

- How many subscribers are there in your area?

- How many primary care doctors are on the provider list? Are they all board certified? If you already have a doctor with whom you feel comfortable, make sure he is on the primary care provider list, or you will have to change doctors if you sign up. If your doctor is a specialist, most likely you will have to see a primary care doctor, known as a gate-keeper, who will decide when and if you need to see a specialist.

  I'm not a cheerleader for HMOs, but my HMO plan allows me to choose my primary care doctor from a list of about 100 and to change primary doctors anytime I want, with a month's notice.

- How are the doctors paid? Are they paid a flat monthly fee per patient? Do they get a bonus or penalty based on referrals to specialists, number of office visits, hospital admissions, prescriptions written, or any other action?

In our area, most of the family practice doctors are paid a set salary with a feature called withholding. They get paid only 90 percent of their salary during the year, and 10 percent of this income is withheld. If at the end of the year you have been an efficient doctor, i.e., you haven't ordered many tests for your patients, you get your money back. Otherwise, you lose it. Our hospital emergency department director calls it immoral. It pits your financial needs against your patient's well-being. Even the most scrupulously honest doctor, trying to do the best thing for his patients, has to think every time he decides not to order a test, "Am I not ordering this because I think it's truly unnecessary, or because I know I'll lose money?"

- Is there a maximum lifetime cap on medical payments? Are there annual limits on the length of hospital stays?

- Must all referrals first have the approval of the primary care doctor? Can the PCP be financially penalized for referring you to a specialist, emergency room, or diagnostic test? Are there economic incentives for the doctors to limit these types of services?

I'm not an HMO doctor, but I think many of them are unhappy. It's very common to hear today, "I wouldn't go into medicine if I had it to do over again" or "I wouldn't recommend it to my kids." When you really try to get underneath that to find out what's going on, I think it's that they don't find the quality of the interaction with their patients satisfying. Part of it is that many of them have abdicated the responsibility for assigning their time to somebody who wants to maximize their income. I think doctors are selling their souls, their professions, and their therapeutic relationships for money. And I think it's a deal that they will very much regret in the future—both as individuals and as a group.

- What hospitals, radiological services, home-health agencies, nursing homes and other facilities does the managed care agency use? Are these facilities located close to your home?

- Is the plan accredited by the National Committee for Quality Assurance (NCQA)? This organization reviews more than 330 managed care organizations annually and gives them one of four ratings: full accreditation (good for three years), one-year accreditation (if the organization is equipped to make recommended changes within one year), provisional accreditation (for organizations with potential for improvement), and denial for accreditation (does not meet NCQA standards). In addition to accreditation status, you can also get a report from NCQA summarizing their findings for an individual HMO. Call the NCQA Accreditation

Status Line at 1-888-275-7585 or order a list of accredited HMOs by calling 1-800-839-6487. The same information is available at the NCQA's web site at *http://www.ncqa.org.*

Treatment varies by region in some HMOs

One key finding in the 1997 NCQA report on HMOs was that managed care organizations vary greatly both within regions and across regions in terms of preventative care, treatment of chronically and acutely ill patients, and member satisfaction. For instance, they found that heart attack patients in the South Central Region (Alabama, Arkansas, Kentucky, Louisiana, Mississippi, Oklahoma, Texas, Tennessee, and several other states) are treated with beta blockers less than 20 percent of the time in some health care plans, but more than 90 percent of patients receive beta blockers in the best performing plans. Beta blockers are a class of drugs which have been shown in many studies to protect heart attack victims from future heart attacks and possible cardiac death. The study also found that in New England, 81 percent of children under age two receive appropriate immunizations, but in the Mountain region, the rate is only 59 percent. Health plans within the Mid-Atlantic region reported mammography screening rates ranging from 30 percent to 80 percent.[6]

- Does the plan pay for a second opinion if you request one?
- Can you change doctors any time?

  Changing doctors in plans can be very complicated. I advise my patients to ask specific questions to learn about all restrictions prior to signing up with a new plan. Typical restrictions include: you can't change PCPs without filing a written request 90 days in advance; can only change physicians during open enrollment periods, for instance, twice a year. I just can't imagine being trapped in a relationship with someone philosophically at odds with me when I'm sick.

- Are the doctors bound by a "gag order" or other contractual provisions that prevent them from fully informing you of all treatment options? Or from disclosing bonuses in the plan if they limit care, referrals, or prescriptions? Ask for a copy of the HMO policy regarding gag clauses and refuse to sign up until you get one. Some states now have laws that prohibit gag clauses for HMO doctors.

- Will you see a doctor at each appointment? How often and in what capacity are nurse practitioners and physician's assistants used? How long will you have to wait to get an appointment?

- Does the plan offer a point-of-service (POS) option to enable you to go outside the network if you think it is necessary to get the best care?

- What is the plan's coverage for pre-existing conditions? If you have a pre-existing condition, federal law (H.R. 3103—effective date: July 1, 1997) restricts group health plans, insurers, and HMOs from denying coverage because of pre-existing conditions if you already have coverage from another health plan. The law has several restrictions, so be sure to check it out if you have a pre-existing condition.

- What is the coverage for mental health care? Are you restricted to picking a mental health care provider from a list? How many visits a year are authorized?

- Does the plan have a formulary for prescription drugs, and if so, are your drugs on it? Is there a way for physicians to make exceptions?

- What is the policy on giving drugs in lieu of psychotherapy? Are providers required to use cheaper drugs first, before being allowed to use newer, more expensive drugs?

Saving money on mental health care

The Wall Street Journal discussed in a front page article how some HMOs save money by enforcing a strict hierarchy of preferred treatments for patients with mental illnesses. They cite situations in which older, less expensive drugs are used to treat depression first. If unacceptable side effects develop (weight gain, dizziness, fainting spells, irregular heartbeat), newer, more expensive drugs—such as Prozac—are given if "the doctor can make a clinical case for it." Talk therapy—the most expensive option— is the last choice. Doctors try to persuade managed care firms to try various antidepressants with patients to see what works best, "But—as in other treatment options—when the managed care firms don't go along, practitioners sometimes have to pursue treatment plans they don't think are optimal."[7]

- What is the coverage for vision care, hearing care, and dental care?

- Will you be limited to selected pharmacies? Is there a monthly drug budget, and are doctors penalized or rewarded for restricting prescription drugs?

- What is the emergency room visitation policy? Are you required to use a specific emergency room? Do you have to call a nurse before you go? Some managed care plans review emergency room visits retrospectively, and decide whether to pay based on outcome. For instance, if you had severe chest pain and were taken by ambulance to the closest hospital, some managed care plans will pay only if a heart attack is diagnosed. If you had gastritis, they will refuse payment. The problem is that you cannot know the cause of your pain until you are evaluated. Some states now have laws requiring HMOs to pay for emergency room visits a "prudent layperson" would consider an emergency.

    I'm a critical care nurse and we take care of many patients who have come in through the emergency room with chest pain. If the patient is a member of a managed care plan, we know that bright and early the morning after admission, a case manager who may not be medically trained will call to find out if the person was "really sick" enough to need to go to the nearest hospital, rather than one approved by the plan. If it turns out that they didn't have a heart attack, we have to argue that need is based on symptoms, not outcomes. I always worry that they might deny paying for these folks' care. Often we have to bundle them up for an inconvenient and stressful transfer to the plan's hospital.

- If you become ill while away from home, will your doctor's or emergency room visits be reimbursed?

- What is the co-payment or deductible for office visits and emergency visits? Does this amount change for evenings, weekends, or holidays?

- What happens if you are laid off or change jobs?

  It's really irritating to have to keep calling and getting things straightened out. Our insurance is through my husband's work. He just changed jobs and our insurance is going from one plan to another, both managed by the same provider. We are having a terrible time keeping Michelle's urologist. He's no longer approved by the plan (but he was when we started), and they want us to take her to someone new. That means gathering up more than three years worth of scans, films, etc., to let this new guy look at them. I really don't want to do this.

- Will you be required to sign a document forfeiting your right to sue and agreeing to arbitration in case of a dispute?

Cancer patient sues for care

Christine deMeurers was a young mother in her early thirties with two young children when she was diagnosed with a rapidly spreading breast cancer by her HMO doctor. She was referred to a noted cancer specialist at UCLA who recommended a bone-marrow transplant—an aggressive and expensive treatment which offered her the best chance for survival. But her HMO refused to pay, calling the procedure experimental. The family sued and the cancer specialist gave a sworn statement supporting the therapy. A vice president from the HMO called the cancer specialist's boss and complained. A less favorable sworn statement was given by the doctor, and this watered-down version was used by the HMO to defend itself in the suit. Arbitrators who heard the case decided that the HMO had interfered in the doctor-patient relationship when it tried to "influence or intimidate doctors." The panel ruled, after Christine died, that the HMO must pay $1.02 million to the deMeurers family.[9]

- What are the plan's complaint and appeals policies? Who is on the appeals board? How quickly are complaints usually resolved?

Do not rely on a salesperson's verbal answers to the above questions. Make sure to get a copy of the contract and read it thoroughly. To see how 150,000 HMO members rate their HMOs, get the *Consumer's Guide to Health Plans* published by the nonprofit Center for the Study of Service (1-800-475-7283).

Preventing problems

There are good reasons for the old adage, "An ounce of prevention is worth a pound of cure." It is far easier to prevent problems—especially in an ever-changing HMO environment—than to try to fix them. Assertive but friendly patients can forestall problems by taking a few basic precautions.

- Don't ever let coverage lapse.

    My husband is self-employed and my son Joe is very ill. We pay around $400 a month for health insurance through a health maintenance organization. We pay a co-pay of $5 per doctor visit and $7 per prescription. Though we can't choose our hospital (our HMO runs their own hospitals) it has been a blessing. With my thyroid cancer and five pregnancies on this plan, well-baby visits, broken bones, and all the stuff of childhood, plus Joe's care, I can't imagine how much we've saved. The $400 a month has been a bargain. My husband was laid off six months before Joe was diagnosed, and I'm very happy we scrimped and saved our medical coverage.

- Pick the best plan and stay up to date on your policy coverage. Make sure you have all supplemental materials. Get a copy of the actual contract (the small print one) not the glossy booklets sent to plan members that provide few details. It is the actual contract itself that governs the plan, not the patient booklets. Evaluate how much you can or cannot get through the plan, how much your physician can or cannot do, and how restrictive the plan is overall.

    My company offers a choice of managed care plans. I'm always amazed by the people who choose a plan based only on which one costs less and/or has lower deductibles. Later, they find out that the plan is too restrictive or that the doctors are dropping out monthly. People need to consider much more than the out-of-pocket expenses. Don't be penny-wise and pound-foolish.

- Pick the right doctor. If you find an ethical, compassionate doctor and you work to establish a good relationship, you will have far fewer problems. It is less likely that your caring doctor will succumb to pressure to give you inferior care if he has a good relationship with you. Use the steps outlined in Chapter 2, *Finding the Right Doctor*, and add the following questions: How are you paid by the HMO? Capitation? Salary? Are there any financial incentives that create ethical dilemmas for you? What would you do if I needed a referral to a specialist, and the HMO said no?

- Add a point-of-service (POS) option to your coverage. This allows you to go outside of the network (approved physicians and hospitals) if you get a serious illness and wish to see an expert not in the plan. The HMO agrees to pay a percentage of the fee from the outside expert (usually 70 percent after you pay a hefty deductible). For instance, if you need a kidney transplant, you may not wish to go to the small hospital in your HMO that has performed only a few such surgeries. Instead, you research the best facilities for kidney transplants, activate your POS, and get state-of-the-art treatment at a renowned transplant center. POS plans are more expensive than basic coverage. However, you buy peace of mind, knowing that you can get the best medicine has to offer should the need arise.

- Don't sign away your right to go to court. Some HMOs have arbitration agreements, in which you lose your right to go to court. Instead, you must go through an HMO-controlled arbitration process. If there is such a clause in the HMO contract, simply cross it out and initial it. If your employer has made such an agreement for his entire workforce, lobby to have that provision changed.

- Always ask if there are other treatment options available for you than those the HMO recommends. If your doctor or a utilization committee denies you treatment or referrals you think you need, or says no other treatment options exist, make them put the denial in writing.

   I was diagnosed with strep a couple of years ago with no real symptoms except a slightly sore throat. The only reason I even had a culture was because I worked in day care at the time, strep was going around, and I thought I was pregnant. The doctor didn't think it was strep, but ran the test to be sure after I insisted.

- Be friendly with doctors, nurses, lab technicians, receptionists, and administrators. Even organizations with strict rules are run by human beings like you. Cheerful greetings and a smile will help the HMO workers see you as a person rather than another package on the assembly line. Friendliness makes it more likely that they will go the extra mile for you if the need arises.

- If you need a referral, procedure, or hospitalization, ask the doctor or hospital if they have any suggestions on how to make authorization easier. There are often key words to use—medical necessity, bad faith refusal, irreparable damage, not within the acceptable standards of care—that may get a quick response. The doctors may suggest strategies that they know from experience will work well.

- If you are referred to a specialist, make sure that the authorization has arrived at the specialist's office prior to your appointment.

> *I had an appointment scheduled with Dr. S. at the UCLA Medical Center. I had received a questionnaire in advance and was asked to bring in any and all records concerning my illness.*

> *I arrived 30 minutes early as requested. After 1 hour and 45 minutes I was informed that they had not received authorization from my insurance. This was a task my doctor was to have done. I then had to sign a form guaranteeing the payment for the office visit ($325). I had driven 2 hours to get there and was now 2 hours into the appointment. I wasn't about to cancel it.*

> *It's been four months since the appointment and the snafu still has not been resolved. The lesson here is that if you need a referral authorization from your insurance company see to it that it is done and a copy is in your hands before any appointment.*

- When you go for an appointment, decide in advance what you want, be clear and concise in your presentation, then be reasonable and persistent.

> *When my pediatrician joined a large group practice, triage nurses began to take calls. Before, I either talked to his nurse or the receptionist. They both knew me and knew that if I called, my daughter was really sick. This nurse wouldn't let me have an appointment. I tried to tell her that, for my daughter, a high fever was unusual and serious, but she didn't listen. So I waited an hour and called back. I told her the fever was higher and I felt strongly that she needed to be seen. I told her that if she felt she'd get in trouble for overbooking, to go check with my doctor for permission. I was sure he'd say to come in. And he did. It's a good thing, because my daughter had pneumonia.*

- Get your HMO doctor on your side. For instance, if you feel you need a specialist, but the quality of the specialists in the network is low, try to get the PCP to side with you that you need a specialist to handle your care. If the PCP cannot get you a referral outside the network, contact well-known specialists outside the network to try to convince the company's medical director that state-of-the-art care cannot be provided by on-staff doctors. Contact national organizations (see Appendix C) or famous institutions (Stanford, the Mayo Clinic, etc.) to see if they will recommend one of the top experts available for your problem. Then send a certified letter to the HMO medical director stating, "Dr. B., national authority on XYZ disease who works at the Mayo Clinic, recommends Dr. A. for neurosurgery."

- Take notes, a tape recorder, or a friend with you to appointments.

My sister, who has had a lot of trouble with her HMO doctors ignoring symptoms, brought a friend with her when she went to the doctor this week. Even though the friend didn't say a word, her doctor's attitude was completely different—he took her symptoms seriously and actually ordered most of the tests that referral doctors had recommended months ago.

- Never stay in a hospital by yourself. Have a spouse or trusted friend present at all times when you are in the hospital, even if that means sleeping in a chair or on the floor. Hospitals are complex institutions, and with nurses and other professional caregivers being replaced in favor of low-wage, relatively untrained laborers, you may be unable to get the attention you require. If you're in a hospital, you may be medicated, or unable to get up easily from the bed. Having an advocate present to monitor what is given you, and to make sure you get the treatment you need, is essential. If something goes wrong, he or she can act quickly to get help.

Dr. Steinberg sums up the consumer attitude you need to adopt in *The Insider's Guide to HMOs*:

The good HMO consumer is someone who is willing and able to search out the best medical care available for her medical problems. If you're shy, don't like to make waves, or are too busy or too passive to take charge of your health care, you'll have to change…First, you have to…fully understand that your HMO may not, spontaneously, provide you with the best possible heath care unless you are willing to prod, cajole, and supervise it and its doctors in the care they deliver. An HMO, inherently, tends to deliver too little care, less costly care, and potentially less effective care unless the consumer knows enough to demand otherwise. It's not that you can't or won't get the best care available in an HMO, it's that you'll have to work to get it.[10]

Types of problems

Problems can arise with any insurance plan. Some of the problems most common with managed care organizations follow.

- Delay in getting an appointment.

- Short appointments.

- Gatekeeper won't refer to a specialist. This is one of the most common complaints lodged against HMO primary care doctors. HMOs strongly encourage primary doctors to handle most medical care themselves to keep costs down. This makes sense for garden-variety ailments—ear infections or bronchitis—but for people with a rare or life-threatening disorder, it can cause major problems.

- Doctors pressured to limit care.

- Specialists in network aren't the best for the problem.

- Restrictions on prescription drugs.

    My daughter was given powerful drugs to fight her leukemia. They made her deathly ill and she vomited continuously. I heard from other people in our support groups that there were some really effective anti-nausea drugs available. I asked the HMO doctors to please give her some, but they refused, saying, "Our policy is to wait until kids have lost 30 percent of their body weight before we give them those drugs. They are terribly expensive."

- Difficulty getting authorization for emergency care. Some HMO subscribers also have difficulties getting their insurer to pay for emergency care if it occurred outside the network, for example, if you became ill on a trip.

    My daughter Belle is seriously ill. We have been pretty lucky (knock on wood!) as far as medical costs are concerned. My husband's union offered us a choice several years ago between PPO and HMO. A lot of negative things have been written about HMOs recently (and I could add my .02), but ours has been very good about paying—we are responsible only for a $10 co-payment for office visits, $10 payment for each prescription, and that's about it. Our costs have been in time and energy spent trying to get authorizations from our primary care physician to the *proper specialist, emergency room, hospital, etc. We have had to sit in offices and emergency rooms for hours (literally) waiting for an authorization to have Belle treated. It's maddening, especially when she is ill.*

- Limited hospital stays.

Heart patient struggles through HMO bureaucracy

Business Week reporter Howard Gleckman wrote of the tremendous amount of time and energy it took to negotiate with HMO doctors and bureaucrats to get his father care for his failing heart. After his father's second episode of heart failure, his mother received a frightening phone call, saying the HMO would no longer cover hospitalization. His father had to go home from the hospital unable to walk, catheterized, medicated, and sick while his mother scrambled to find help. Once home, he couldn't see his heart specialist without first visiting his primary care doctor. Both trips required an ambulance. Then, when the family complained that the primary care doctor was slow in responding to problems, the company told them to change doctors. The family called three: one wouldn't take any more HMO patients, the others never called back.[11]

- Limitations on care.
- Refusal to pay for treatments deemed experimental by the HMO.
- Refusal to pay for care at noncontract facilities.
- Automatic refusals.

It is very easy for HMOs to reject a claim, and they know a certain percentage of patients will take it lying down (some literally, sadly enough). They also know if they have to explain their rejection, it may be tough. There may be a gray area, in which, when push comes to shove, they can't defend themselves. I remember trying to get pre-approval for a procedure at a nearby hospital. My doctor told me I shouldn't panic, as the insurance company turned everyone down the first time—that was their procedure. Then, when you wrote an appeal, they would take your request seriously, and usually they honored it. I guess it was their way of weeding out the nonfighters.

Solving problems

The types of problems encountered by patients in managed care systems range from having to wait weeks for an appointment to refusal to pay for emergency room visits. Each managed care organization has a complaint and appeals procedure to follow, and they are required to provide this information to you. Get a copy of your group's policies. Don't rely on the information given to you on the phone—you could waste precious time following the wrong rules. As one patient said, "One thing I learned in the HMO, you can't be a wimp."

Problems fall into two broad categories: grievances and appeals. Grievances are complaints about service, such as a rude doctor or waiting too long for an appointment. Appeals are a procedure used when the plan denies or terminates a service you think you need, or refuses to pay for care you've already received. To file a grievance with your HMO, take the following steps.

- Talk to the person with whom you had the problem to see if it can be resolved.

- Call the member services department and explain the problem. Make sure to write down the date and time, the phone number, and the first and last names of the person with whom you spoke. Keep a record of what was said and note the person's direct phone line number.

- If the problem is not resolved, write to the plan to ask for an investigation. Different states (as well as each plan) have varying amounts of time during which they are required to respond. To find out your state's regulations, call your state department of insurance.

- Call frequently to ask about the status of the investigation.

Take the following steps to begin the appeal process.

- First, make an appointment with your PCP to explain your problem and ask for help. For example, if the problem is refusal to refer you to a specialist, ask her for the reasons (medical and economic) why she refuses to refer you. Tell her clearly why you think the referral is necessary. You may just change her mind.

    Here's what I do when my HMO refuses to do something I think I need. Let's say I have a lump in my breast I want biopsied, but the mammogram is negative. I want the biopsy, but the doctor says no. I whip out my pen and notebook and say, "I want to be sure I understand you correctly. You are saying you will not do a biopsy on this lump which has doubled in size over the last ten months, is that correct?" When he says yes, I tell him, "I will be writing a letter for your file containing that exact information." I'd send this letter to the head of the medical staff, the administrator, the local medical society, and anyone else who might be a big gun.

I'd tell them what I want to happen, for example, "I want my biopsy by Friday the 23rd or I will have it done by an outside physician, and I will bill the HMO for all associated costs (including travel time)." I'd include my phone number, and give a specific time when I will call for their final decision. I'd send the letter by registered mail, so they have to sign for it and I get the receipt. It may be that the doctor is under orders not to do a biopsy without a positive mammogram. He may welcome me going toe to toe with the administration so he can do his job. He may not be the bad guy here.

- Your plan is required to notify you in writing about any denial, reduction, or termination of services. If you have not received it, ask for a written response explaining the medical and financial reasons for refusing the treatment or payment. Demand that the names of all persons involved in the decision, including any "medical advisors" and their qualifications, be included. You should also ask for articles from the medical literature that support the plan's position. If the administration can't or won't provide any, your case is strengthened. In the meantime, locate articles that support your position (see Chapter 13, *Researching the Medical Literature*) and attach them to your appeal.

- Take the written denial to your primary care doctor to ask him to write a letter of appeal on your behalf. For instance, if your doctor thinks you need a sophisticated diagnostic test, but the HMO refuses to pay for it, he might be willing to go to bat for you. If he refuses, try to get the plan to send you to another doctor in the network for a second opinion. If they refuse, or if you feel it is important to get an out-of-network view, pay for an independent second opinion yourself.

I have a rare cancer called leiomyosarcoma. I was first treated with chemotherapy, but found out several months later that I had one or possibly two new lung metastases. However, my HMO said I could no longer visit the University of Iowa. They put "CLOSURE" on my case. I went over a year with no treatment while we fought it out. I did not have any traditional treatments during that year, and my lesions grew from two nongrowing lesions in my lungs and a possible residual kidney tumor to over thirty throughout both lungs, a far larger residual, three in my liver, one on my scalp, and possibly one in my right arm and one in my right leg.

I'm not really sure who was at fault. My primary care physician's nurse implied that the HMO was at fault, and my local oncologist said that the HMO was not responding to any messages or phone calls related to my case. However, I really feel that, had either office been a bit pushy, I would have had care prior to the time in which I finally succeeded.

The problem was eliminated after I took the matter into my own hands. I told my oncologist's nurse that I wanted all correspondence between their office and the HMO office to be via registered letter and that I wanted copies. Then I researched my options, and visited the University of Michigan to discuss a gene therapy treatment. One of the oncologists I visited wrote a very long letter to the HMO and informed them that he had read my case very carefully and that he knew how long I had been without care.

HMOs seem to respond to strong-arm tactics. I was told by several nurses at several clinics that the gatekeeper at my HMO had no medical training at all, but that it was her job to keep me from care. The nurses seemed to resent the fact that the person wasn't medically trained, and I don't blame them.

I have been on the new therapy for six months, my disease has stopped progressing, and I'm doing well. All of the above is my case as I know it. The HMO might see it differently.

- Write a letter of appeal yourself and send it to the insurance carrier and your employment benefits manager. Send the letter by certified mail and get a receipt with the signature of the person who accepted the letter. The letter should include a clear and concise definition of the problem as well as your name, policy number, doctors' statements, lab results, and other pertinent materials. Make sure to state in the letter what action you want the group to take to resolve the problem. Don't delay writing the letter: your right to start an appeal may expire in as few as 30 days. Keep copies of all correspondence for your records.

There are two things that I emphasize when I talk to my patients. First, strive to keep the problem in the medical domain to the degree possible. Work to make your doctor your ally. Once you go to appeal, it becomes a contractual process, further and further removed from the human need. Second, I give people permission to challenge the authority of these decisions. The idea of appeal is really foreign to most people and very few actually appeal decisions, even when they clearly should.

- The appeal process begins when you write the letter asking for reconsideration of the HMO's decision. The plan generally must complete this reconsideration of their decision within 60 days. Keep calling to find out the status of the appeal. If you need an expedited appeal because your health could be in peril if you wait the 60 days, request it in writing, and enclose supporting documentation from a doctor.

- Consider hiring a medical claims assistance professional. She will organize paperwork, research appeals procedures, and gather medical reports.

- To go outside the HMO for help, send a copy of your written complaint and related documents to the state insurance commissioner as well as your local and state medical societies.

Outside-network expertise

Harry Christie's nine-year-old daughter, Carley, was diagnosed with a rare cancer called Wilms' tumor. He wanted his daughter treated by physicians with extensive experience. However, he found out that the HMO surgeon had never performed the necessary surgery on a child. The Christies went outside the network to a pediatric surgical oncologist and had their daughter treated. Carley is now twelve with no signs of cancer. Her parents' refusal to allow the inexperienced surgeon to operate led to a nearly year-long court battle resulting in a ruling that the HMO pay all the medical bills.[12]

- Send your appeal to your state senators and representatives and your U.S. senators and representatives. These elected officials have staff members who try to help their constituents. In addition, it helps them, as they ponder how to vote on health care-related bills, to know the struggles that members of managed care organizations sometimes face.

- If you are insured through your place of employment, contact the benefits department or union benefits manager to see if they will support your position. If enough problems arise, your company may threaten to find another health care plan, and this threat may help resolve your problem favorably.

- Don't pay a bill that your insurance or Medicaid should pay, even if the claim is taking a long time going through the system and you are being hounded by collection agencies. Many public assistance programs like Medicaid have no provision for reimbursing you once you have paid. Keep your providers informed about your efforts to get payment. A lawyer suggests :

  People are afraid of ruining their credit rating, but it takes years for medical bills to hit credit reports. As long as an investigation is open, any adverse reports can be explained to creditors. There are federal laws— including the Fair Credit Reporting Act—which govern this.

- If you still have the problem, tell the HMO staffers that you will go to the local and national press after a certain date if the problem is not resolved. Sometimes the threat of bad press will help, while other times it hurts.

- Contact Physicians Who Care, an advocacy group of more than 3,500 doctors. Call their complaint hotline (1-800-800-5154) and leave a message about any abuse or ill effects (denials of access to specialists or procedures, reimbursement problems, denials of needed treatments, etc.) resulting from your HMO care. They will contact you by letter within a week. All information is confidential.

- Contact a consumer advocacy group such as the Consumer Federation of America's insurance group at (202) 547-6426, or the Center for Patient Advocacy at 1-800-846-7444 or on the Internet at http:// www.patientadvocacy.org. Families USA provides a list of state agencies regulating health care and information on state managed care laws at (202) 628-3030 or http://www.familiesusa.org.

- Get a lawyer. Lawsuits can take years, and involve endless maneuvering. Most who go through the process say they underestimated how hard it would be, especially to relive the medical trauma. And then, of course, there is the possibility that you have a legitimate case but will be unable to prove it in court, or state laws may limit your right to collect. Nevertheless, legal help may be your last chance to get the care you need.

Contact your local bar association to find an attorney skilled in insurance litigation. If you need a bone marrow transplant, call the Blood and Bone Marrow Transplant Newsletter's attorney referral service at (847) 831-1913.

Remember that such cases are taken on a contingency fee basis, with no cost to the patient unless/until the case is won. The attorney is paid from the damages awarded. Finding an attorney who feels that your case is worth his time (or money) can be difficult, however. This is when law library research can divulge names of successful attorneys in this field.

Try to remember that many managed care organizations are used to passive consumers. Proactive, savvy HMO consumers can get excellent and comprehensive health care from an HMO if they choose wisely and have a good relationship with their doctor. Even when you are happy with your care, check the status of your HMO periodically because they are being bought, sold, and merged at a rapid rate. Make sure that economic forces have not changed the quality of the care provided by your plan.

Our experiences with an HMO since Belle's leukemia diagnosis in 1996 can be divided into two categories:

1. Financial: very good

2. Authorizations: mediocre to downright scary

Through my husband's union, we were switched from a PPO health plan to an HMO several years ago. At the time, I was very glad because the cost to us, after the PPO plan paid only 80 percent of what they thought was appropriate, got very large after the birth of our second child.

As far as financial impact goes, the HMO has paid (to date) all of Belle's hospital (inpatient, outpatient, emergency room) bills; all but a $10 co-payment for office visits; home health care (from Broviac care to IV antibiotics); all but a $10 co-payment for prescription drugs. On the down side, there is this matter of authorizations: technically, nothing can be done by anyone except the primary physician (Belle's pediatrician, in this case) without an authorization. In order to get one, someone must call the pediatrician, explain why the authorization is necessary, get her to write up an authorization and give it to the person who processes them and who will then (you hope) get the authorization to the relevant doctor, clinic, etc.

Sometimes, a simple phone call suffices. Other times, I have to double-check the process every step of the way. More than once we have arrived for an appointment and have had to wait (sometimes with a sick child, always with an anxious and bored one) while we tracked down the authorization.

Another complicating factor is the conflict between the pediatrician, who wants to stay on top of things and direct Belle's care, and the specialist, who feels that he/she should be the person in charge. This has led to shouting matches, recriminations, etc., some of which we were forced to be involved in. This has not improved Belle's care in any way I can see.

Finally, a relatively minor, but very real problem for us parents: we have had to listen to literally hours of badmouthing HMOs by the doctors. This (1) placed us in an awkward position, since without the HMO we would surely be bankrupt and, despite the many glitches, Belle has received excellent care, and (2) wasted our valuable time—time in which we could have slept, eaten, taken care of our daughter, written thank-you notes to all those who helped us out, etc.

We have been very lucky that Belle contracted a disease for which there is a pretty straightforward protocol; even so, we have had to fight to extract every single authorization for the most mundane and predictable things, like regular blood tests. ("Why does it have to be done there? Why can't you do it here? Why do they have to use the catheter?" and so on). I just pray every day that we don't get into some of the murky areas that HMOs are notorious for fighting over. Would that everyone could be so lucky!

CHAPTER 4

Communication

It is often said by way of excuse that doctors are insufficiently trained for humane relations...but what I wanted and needed badly, from that man then, was the frank exchange of human concern. When did such a basic transaction between two mammals require postgraduate instruction beyond our mother's breast?

—Reynolds Price
A Whole New Life

LANGUAGE CAN ILLUMINATE OR OBSCURE. It can present the facts, camouflage ignorance, or influence the unwary. Your job, as an assertive recipient of health care, is to ensure that your medical communication is an exchange of information. What you tell your doctor is the foundation on which diagnosis and treatment rest. Clear explanations of symptoms, combined with relevant context from your personal life, allow the doctor to begin his examination armed with all pertinent data. You are the expert on your symptoms, feelings, and medical history. Without this vital information, the doctor, despite the availability of a high-tech arsenal, cannot give you the best possible care.

On the other hand, the words spoken by the doctor to you not only explain the probable cause of your illness, but help you interpret this information as well. Clear, meaningful conversation determines whether you will buy and take medications appropriately or make lifestyle changes necessary for your continued well-being. How the information is presented can determine what treatment choices you make and how you feel about them. Clear, honest discussions with your physician are an important health resource, enabling you to understand the complexities and ambiguities of treatment options and make informed decisions. Such discussions help you feel better and give you power. The words spoken by a doctor can bestow the gift of hope, or rip it away. Louis Nizer once said, "Words of compassion, skillfully administered, are the oldest therapy known to man."

Thus, in medical talking, both sides of the dialogue are essential for good care to result. This chapter will help you form a satisfying partnership with your doctor by exploring different models of patient-physician interactions and discussing effective strategies for improving communication. Methods are presented to prevent jargon from interfering with understanding and to equalize power with your doctor. Many veteran patients share their stories on how they elicited information from and shared decision-making with their doctors.

Types of relationships

Once you and your physician enter a relationship, you each have expectations and hopes for the conduct of the other. Central to the roles of both patient and doctor are authority and autonomy. The likelihood of conflict diminishes if you both have similar views about who is in control and how much freedom you have to accept or reject your doctor's suggestions.

There are many types of doctor-patient relationships, but they can be grouped into three broad categories: paternal, adversarial, and collegial.

Paternal

In a paternal relationship, the patient tends to be submissive, and the doctor assumes a parental role. Patients in such relationships with their physician are often afraid to disagree or offer suggestions concerning their treatment due to a misplaced sense of deference. A surprising number of patients feel intimidated by their doctor and express fear that if they question the doctor, their care will suffer. These patients feel that "good" patients always defer to their doctor's superior education and experience. In fact, paternalistic doctors place a high value on compliant patients—those who reliably do what they are told. Max Lerner describes this model of doctor-patient interaction as "drenched with authority."[1]

Part of the regression common when dealing with serious illness is the tendency to view the doctor as a trusted parent, able to heal, soothe, and make it all better. While this submissive role is comforting for many patients, the problem remains that, although medical personnel never intend harm, they are human and sometimes make mistakes. If you don't monitor your own drugs and treatment, these mistakes may go unnoticed.

In addition, most patients are the experts on their bodies and symptoms. If communication is only one-way—from doctor to patient—crucial information can be overlooked. The leave-it-to-the-doctor model dispenses with patient responsibility. It occurs if patients are awed by the doctor's expertise, think they don't know enough, or are frightened about the possibility of conflict if they express any opinions. Even members of the medical profession find themselves sometimes reverting to a childlike role when they are ill. In *Equal Partners*, Jody Heymann was a medical student when she was diagnosed—eventually—with a brain tumor:

> As the headaches grew more frequent and harder to ignore, I called an internist... Over the phone he diagnosed stress because I was writing both a master's and doctoral thesis. Sensing the headaches were more severe than stress-based headaches, but needing to place my trust in the physician caring for me, I traded trusting myself for trusting him.[2]

Adversarial

Some patients and physicians adopt an "us against them" attitude that is counterproductive. A small number of patients seem to feel that the disease and its treatment are the fault of the medical staff, and they blame staff for any setbacks that occur. This attitude prevents the development of trust and confidence in the doctor—one of the crucial components of healing. Some doctors, as well, help create an adversarial relationship by failing to recognize the needs of the patient and refusing to negotiate an acceptable middle ground.

> I was in the hospital after surgery, but in a panic waiting for the results of a bone scan. The covering surgeon came in and with a broad smile asked if I was ready to be discharged. "What's with the bone scan?" was my reply. He got arrogant (obviously hadn't bothered to check for the results) and yelled, "Do you want to go home or not?" I responded, "Frankly, my concern at the moment is not whether I go home now or later. I want to know the results of the scan." Well, he had had enough. He stormed out, tried to slam the door, but hospital doors don't usually slam very well, and raced down the hall. A lovely nurse had observed the whole scene and said she was absolutely shocked at this behavior and she would get the results of the scan. They were fine. I went home.

Other patients are pushed into an adversarial stance by inconsiderate or inappropriate treatment, as the following story describes:

> Ultimately the pain brought me to the emergency room, where I could hear the emergency room physician on the phone with my doctor upstairs telling him, "She clearly has a benign abdomen, I don't think it is anything, I will send her up." I was furious. I was doubled over in pain

and I am hearing a doctor tell another that there is nothing wrong with me. Do they think that the walls are soundproof and that we are all deaf and dumb? If doctors are going to be talking about a patient they should be sure that what they are saying will not be harmful to the patient if they hear it or they should be sure that the patient cannot hear them.

Once upstairs my fury led to a very unpleasant exchange. I overheard the doctor and resident in the hall and heard the doctor tell the resident, "Well, let's just look at her and get this over with." I had lost 20 pounds, looked cadaverous, and was doubled in pain and I was just someone to get rid of. That was twice in a period of 10 minutes that I was allowed to overhear doctors discussing me in derogatory terms as if I were no more significant than a sack of flour.

My anger was clearly obvious and I informed them upon entering the room that I was not interested in anything they had to say. I was there under protest and wanted only a referral elsewhere.

In other cases, some patients react to the adversarial doctor as they would to a paternal one. The doctor becomes the scolding parent and the patient shrinks into submission. These failed relationships result in patients changing doctors or dropping out of medical care completely. Often, doctors are not even aware that the relationship has failed: the patient simply doesn't return.

Collegial

A true partnership exists when patient and doctor are able to engage in mutually respectful dialogues and defer to each other's areas of expertise. Here the doctor recognizes that the patient is the expert on his own body and symptoms. He creates a climate in which the patient feels comfortable discussing various treatment options or any concerns that arise. In turn, the patient treats the doctor with respect. This collaboration leads to a healthy and mutually beneficial relationship. Honest communication, and a commitment to work through disagreements, is essential for the partnership to work, but the effort is well worth it. The patient has confidence in the doctor, stress is lessened by the supportive nature of the relationship, and the physician feels comfortable that the patient will comply with the treatment plan, thereby ensuring herself the best chance for recovery.

I had a wonderful relationship with the specialist assigned to me. He blended perfectly the science and the art of medicine. His manner was warm, he was extremely well qualified professionally, and he was very

easy to talk to. I could bring in articles to discuss with him, and he wel-
comed the discussion. Although he was very busy, I never felt rushed. I
laughed when I read in the chart, "M. asks innumerable appropriate
questions."

One doctor remarked on the change over time in doctor attitudes:

I think that, in America, the younger physicians try to be a different
breed from the ones who trained twenty or thirty years ago. We've gone
from being paternal to working together. We tell you your options, make
a recommendation, and then you need to make the decisions.

It is not just a bit of folk wisdom that the patient is expert on himself. Many studies have assessed the patient's "subjective" feelings versus the doctor's "objective" findings, with the assumption that clinical, science-based physician opinions would be more accurate than patient intuition. On the contrary, one study from Yale that followed 23,000 people for up to 17 years, found that patients' self-evaluations of their health were far more accurate than those provided by physical exams or numerous tests. [3]

Sharing your knowledge of yourself and your symptoms will help you and your doctor work together to improve your health.

Equalize the power

The doctor brings specialized knowledge and experience to the medical encounter, but you live with the results. Taking action to equalize the power may not only make the medical relationship more satisfying, but might also improve your care.

We will never have the broad-based knowledge of a medical profes-
sional, but I find that medical professionals continue to be unaware or
unappreciative of the fact that in narrow areas patients are often better
informed on the most current literature, issues, etc., than they are.

It seems to me that with a patient who has the skills and time to
focus in on the information relevant to her own situation and a doctor
with his/her general knowledge we have the best possible combination for
teamwork. But it does take a doctor who isn't threatened by the patient
knowing something he/she doesn't and who respects the patient as an
equal partner in practicing medicine.

What do you want to be called?

Persons of perceived higher status are usually mentioned first in conversations, hence, king and queen, husband and wife, doctor and patient. See if you are uncomfortable saying them out loud in the reverse order: queen and king, wife and husband, patient and doctor. Some of the discomfort comes from changing a habit, but there's more at work here than that—the discomfort also stems from upsetting the social apple cart. In contrast, the order does not establish the status in power-neutral word pairs—such as day/night or right/left.

Think about how the use of titles establishes power sharing—or lack thereof—and decide how you want to be addressed by your doctor. What is important is not so much what you end up calling each other, but that you feel the issue was addressed as two adults and not just assumed that it would be Dr. Smith and Pat.

> If they stand, then I stand. I am polite but meticulous and careful about what I say. I often repeat back what they say and then ask if I understand correctly. I don't believe thinking of them as a plumber is good nor is it good to think of them as a super-person. They are peers, who have specialized knowledge on a topic of importance to me. I want to treat them courteously and professionally just as I generally expect persons to treat me. I don't know if the use of first names is a generally good rule or not, but since I hold a Ph.D. then it's appropriate for us to both use first names or both use Dr. If they introduce themselves as Dr. ___, then I say I'm Dr. ___. I may then say, "Are first names okay with you?" My experience is that the best don't need their egos fed by use of the Dr. title.

The mother of a frequently hospitalized child adds:

> I ask right off the bat what the doctor wants to be called. Then I suggest equal billing. We either both go by titles (Dr. and Mrs.) or by first names. I actually prefer first names, but realize that some doctors aren't comfortable with this social etiquette. I do not let them call me "mom."

Another patient has a different view:

> I've had doctors that prefer to be called by their titles and I respect that. However, I still like to be called Carol because that's what I'm comfortable with. As long as he offers to call me what I want—and doesn't presume to use my first name and his title—I'm happy.

Tell the doctor how much you want to know

Before you can share your information needs with your doctor, you must know what those needs are. To help identify your needs, think about what level of information sharing makes you comfortable. If, for instance, you are someone who likes to discuss the scientific aspects of illness—current studies, statistics, probabilities—look for a doctor comfortable with that type of information sharing. If you need to talk with your doctor about your feelings related to the illness and its impact on your life, find someone who is warm, caring, and interactive. These are not necessarily mutually exclusive traits.

Part of the doctor's communication style depends on personality and training in interpersonal skills, but gender can also play a role.

Sex of the doctor affects amount of conversation

A study from Johns Hopkins reported the results of 537 audiotaped medical encounters. On average, female physicians spent more time with each patient, especially female patients, than did their male colleagues. The extra time was spent on positive talk, partnership building, question asking, and information giving. Particularly striking, female doctors spent 40 percent more time in conversation while taking a history than did their male counterparts. Female patients talked almost twice as much with female physicians than they did with male doctors.[4]

If you don't tell your doctors how much you want to know, they try to ferret out what level of information you want, and provide only that. Unfortunately, their interpretation may not be correct. For instance, in the book *Doctors and Patients*, author Peter Berczeller, M.D., presents his view:

> *Of course, patients have to be told what is going on if they require an operation, for example. You cannot recommend removal of part of the colon and yet not tell the patient that he has colon cancer. But if, later on, the tumor has spread, it is not necessary to go over the whole list of organs that are affected. This excessive frankness can only make him even more discouraged... I am not suggesting that we lie to patients or that we give them empty assurances. What I am suggesting, though, is that doctors fulfill their function as interpreters for their patients. It takes courage and the willingness to take responsibility to do this, as well as the ability to keep things to themselves if necessary.[5]*

Unless you are willing to have a doctor assume responsibility for the amount of information you should have about your own illness, you need to speak up. Each of us is different, and we need to share with our doctors what types and amount of information makes us comfortable.

Accept that doctors cannot read your mind. They have widely varying abilities to elicit information from you concerning your preferences. Also accept that there is no one right way for doctors to give information. All patients do not have identical preferences. One patient wrote to a computer cancer discussion on the Internet of her anger at the impersonality of receiving her diagnosis on the phone. Another patient wrote in response:

> And I was annoyed that I had to pressure my surgeon to give me the diagnosis over the phone! Just goes to show that our poor doctors have to deal with very diverse preferences. That's why I think it's a good idea to have a little heart-to-heart with your doctors about how much and in what manner you want to get information. In my case I'm clear: as much as they have time to tell me and ASAP!
>
> Also, this is something that you may need to change from time to time. Keep an eye on your own reactions to information and if you find yourself either more or less eager for the information, it may be time to review your preferences with the doctor. I've noticed, for example, that as a patient's disease progresses, their need for information sometimes dramatically decreases. I think that's reasonable—other things are simply more important when the war is being lost than the details of how it is conducted in the final battles.

Learn the language

When doctors slip into medical jargon, patients react with a variety of feelings, including confusion, annoyance, and bewilderment. A woman going to the doctor because of heavy periods probably will not be reassured to know she has menorrhagia, if no further discussion ensues on causes and treatment. Often, in the world of doctors, hair loss is alopecia and heart attacks myocardial infarctions. As one patient aptly noted, "A rose by any other name would likely be a 'deadly thorned assault vegetation.'"

> During my residency I took care of a woman who came into the renal clinic. She told me she had polycystic kidney disease. She'd been treated at the clinic for over three years. I thought her kidney functions looked suspiciously normal, so I thought maybe there had been a misdiagnosis made long ago. I looked back through her chart and found that

the internal medicine clinic had told her years ago that she had Paget's disease of the bone and she had misunderstood what she had. What probably happened was she came back in and said something that sounded like polycystic and she was funneled to the renal clinic and just stayed there. Her Paget's disease had never been treated. I always recommend that patients ask their doctor to write down the diagnosis so there is no confusion.

Doctors learn to speak medical jargon during their long apprenticeship. While scientific language between doctors or in patients' charts allows precision and clarity, it often causes confusion when used with patients. If a doctor tells you, "You have atrial tachycardia" without any further explanation, it seems much more frightening than if he added that the term means your heart was beating much faster than normal. If he went on to explain the cause of the rapid heartbeat and his plan for treatment, you would probably be less worried and your heartbeat might even slow down a bit as you relaxed. If your doctor then asked your opinion of the proposed treatment plan and discussed any problems you might have with the pill schedule or follow-up appointments, you would probably walk away feeling respected and empowered. Dr. Edward Rosenbaum describes his altered perception about communication in *A Taste of My Own Medicine*:

> *At my first visit [with] Dr. Duvall…he'd shaken my hand and said, "I'm sorry to meet you under these circumstances." At that time, I'd taken his expression to mean that he was saying good-bye—a final good-bye— when in fact what he was doing was expressing sympathy. I used to think a little condescendingly about patients who misinterpret doctors' words and expressions. Yet, with all my experience, I did the same. Patients are vulnerable. They need good, plain language to explain their situations. Even so, they are watching for every sign from the doctor. Maybe there's nothing to be done about that, but a spoonful of empathy might help.*[6]

Some doctors use scientific shoptalk to maintain their position of authority, while others simply think in those terms and forget to translate into plain English when speaking to patients. Jargon can also be used as a way for the physician to distance himself from you. Whatever the reason, you don't have to be the target of language that hurts rather than helps. You could take any of the following actions to deal with jargon.

- Any time the doctor uses a word that you are not familiar with, say, "I don't understand, could you describe it another way, please?" Pleasant persistence can work wonders.

- Write down what he says and ask him to spell any unfamiliar words. Pretty soon he'll use lay terms, if only to save time. Use a medical dictionary such as *Mosby's Medical Dictionary* or *Taber's Cyclopedic Medical Dictionary* (usually found in the reference section of your local library or a bookstore) to translate any unfamiliar terms that you wrote down.

- Bring along a friend or relative to write down or tape record the information.

  Demand that they make things as clear as possible. If needed, call back and leave a question with a nurse. Write out a question and send it to them. A good trick is send them a fax. They get very few of these and this has been effective for me. In a recent conversation with a doctor, she said she was going to have to get more computer literate as she had more and more patients coming in with computer printouts. Information is power. Get all you can and use it.

- Try to ignore their odd use of common words. For instance, their definition of a "tolerable" treatment might differ greatly from yours.

  The chemotherapy treatment was "tolerable." To a patient, the word means the treatment was extremely rough. The medical world uses this term when the patient survives.

- Ask if the doctor has any preprinted information sheets on your condition. These can be invaluable sources of understandable information and sometimes serve as a starting point for more conversation.

- If you are having trouble trying to interpret your medical chart or other records, call the American Health Information Management Association at 1-800-335-5535 and ask for their brochure called *Understanding Your Medical Records*. The brochure helps you to obtain and understand your records and also contains a list of common medical prefixes, suffixes, and root words.

Rather than thinking that you shouldn't ask for clarification because you might be taking too much time (the passive patient viewpoint), shift your focus to thinking, "Why is he wasting my time (and his) by speaking a language that there is no reason I should know?"

Remain a person, not an object

Many of us have been shocked to hear a doctor refer to a hospitalized person as "the liver in room 103" or "the tonsillectomy down the hall." Students learn to call patients by the names of their disease, as if the disease and its treatment are more important then the person suffering from it. This tendency is increasing in this age of subspecialization, when it is common for one patient to have several doctors, each caring for only one part of the body. A crucial part of healing is the need to feel cared for as a person. Both subtle and direct methods can be used to remind doctors that you are a person, not an object. Some suggestions from assertive patients are:

• Wear your own clothes while hospitalized or when being examined.

> *I feel uncomfortable and, yes, even awkward wearing a paper vest in the doctor's office. To me it is a question of dignity. I don't mind the vest when I am actually being examined. But the examination takes just a few minutes; the rest of the time I spend just talking to my doctor. And I have a hard time talking to a fully dressed doctor as an equal when I am dressed in a piece of paper. When I decided to just wear my own clothes—a loose, button-down blouse—it made a big difference in my comfort level and confidence. My doctor actually agrees with me on this, and he tried to get cloth gowns for his office. But his partners voted to keep paper vests because it would cost too much to have the gowns cleaned and ironed.*

> *Last summer I started going to a new internist, and I was given a regular hospital gown to wear. I told the doctor how much I appreciated not being handed a paper vest. He replied that two women had recently joined the practice, and they insisted on cloth instead of paper gowns. So some doctors do realize that the dignity of the patient is important. And all the nurses and female technicians at my doctor's office said, "Good," when I told them I wouldn't wear the paper anymore.*

• Don't let medical caregivers blame you for your diagnosis through the use of guilt-inducing language. In her book *A Not Entirely Benign Procedure*, Perry Klass wrote, "You never say that a patient's blood pressure fell or his enzymes rose. Instead, the patient is always the subject of the verb: 'He dropped his pressure.' 'He bumped his enzymes.'"[7] One husband who was told that his wife's premature delivery was due to her "incompetent cervix" responded sharply, "The only incompetent around here is the doctor who didn't diagnose this problem that resulted in the death of our firstborn child." Another patient describes the blame game:

> *My doctor made me feel like I was not even a person but a statistic. Frankly, he told me that I had failed the treatment and that was why I had a recurrence. I left the clinic so shaken that I was willing to give it all*

up and take my chances. But, instead, I went back in and demanded to see a new doctor.

Simply refuse to accept blame. You could say, "I feel blamed by your language. Perhaps we could just agree that the medicine you recommended did not work as well as either of us hoped it would. Do you have any further suggestions for treatment?"

- Remind the doctor that your illness is not affecting just one organ, but many aspects of your life: level of activity, friendships, marriage, career, frame of mind.

My gynecologist is great at discussing treatment options in terms of how they will impact my life. After a recent surgery, my estrogen levels declined resulting in drying membranes and much discomfort. We talked about how this was affecting my life and what the benefits and problems might be from hormonal therapy. I have a lot of personal problems, and she was worried how I would respond emotionally to the hormones. We discussed it in depth and chose a plan based on me and my life—not some cookie-cutter approach to all low-estrogen premenopausal women.

- Talk about nonmedical portions of your life. It's often surprising how an emotional connection can be forged just by establishing a shared hobby or chatting about grandchildren.

I once told my daughter's doctor that I had a dream in which she (the doctor) was a Shakespearean actor. I just expected her to laugh and get back to business. I was surprised when she started telling me that her daughter was an actor currently appearing in "A Midsummer Night's Dream." With every appointment, we learned more about one another's outside lives. We no longer need to see her professionally, but we send Christmas cards and occasionally correspond.

Making sense of statistics

Doctors are trained to treat disease. They decide on the best options for treatment by learning how large numbers of people respond to it. You, however, are an individual.

Stephen Jay Gould, an evolutionary biologist and author who teaches at Harvard, is a long-term survivor of a type of cancer that has a median survival rate of eight months. He knew from his scientific training that, according to the statistics, half of those diagnosed would be dead by eight months, while half would live longer. His research revealed what he had hoped: the survival curve for the half who survived longer stretched out for years, in some cases, many years. He wrote a wise and humane essay called "The Median Isn't the Message" (electronically printed at *http://www.cancer-guide.org*) that explains a valuable approach to applying statistics to individuals.

If you choose to learn about the probabilities associated with your medical treatment, make sure that the numbers cited are current for your age, disease, amount of disease at diagnosis, condition, and proposed treatment (if you are going to participate in an experimental treatment, there may be no statistics on success rates). Also, consider the qualifications of the person providing the numbers. A professor of computer systems engineering describes his way of dealing with statistics:

> *Always have a notebook or paper to write down things. A tape recorder is OK, but may be intimidating to the doctor. I think paper is better. When they spout some numbers, force them to slow down. First write down the number(s), that's the easy part. Then ask them again what these numbers mean and write it down. Then repeat it back to them as in: "If I understand you correctly, then you are saying that if I do this procedure that my risk of _____ will be 15-30 percent. Is that correct?" You can also ask (at the risk of making them mad): "What is the source of these numbers? Can you give me the references so I can read them?" I would only do this if I truly intended to check the reference. But, then, I often check references.*

Steer clear of asking for statistics on how long you will live. No doctor knows.

> *My own doctor is an optimistic man who always tries to find the bright side, but he doesn't give false hope either. He just doesn't give statistics unless asked. For instance, he has never given me a prognosis, and I have never requested one. If I thought he knew when I would die, I would ask him about it. But he doesn't know what will happen to me, so I see no need to ask. When I do want his honest opinion about something, I ask and he tells me. I like his positive approach. He doesn't ignore the negative; he just doesn't stress it.*

When writer Norman Cousins was diagnosed with a degenerative disease and given a one in five hundred chance of recovery, he wrote in *Anatomy of an Illness*, "Up until that time, I had been more or less disposed to let the doctors worry about my condition. But now I felt a compulsion to get into the act. It seemed clear to me that if I was to be that one in five hundred, I had better be something more than a passive observer."[8] He used a dire prediction to take control of his medical care. Others, however, are crushed by hearing dismal statistics. Once again, it is your right to tell the physician what, and how much, you want to know.

There are two statistics that I believe.

At this moment I am alive. Certainty: 100%.

I will die sometime. Certainty: 100%.

I find both equally comforting and challenging.

Establish effective communication

Clear and frequent communication is the lifeblood of a positive patient-doctor relationship. Doctors need to be able to explain clearly and listen well, and patients need to feel comfortable asking questions and expressing concerns before they grow into grievances. Nurses and doctors cannot read patients' minds, nor can a patient prepare for a procedure unless it has been thoroughly explained. The following sections contain patient suggestions on how to establish and maintain good communication.

Recognize that we can't walk in each other's shoes

Unless your doctor has actually had your illness, she can't imagine what you are experiencing. Given that, we need to extend sympathy and understanding to one another, while recognizing the gap between our realities. She's trying to stay on schedule, worrying about one of her patients who just went to the emergency room, thinking about whether she's going to fit in lunch, perhaps wondering about when she'll get home to her kids. You may be worrying about whether your shortness of breath means that you'll die of emphysema like your Aunt Maude and you're too terrified to describe your feelings. James Payne, in his book *Me Too: A Doctor Survives Prostate Cancer*, captures this duality:

> "*Dr. Payne, I got the results of your blood test back and everything was OK except that your PSA was slightly elevated. It probably doesn't mean a thing, but I think we ought to get a urology consultation to evaluate your prostate. I hope this news doesn't spoil your weekend.*"

> "*Not at all, Judy. I appreciate your interest and concern. By all means, let's proceed with the urology consult.*"

Translation: "Not only have you spoiled my weekend, but every day and night for the foreseeable future until some knowledgeable specialist can truly say, 'Well, Dr. Payne, we've run every test, X ray, scan, and gadgetry known to God and man, and we find that your only possible problem is an overactive libido. Further, although each test was uncomfortable, expensive, and completely dehumanizing, and the normal findings were reported agonizingly slowly, we declare you healthy and free of all forms of cancer.'"9

Patients and doctors truly occupy different worlds; but together we control whether the intersection of these worlds heals or hurts.

Befriend the staff

Your doctor's staff will make appointments, determine how long the appointment will be, answer your phone calls, resolve billing problems, and track down lost test results. They can be incredible allies or formidable opponents. Learn their names, smile, and chat briefly whenever you are in the office. Some patients who require frequent appointments often show their appreciation in tangible ways.

Early in my daughter's treatment for cancer, we changed pediatricians. The first was aloof and patronizing, and the second was smart, warm, funny, and caring. He and his staff were absolutely wonderful. So every year, she and her younger sister put on their Santa hats or their elf outfits and take homemade cookies to the doctor, nurse, and staff. The first year, I carried her in and she sang, "We Wish You a Merry Christmas." The entire staff crowded around, but her nurse went in the back room and cried, and her doctor got misty-eyed.

Talk about money

A persistent taboo in patient-doctor relations is talking about money. You hire your doctor for his expertise just like you use a lawyer to write a will. But culturally—at least in the U.S.—doctors have acquired a higher status, making it difficult for many patients to broach mundane matters such as fees. However, if you are thinking about how much the visit is going to cost you while he is describing a test, you might miss some important information. Likewise, the doctor may also be constrained by his employer to limit his medical recommendations based on cost—a fact you need to know. So how can you broach this sometimes delicate subject?

- Ask about fees during your first appointment, for example, "Could you please explain the fees you charge for the different types of appointments?"

- Discuss with your doctor the option of substituting generic medications for name brands.

  Every time I get a prescription, I have them check the box at the bottom of the form that says generics can be substituted. I'm on a limited income and I count my pennies. I make sure the pharmacist knows to give me the cheapest medicine, too.

- Ask your doctor if he has any free samples. Drug companies give doctors many samples and often you can get these free if you ask.

- Tell your doctor how your finances might affect your ability to pay. Some doctors work out payment plans for financially strapped patients.

- Prevent your doctor from making assumptions about your financial status and its impact on your treatment choices.

  I was diagnosed with an ulcer and my H. pylori count was 72 (normal 12). A new multi-drug protocol had just been approved by the FDA, so my doctor prescribed it. It cost $96 for a two-week course. It's been three months and some of the symptoms have returned. They did another blood test and the count was 36. This time they prescribed tetracycline and Pepto Bismol tablets—total cost, $10 for two weeks. I asked the nurse (who called to tell me the results of the blood test and the prescription) why he chose this treatment rather than the last and she didn't know. There are so many layers of people before I ever get to the doctor that I just never seem to get my questions answered. Does he think money doesn't matter? Does he think I am too stupid to arrange my drug intake around my eating schedule (as is required by tetracycline)? Or was he just initially intellectually curious about the new treatment but has now gone back to the old standby? Or did he simply make a value judgment about the cost versus ease of use and decide for me? Did he even know the cost?

- If there is a problem with billing, find out who is responsible for the problem: doctor's staff, insurance company, managed care plan. Go to the source of the problem for resolution.

Stop the interruptions

Doctors are notorious for interrupting, and it is only going to get worse as pressure mounts on doctors to cut visits short. Interrupting is not only disconcerting, but it can prevent you from sharing the primary reason for the visit. Often, due to embarrassment, anxiety, or fear of the diagnosis, patients don't immediately state their major concern. If you allow the entire visit to focus on what is, in reality, not your true problem, you may very well leave the office misdiagnosed or inadequately treated. On the other hand, if you ramble on about a multitude of complaints, the doctor will need to interrupt to get you to explain the actual reason for the visit.

Incessant interruptions

During the first ninety seconds of the medical visits studied, the doctor interrupted the patient 69 percent of the time after fifteen seconds on average. After interrupting, the doctor asked about the first specific concern mentioned. When the patients tried to respond to the doctor's opening question, only 23 percent completed their reply without the doctor interrupting. Of the patients who were allowed to continue talking, none took more than two and a half minutes to complete their response. The study concluded that the physician's use of closed-ended questioning and controlling style resulted in "the potential loss of relevant information."[10]

To help prevent interruptions, experienced patients made the following suggestions:

- Prior to each appointment, write out a list of problems that you wish to discuss, with the most important items first. Since most of us do not reveal our hearts in just a few minutes—and the average doctor's office visit in the U.S. is only twelve minutes—thorough discussions are difficult, especially for complicated problems. Stating your primary concern first prevents the doctor from focusing on the wrong issue. Stating the major problem early also prevents what doctors dread: a patient who is walking out the door and turns to say, "Just one more thing. Can you think of a reason why I get dizzy several times a day? It's probably nothing, but..."

- If you are interrupted, say in a polite tone of voice, "Excuse me, although I am interested in your thoughts on this, I'd like to finish my explanation. I'll be brief."

- If you are frequently interrupted, you could say, "I feel frustrated when you interrupt me so often. I try to be as brief as possible, yet you continually interrupt. Could you please let me complete my explanation?" You may actually do your doctor a favor by pointing out this habit. Your comment may cause him to re-evaluate his history-taking skills, resulting in better communication. After all, conversations involve two people.

Tell the whole story

Clearly describing your problem or illness enhances communication and saves time for the examination and discussion of treatment options.

> My father, a very active man in his late seventies, developed severe chest pain whenever he was exerting himself. I found him, many times, leaning against his trailer, clutching his chest and panting. He went to the doctor, but didn't tell him when he had the pain. Many wild goose chases followed. He was on all sorts of different medicines. I finally told him, "Dad, it's your heart. Every time you exert yourself you have chest pain. Tell the doctor the whole truth." It turned out that several coronary vessels were blocked. He had a bypass, and he is now pain-free.

Other information to include in your story are answers to the following questions:

- What is the location of the complaint, when did it begin, and is it constant or intermittent?
- Does the problem stay the same or get better and worse?
- Describe the pain (sharp, dull, crushing). Does it spread to other areas of the body, for example, down the arm or leg?
- Is there anything that makes it start, get worse, or improve, such as food, exercise, or stress?
- Are there any other sensations or symptoms that accompany the main problem?
- Have you had this before, and, if so, how was it treated?
- Have you had any significant life changes lately?
- What have you done about this problem, e.g., over-the-counter remedies, homeopathy, or acupuncture?

Use extremely clear language to describe the problem. The less room you leave for misunderstanding, the better. Use concrete terms, and describe how your job, activity level, sex life, or general sense of well-being is being affected by your illness or treatment.

I think fatigue is a particularly difficult problem because it's often not acknowledged or understood, and as a result, there is frequently no treatment. One way to address this issue is to stop referring to your condition or symptom as fatigue. Instead give specific, measurable details which cannot be ignored. For example:

"When I wake up in the morning, I have to sit on the side of the bed for five minutes to gather the energy to walk to the bathroom. I have to hold onto the wall as I walk to the kitchen to prepare breakfast. I sit on a stool to cook, as I cannot stand upright for ten minutes. I go to bed at 7:30 PM and wake up at 7:30 AM."

As compared to:

"When I get up in the morning, I am already exhausted."

After sharing the above information, end with a statement that puts the problem in a life context. One example is: "This is causing me problems because..."

Doctors can help get the full story from patients by asking questions such as:

- What's been going on since the last visit?
- What do you think your problem is and what do you think caused it?
- Is there anything else you would like to discuss?
- Have I answered all of your questions?

It also helps if both parties compliment one another whenever the occasion arises. For instance, you could tell your doctor, "I was really impressed at how you diagnosed my problem last visit. I feel so much better. Thank you." Your doctor could reply, "Well, I'm impressed by how well you've managed that complicated drug schedule and made so many lifestyle changes. That must have been hard."

Use humor

Nothing eases tension and smoothes over the rough spots in relationships better than humor. But levity is missing in most health care relationships.

Hospitals tend to be depressing, serious places and doctor's appointments often end without either party cracking a smile. Anything you can do to lighten up the atmosphere helps.

Humor not only makes an appointment or hospital stay more fun for both doctor and patient, but studies show that doctors who have warm, friendly manners and laugh a lot during office visits get sued less than their more stern colleagues.[11] The father of a young girl who was hospitalized for months describes how he tried to "make leukemia so much fun that all the kids would want to have it."

> The humor was not used to make the illness go away, but I used it just to make us feel good. (His wife at this point said, "I disagree. I think it helped her get better faster.") I just figured that no matter what happened, we might as well not be miserable. We were stuck there twenty-four hours a day and I wanted to make it a positive experience.

> I told her that there were three classes of people in the hospital: the nurses, who must be adored and obeyed; the attending physicians, who must be respected because they are big shots and will help you get better; and residents, who are cannon-fodder and will be gone in a month anyway. "Adele, you can do anything you want to them." She actually developed resident radar, she could identify them on sight. Before one surgery, a resident was explaining the consent form, and she stared at him and said, "Daddy, it's a resident, let's diss him." The resident went along with the gag: Adele pulled the consent form from him and signed her name in all big, shaky uppercase letters.

> We had gratuitous praise days on which we'd pick (on) a different staff member every day and constantly tell her how great she was. We'd really load it on, for instance, "Oh, Robin, wow, what have you done with your hair? And your jewelry is fabulous." They'd laugh—and some even asked for extra days.

Mutual decision-making

Times have changed since the first code of the AMA, written in 1847, included these words: "There is a class of patients much dreaded by physicians, namely, those who insist upon being taken into a medical consultation with regard to the treatment. Such patients desire not only to know what medicines are prescribed, but to discuss the reasons therefor; they are not content without exercising their own judgment concerning therapeutic indications and the means of fulfilling them."[12]

Knowledgeable patients no longer blindly follow the advice of their physicians, and with good reason. With the explosion of medical knowledge in the last few decades, one doctor cannot know it all. In addition, doctors are trained to treat disease, not balance the beneficial with the detrimental consequences of treatment for individuals. However, if you think of the proposed therapy in terms of your philosophy of life, family situation, and job, and discuss the therapy with your doctor in that light, your treatment will be personally tailored for you. This process can be easy or difficult, depending on what you find out in your research, and the personalities and communication skills of both you and your doctor. The following story from a breast cancer patient clearly explains the conflicts that sometimes arise over medical information sharing and decision-making:

> I had gone for a routine mammogram and found out that it indicated the need for a biopsy. The preliminary results showed cancer and my husband and I were told to come back in ten days for the full pathology results and treatment discussion. Shocked, we left the office and went straight to a bookstore and the library and collected many books concerning breast cancer. My stepfather is a retired pharmacology professor, so we traveled to his home and spent ten days studying. We then went to see the surgeon who had been recommended by my gynecologist.

> He had already decided that I should have a mastectomy and reconstruction. In fact, he had already made an appointment with the reconstruction surgeon and the only decision that I was expected to make was one of timing—whether to have the reconstruction immediately after the mastectomy or at a later date. When we questioned why he was recommending a treatment at odds with the guidelines set by the National Cancer Institute and many other sources, he started backing his chair further and further into the corner. He didn't even have the copies of my tests or lab reports to discuss. He was unbelievably unhelpful.

> I wanted to get a second opinion so I asked my OB/GYN for a name. She told me to get the mastectomy. I was shocked and said, "But Jody, why?" She replied, "Because if it gets in your lymph system you're fu**ed." I was speechless.

I went to see another surgeon who also recommended mastectomy. I was fairly angry by this point. I am not stupid and resent being treated as if I am. I am perfectly capable of reading the literature and understanding it. I was very concerned about my health and eager to begin treatment. It was hard to keep making appointment after appointment trying to find a doctor who would discuss my options rather than just their own foregone conclusions.

Luckily, I have portable insurance, so I sought out doctors at the University of Michigan Hospital. There, I met with a team composed of an oncologist, a radiologist, surgeon, and a social worker. After carefully reviewing my case, we worked together and came up with options that were within the range of treatments that were acceptable to me. Finally, I had found a patient-centered system which empowered and informed me while providing options for excellent care. I had my lumpectomy and my radiation treatment there.

Unlike the first doctors above, some doctors care a great deal about discussing all the options and truly communicating with their patients.

At any moment, you are interacting with another human being. This is where medicine is really and truly an art—your ability to communicate with a patient and reach out to meet their needs. And that's where the art of medicine comes in and where the good doctors are well appreciated. There is no cookbook technique. There are many different ways to do it, depending on who is sitting in front of me and how well I know them.

Some strategies for improving understanding prior to making joint decisions are:

* You and your physician should compare definitions of the problem, goals of treatment, and preferred methods of treatment.

My son was diagnosed with histiocytosis, a rare disease. We were assigned a third-year resident to be our primary doctor at the children's hospital. We told him that we were not just going to hand our son over and say, "Fix it." We wanted to be truly involved in the research and decision-making. Our doctor was a real sweetheart. He fed us research information by looking up articles and copying them for us. We would all study the information, have a meeting to discuss treatment options, and make a decision. Because this was such a rare disease, he would then present the case and treatment options to the tumor board. It worked out quite well.

- Ask the doctor why she thinks the recommended treatment is best, and if there are any guidelines for treating your illness or condition. See Chapter 10, *Questions to Ask About Tests, Drugs, and Surgery*, for information on national treatment guidelines.

I've evolved a simple method of separating competent people in any field from the phonies...I ask them to explain how they arrived at a conclusion. Whether it is a carpenter giving you a kitchen remodeling estimate or a physician giving you a treatment plan...real pros love to discuss their work, are happy to explain how they arrived at their decisions, what the variables are, etc.

So my first rule is if you can't/won't explain how you arrived at a decision, suggestion, bid, I won't do business with you. My second rule is you must understand and respect the fact that I know more about my body than you do. I tell new doctors, "I have a weird body that does not react in standard ways to medicines. If you are not prepared to discuss the family history of allergic reactions to medications before each treatment is started say so now and recommend someone else." Two have passed me on to others and I'm happy with my current doctors. It's time well spent: if you don't trust or are uncomfortable with your doctor it can be bloody hell.

- Explain as clearly as you can your life circumstances that make one treatment more appropriate than another. If, for instance, you have three preschool children at home, you might not want to take a pain medication that would cause you to sleep most of the day.

While in graduate school at the American University in Washington, DC, my migraines were almost eliminated after a series of long talks with a physician's assistant at the Student Health Center. She gave me a fact sheet about foods that trigger migraine and also suggested I cut out caffeine and aspartame. She worked with me to try various types of birth control pills (the original purpose of my visit), to try and eliminate the migraines they triggered. I remember her looking up in a medical/drug dictionary the various types of pills and dosages of estrogen versus progesterone to check possible side effects (especially migraine) and to discuss them with me. It made me very comfortable that she wasn't just relying on memory.

She described several new migraine medications and we discussed the merits of each. She also suggested that I come in for a special injection if I was hit again by severe pain and nausea that would keep me from taking the pills.

This ongoing, rather holistic discussion (i.e., my sleeping, behavior, eating, sex life, habits, and concerns were taken into account) helped me vastly reduce the negative effects of a problem I've had since the onset of puberty. I can now recognize the behaviors and foods likely to trigger a migraine and have changed my lifestyle so that I rarely get one and can usually eliminate it quickly with medication if I have an attack. Also, this physician's assistant really knew her stuff, educated me (and herself in the process), and made me feel like a partner in my conquering of this hereditary problem.

- Repeat back instructions and explanations to make sure you understand. One way to do this is to say, "Let me see if I fully understand. You think the problem is _____, caused by _____. You want me to take _____ medication and call you back in a week if things improve, and sooner if they get worse."

- If you find yourself getting overwhelmed by information during an appointment, say so and ask to come back another time to complete your discussion.

- Bring a list of all of your medications, prescription and over-the-counter, with you to each appointment. Your doctor can be tired or hurried just like you are on hectic days, and she may forget one or more of your medications or conditions. Whenever your doctor writes a prescription for a new medication, take out your list and go over it together to make sure that all of the medications are compatible. At this time, remind the doctor of any chronic health conditions you have, such as diabetes, congestive heart failure, or asthma.

Keep asking questions

If you ask pertinent questions every time you see your doctor, it keeps the lines of communication open as well as prevents an unhelpful routine from developing. Even if the only thing you can think of is, "Anything new on the horizon for treating my illness?" ask it. In addition to gathering information, asking questions has been shown to actually improve patients' response to treatment.

Immediately before their doctor's appointment, patients read their medical records and were given explanations of parts they didn't understand. They were coached to ask questions and negotiate medical decisions with their doctor. The coached patients were compared to a control group who received educational counseling only. The patients who had read their record and learned rudimentary questioning techniques had fewer physical limitations, preferred a more active role in decision-making, and were more satisfied with their care than the control group. Examinations of the audiotapes of the appointments revealed that the coached group was twice as effective in obtaining information from the doctor.[13]

If you are not used to asking questions of your doctor, it can be intimidating to start. Think about it this way: for most doctors, medicine is a passion and consumes virtually all of their time. Just like anyone with a passion, they tend to enjoy talking about it. So keep asking questions—it's one of many ways to learn what you need to heal.

Asking questions also helps you detect if your relationship with your doctor is changing due to an economic shift in the relationship. A doctor explains how this happens.

Long-standing relationships with doctors can change due to economic changes, often without the patient even knowing. For instance, she'll sell the practice to a practice management group or she'll become an employee of an HMO unbeknownst to the patient. The patient is still thinking that the doctor is acting solely in their best interests, when in fact subtle changes are occurring. People need to be aware that even long-standing relationships change. Ask questions about whether she is being paid differently or if practice management has changed. You need to be polite but direct. Don't challenge. Try to keep the physician as your ally. But if the doctor gets defensive or refuses to answer, go somewhere else. If you can't discuss those things, what will happen when you need to discuss very difficult subjects like end-of-life decisions? You need someone with whom you can communicate freely.

Change how you talk to your doctor

Communication is truly a two-way street. Many patients consciously change the way they interact with their doctor, and the relationship shifts. One mother of a child with a serious illness was irritated when the doctor said at every visit, "I'm surprised to see him doing so well." After several variations of this gloomy comment, she finally responded, "Really, we rejoice in each day, and expect many more." The mother continued to talk in a positive manner and saw a gradual shift in her doctor's outlook.

> One thing that I have been doing lately is talking to my doctor about my feelings and philosophies. I got sick of just talking about side effects of medications, so now I talk about other things and it is just great.

> This doctor is particularly wonderful and easy to talk to, but in the past he didn't talk like this. I think that was because I wasn't giving him any signals that I wanted to be more personal. So I think that we as patients need to work at communicating better with our doctors, and not just leave it all up to them. When you get sick you feel like you lose control of your body, your life. So, for me, regaining some control made me feel better. And now I feel like I have some control over my doctor appointments, because I choose some of what we talk about. It's a small thing, but I get a lot of satisfaction from it.

· · · · ·

> Although I have been fortunate to have a very personable doctor from the start, I have noticed that as I have been freer with my feelings, he has been freer with his. Recently he suggested a course of treatment that I wasn't comfortable with—I wanted to be more aggressive. He agreed to the change, but afterwards confessed that he wasn't sure how he should play his doctor role. On the one hand, he wanted me to be comfortable with my treatment, but he was concerned that I would really suffer badly from the side effects—he was basically thinking out loud as he expressed his doubts if he was doing the right thing in letting me decide my treatment or if he should be more insistent in his preference. It was such an honest, human thing for him to share this, and it made me all the more appreciative of the partnership relationship that we have.

Show appreciation

Doctors, like patients, are grateful for encouragement, expressions of appreciation, or a pat on the back. Thank-you notes for kind deeds or excellent work are treasured by doctors because they don't often get such tangible expressions of thanks. Patients who show appreciation for their doctors and nurses help smooth over the rough spots that are inevitable in relationships and bring some much-needed pleasure into the sometimes grim work of medical caregivers. Praise shows that you appreciate the difficulty of their jobs. Feedback also gives doctors vital information on how their actions help or hurt their patients. Rewarding good deeds is one of the most effective methods to alter behavior.

My daughter Casey was treated for bone cancer by Dr. W., an orthopedic oncologist. As soon as she stopped vomiting from chemotherapy, she returned to her beloved cheerleading, took up jazz dancing (she claims it was the very best physical therapy), and is now on the varsity springboard diving team at her high school. She sends Dr. W. photos and videotapes of her doing these things that he claims give him heart pains. But, one day, when he observed her sitting cross-legged in his examining room (which he claims no one with her type of surgery could physically do), he finally admitted that she has had the best physical response of any of his patients and he took a picture of her sitting that way for a brochure. I can't explain to you how wonderful it makes me feel to see this doctor actually glow when he sees Casey (now only once a year)—he calls the whole office together to behold her!

* * * * *

Our pediatrician is wonderful. He helped us so much during my daughter's lengthy life-threatening illness, as well as the ear infections, illnesses, and stitches that normally occur during childhood. Every year my children design our Christmas cards and we send him one with a picture of them and something mushy written inside. One year I wrote, "You've been a constant bright light during some dark times. You'll never know how much we appreciate you." Another time I saw him at a child's funeral, and we just put our arms around each other and hugged. I told him I knew how hard it was for him to take care of so many really sick kids, but that we all couldn't do it without him. I said, "You'll never know what a weight it lifts off our shoulders knowing that you're there—to answer questions, keep track of treatments, and make us smile. We think you're the greatest." We both got a bit teary. His nurse called me to tell me how much it means to him to hear such things.

Not only are such expressions of thanks appreciated, but they help establish a more balanced relationship. You are relating in an active, human way, rather than being a passive recipient of an exam and medical advice. It also creates a "goodwill bank." When you make many deposits, an occasional withdrawal will not be as noticeable.

The birth of my first child was hospital-controlled and not terribly pleasant. I resolved that the second time around would be different. My new OB was a woman about my age. We just liked each other from the start. I told her that I had lots of questions and she said to keep a running list, and she would get them all answered before the delivery date.

So, every appointment, after my exam, I'd dress and meet her in her office. I'd pull out my little notebook and pen and start to ask questions. She always told me her time constraints ("I'm running late, I'll just answer a couple" or "Someone canceled, we have 15 minutes"). She always ended the visit with a smile and a cheery, "We'll have them all answered by the big day, I promise."

I asked all about her views on episiotomies, cesareans, anesthesia, husband involvement, birthing rooms, positions, etc. I asked her many "What if" questions. By the ninth month, I really knew what to expect from her, and she knew how I felt on all birth-related questions. As a matter of fact, I joked with her that I was only hiring her for the 5 percent chance that I would need expert assistance, otherwise, just leave it to me and catch the babe.

During labor, the birthing room was dark and classical music played. The nurse was supportive but nonintrusive. My doctor phoned over every so often to see how things were going. She was on the floor the last hour or so, and at one point came over and whispered, "Am I staying out of your hair enough?" It made me laugh.

I think we both benefited immensely from my questions. She grew to understand and appreciate my views, and I was comforted that there would be no surprises. A deep mutual respect and affection developed. All because I asked a lot of questions and she answered them.

CHAPTER 5

Physician Rights and Responsibilities

It is our duty as physicians to estimate probabilities and to discipline expectations; but leading away from probabilities there are paths of possibilities, towards which it is our duty to hold aloft the light, and the name of that light is hope.

—Karl Menninger
The Vital Balance

DOCTORS HAVE RIGHTS as well as responsibilities. Although patients are sick or hurt when they see doctors, they still owe them courteous and respectful treatment. Doctors also have a right to an honest history from their patients, as well as good faith efforts to comply with a mutually agreed-upon treatment plan. Having patients show up on time for appointments and pay bills promptly are critical for a doctor's practice to run smoothly. These rights are discussed first in this chapter because they are so often overlooked.

The cornerstone of medical ethics is "First, do no harm." Beyond this basic guiding principle are several legal and ethical standards that rule doctors' everyday encounters with patients as well as help resolve tricky ethical dilemmas. Doctors' conduct is guided by professional codes of conduct based on moral principles such as confidentiality, informed consent, equal access to health care, and the right to be helped, not hurt. Respect for patients' autonomy and promotion of patients' rights to full disclosure of all information are essential ethical concepts. The American Medical Association's *Principles of Medical Ethics* are contained in Appendix A.

The following lists of rights and responsibilities were compiled by both patients and doctors, and the stories they share show the difficulties that can arise between patients and doctors when both are not clear about their roles and the rules that define them.

Physician rights

Physicians have several legal rights, as well as rights that flow from the respect and kindness that should mark all worthwhile human relationships.

Be treated courteously and respectfully

Doctors and their staffs have a right to courteous treatment even when patients are feeling sick or emotionally distraught. While most compassionate doctors understand if a patient blows up at them out of fear or anger about an illness, they don't deserve to go through each working day on the receiving end of misplaced anger. Rude behavior has no place in medical partnerships.

One emergency room doctor describes most patients as generally pleasant, with a few exceptions.

> It's funny you should ask me about courteous behavior, because just today my wife and I were walking through a store and heard a woman say, "There's that damn doctor." But, on the whole, most people are really nice. If they do get angry, there is usually something else going on. For instance, one night a father brought his young daughter in who needed blood work and an intravenous line. It was one of those awful situations where she was just so dehydrated it was hard to find a vein. The man said, "I want the best person available. Call them in if necessary." I said, "Believe it or not, that's me, and I'm doing the best that I can." He was pretty angry and it got really tense. But it was clear he wasn't really mad at me; he just couldn't stand watching his daughter get stuck multiple times. So, once again, there's usually a reason. And occasionally, the doctor precipitates it with his attitude, which I have done on occasion, but far less often as I get older.

Expect patients to show up on time for all appointments

Doctors have a right to expect you to not be late for your appointment. Unless they are employed by a hospital or HMO, they are running their business as well as trying to restore or improve your health. Their business requires that they see all of the patients who have appointments with as little delay as possible. Common courtesy demands that if you are going to be late or miss an appointment, you give as much notice to the doctor's office as possible.

> My standard practice (and most other doctors' too) is that if you are fifteen minutes late, you lose your slot. We will try to fit you in, but often it's necessary to make another appointment.

Have patients provide all pertinent information

Doctors have a right to full disclosure of all information related to your illness or injury. Your doctor cannot make a reasonable suggestion for treatment if she has not heard all of the pertinent information. If something is embarrassing, you could state your discomfort ("This is really hard for me to talk about"), then just forge ahead and say it. You may neglect to mention a fact to your doctor because you think it's not important, but your doctor may need just that bit of information to correctly diagnose your problem. For instance, you might not connect frequent nosebleeds to your new medication, but your doctor would investigate immediately if the new prescription was a blood thinner. Try to be concise in describing the reason for your visit, but be sure to include anything out of the ordinary in your life, whether you think it's related to your problem or not. One doctor remarked:

> I run into this problem all the time, especially since I work at a college and deal primarily with students who are less sophisticated than some older adults and are not used to seeing a doctor on their own. They come in thinking that they are dying of a heart attack or a brain tumor, when really they are hyperventilating or getting headaches from stress. Sometimes the real problem is even more deeply hidden—like sexual or domestic abuse. I've become more aware about picking up clues. I also realize that it often takes more than one visit to really find out what is going on. It's all part of the challenge of being a doctor.

An emergency room physician underscores the need for information in the following story.

> It's important for us to know what medicines people are on. Sometimes in the hurry of getting to the emergency room people forget to bring their medication, but other people just assume there's some database we hook into that can tell us about their medications. But that's just not the case. If they could just throw their medicines into a paper bag and bring them it's very helpful. Some people who have oddball EKGs carry them along when they travel and it's great to have them if they end up in the emergency room. There are new microfilm histories that some people with health problems carry that are also helpful in emergencies.

Expect compliance with a mutually acceptable treatment plan

Doctors have a right to expect you to comply with a mutually acceptable treatment plan. Of course, this requires that the decision be made together and be agreeable to both you and your doctor. This joint decision-making is based on a principle of medical ethics known as autonomy—the right to be informed in language you can understand about the illness or injury and your options. You should not be pressured to make decisions or influenced through incomplete or biased information. But, once you do agree to an approach to treatment, your doctor has the right to expect you to stick with it, or tell the truth if you don't. One doctor explains how his patients sometimes aren't aware of what they realistically can do.

> Compliance is a hard one. Even if you've talked over the treatment plan, some people don't know what they are capable of complying with. Sometimes people feel guilty that they didn't comply; they feel they should have done it to please me. It's especially a problem with some older folks because they are so interested in being polite. Sometimes I have to break through that reticence to really communicate.

Another doctor says that he expels patients from his practice over the issue of compliance.

> I have a right to expect the patient to do the things they have agreed are important to do. One of the few things I kick patients out of my practice for is not doing—consistently over time—what they agreed to do. If they say they are going to walk 30 minutes every day and increase the amounts of grains and vegetables they eat and decrease the amount of fat and sugar in their diet, I expect them to do it. If they are overweight and diabetic and have heart disease, I treat those things, but, in addition, I expect them to make the lifestyle changes they've agreed to. If they don't do them despite the loving, caring, supportive environment that I provide, then I ask them to leave. I think it's important to do that, otherwise it's a charade.

Another doctor expresses her concern about judgments made if patients do not or cannot maintain a healthy lifestyle.

> For all the emphasis on health standards, we each remain mortal and imperfect. Some persons can't lose weight, no matter how hard they try. Some people have unhealthy habits because of other conditions in

their lives. The last thing these people need is someone—especially a doctor—who attempts to change behavior through threat, intimidation, or righteousness. One's doctor should accept you as you are, help you to find ways to overcome unhealthy habits and conditions, but never abandon or treat you less when you do not meet his/her or some health plan/employer standards.

Limit social conversations that interfere with patient care

Doctors have the right to limit conversations if they interfere with the care of other patients. You really shouldn't expect a leisurely chat when you're in your doctor's office. He needs to treat you then see the next patient promptly. This does not preclude the doctor from asking pertinent questions about your family, job, or hobbies in the course of obtaining a history, nor does it prevent him from chatting if he so chooses. But he does have the right not to be detained by social conversation if he doesn't have the time or the interest.

You can define social interactions in a variety of ways. I don't see the doctor-patient relationship as a friendship relationship; neither do I see it as a strictly business relationship. In order to achieve healing, often it requires more talking. For instance, I had a wealthy community leader spend a day with me at work once as part of a medical society internship program. That day I was working at a low income clinic, and I had a woman patient scheduled for a 45-minute appointment. She has hepatitis C, and is a recovering alcoholic and drug addict. One of the things about hepatitis C is that your immune system gets damaged fairly substantially. Since the stronger your immune system, the better response to treatment you'll have, part of the treatment protocol I use is to include diet and smoking interventions. So, I spent 45 minutes talking to her about her life. At the end of the day, this very well-to-do fellow was most impressed by one thing. He said, "How can I come here as a patient? My doctor never treats me like that." I don't think you should focus on social things, but in order to be healthy there's a lot more needed than a simple exchange of technical information. People have to know each other, they have to trust each other, and they have to know each other's values. I really need to know what they are willing to do and not willing to do.

Be paid for services promptly

Doctors run businesses with high overheads that require prompt payment of bills. They must pay their office staff, pay their mortgage on office space, keep up their malpractice and other insurance, and buy all office supplies. They rely on prompt payment, both from insurance companies and patients. So try to pay your bills promptly, and intervene if your insurance is slow in processing claims.

Be recognized as human beings

Doctors have good days and bad days just like the rest of us. Some days they are patient and some days curt. If they are short on sleep, they may make a mistake that they would never make when well rested. They may be worrying about family problems when you are trying to describe your concerns. One doctor requested a bit of compassion from patients who place him on pedestal by saying, "Doctors are human. There are no perfect doctors out there; we all make mistakes sometimes." Another doctor describes a mistake she made during her residency.

> *During one of my first deliveries, I asked the mom not to push for a moment because the baby's head was covered with meconium. I reached for an instrument to clear out his mouth and nose, she pushed, the baby popped out, and he dropped into the trash can. I was worried sick and totally mortified. One of the more senior residents came in and said, "I always pull the tray out." Nobody had ever told me there was a tray. I fished him out of the trash and checked him over. He appeared to be fine. So, while a nurse wrapped him up, I explained to the mother what had happened. She was very blasé and said, "Oh yeah, the doctor dropped my sister's baby, too." I called the pediatrician to tell him what happened and asked him to check the baby over carefully. He was very reassuring and told me it happened all the time because, "Babies are really slippery."*

Physician responsibilities

Numerous ethical duties guide the day-to-day actions of physicians. Among these are justice (including fair distribution of resources and burdens), beneficence (to promote good and prevent harm), and respect for patient's autonomy (protection and encouragement of free choice). The ethical requirement for patient autonomy also includes full disclosure of all facts, telling the truth, and promoting informed consent.

Responsibility to serve

Justice is the guiding principle in medical ethics that governs doctors' responsibility to serve. All citizens have a right to equal access to health care and a slice of the available resources. Doctors have a responsibility to provide that care in a just and fair manner. This distribution of shrinking resources is the focus of intense discussion in the U.S. today. More than ever before, doctors struggle with their duties as advocates for all patients while facing economic constraints.

> I'm a public health doctor and I feel strongly that we have a responsibility to serve all of the people in our community. We enjoy that privilege. Every single medical association—whether it be OB/GYNs, cardiologists, orthopedists, family practice doctors—at the national level say we need to provide uncompensated care to all members of the community. Some of them even quantify it, such as a day a month. It's explicit. So it's interesting to me to see which doctors really do it. It's actually very heartening—we have ninety doctors who routinely give generously of their time to our clinic. Every day I see people doing what's right. Even when the big managed care outfit in town told their doctors not to give any free care on company time, some find ways to work around it: some still read all of our EKGs for free, some donate their days off to the clinic.

Exercise reasonable care and skill

Doctors have a responsibility to exercise reasonable care and skill in treating their patients. The ethical principle involved is called "beneficence," the duty to do good, not harm. Each area of medicine has "standards of care" that knowledgeable, reasonable physicians are expected to meet or exceed. The skills are defined as those of an average, prudent, reputable professional in the medical community. After choosing your physician carefully and evaluating his credentials, you should expect skilled treatment of your condition. Your welfare and best interests should be your doctor's primary concern whether your care occurs in a fee-for-service setting, managed care, hospital, or military setting. The *American College of Physician's Ethics Manual* third edition states:

> Whatever the treatment setting, at the beginning of the relationship the physician must understand the patient's complaints and underlying feelings and expectations. After they agree to the problem before them, the physician presents one or more courses of action. If both parties

agree, the patient may then authorize the physician to initiate a course of action, and the physician accepts this responsibility. The relationship has mutual obligations: The physician must be professionally competent, act responsibly, and treat the patient with compassion and respect. The patient should understand and consent to the treatment and should participate responsibly in the care.[1]

Part of providing reasonable care and skill is to do only what is necessary, and no more. Recommending unnecessary tests or surgery violates the basic ethical concept of "do no harm." The following report dramatizes the extent of the problem in the U.S.

Unnecessary pacemakers

The *New England Journal of Medicine* published the finding of researchers from Pennsylvania who studied the records of 382 patients who received pacemakers. In more than one-third of the cases, the reasons for the surgery were "unclear," and in another one-fifth of the cases, the pacemaker was not needed at all. More than 120,000 pacemakers are implanted annually in the U.S., at a cost of $2 billion. If the Pennsylvania findings were extrapolated to the entire U.S., more than half of the pacemaker implants and $1 billion in expenditures were unnecessary.[2]

Treat people with respect and kindness

The ethical concept of beneficence obligates doctors to treat patients with compassion, respect, and kindness. If you read books by patients or doctor-patients, you will discover that simple acts of kindness are a recurring theme. Gestures that take almost no time—a smile, a hug, a telephone call at home—are treasured memories, partially because they are becoming increasingly rare in our time of mechanical medicine. One patient talks of how comforting it was when her doctor told her with passion, "I hate this disease," while an ill doctor mused, "Only one of my many doctors smiled at me. It seemed as if they couldn't look me in the eye anymore because now I was sick." A caring, sensitive, empathetic manner can make a world of difference. As one doctor stated, "Kindness shouldn't be extra."

When Casey's family doctor decided her knee pain needed to be x-rayed and evaluated (we all still thought it was a common sprain), he sent us to a group orthopedic practice I had had much experience with (many broken bones with many kids). However, the particular doctor we saw was not one with whom I had had a previous relationship. Still believing nothing was amiss, I dragged Casey and her best friend to the appointment on the Friday before Labor Day weekend. The doctor examined Casey's knee (and hurt her in the process, which I saw no necessity for) and had X rays taken. After reading them, he came into the examining room and told her she had a "bone abnormality" that needed a specialist. He knew of only three in the state and wanted to send us to the farthest one (four hours away). Still clueless, I smiled and said fine. Then he said he wanted to show me something while Casey was getting fitted with a brace. He took me into his office and pointed to an X ray on the light box and said, "There it is." I, still blissfully ignorant, said, "There is what?" "Why, the tumor, of course." Stunned and still not fully cognizant, I asked, "Is it cancer?" The doctor looked at me as if I were insane and declared, "Of course it is," walked out of the room, and never said another word to me, not "good luck" or "I'm sorry," not a single word!

Casey's mother quickly marshaled her forces and found an orthopedic oncologist in a nearby city to treat Casey's cancer. It was quite a different experience from the diagnosis.

And, as it turned out, the closest specialist (not the one he recommended) was that bright guiding light I needed. The very first thing he did when he introduced himself was to hand me his card with his home phone number on the back and a demand that I call him or his wife (his nurse) at any time to ask anything. Can you imagine an orthopedic oncologist (with mostly adult patients) giving out his home phone number on the first visit? I would have followed him anywhere at that point! And then he spoke mostly to Casey, which I really appreciated. She was only 12, but he told her everything in detail and explained that she would soon know as much as he did about her disease.

We didn't see Dr. W. as often as we saw the medical oncologists at the local children's hospital that was providing Casey's protocol, but we always knew he was around. He consulted often with the oncologists and made sure they understood what he would be doing during the surgery several months hence and why. The oncologists thought he was as wonderful as I did.

Dr. W. did all the things that ease patients' fears and engage them as allies in the fight against disease: He showed he cared, he kept in touch with the treating physicians, he spoke to Casey rather than just her mother, and he forged a bond.

In contrast, consider Arthur Frank's experience recounted in *At the Will of the Body*:

> Here I had half good luck—an excellent technician who was a terrible communicator. The physician told me he observed massive lymphadenopathy, or enlargement of the lymph nodes, behind my stomach. When I asked what would cause this, he abruptly told me it was either a primary or a secondary tumor...Looking back, I respect what the physician was able to discover. But at the same time, in that basement laboratory, all I could think about was being told I had massive tumors. The physician added nothing to his abrupt statement. He would send a report to my family physician; that was it, not even a good-bye or good luck, just over and out. It was a triumph of science and a lapse of humanity.[3]

Patients want to be treated as valuable people and not things. They shrivel inside when doctors overlook who they are and how they are feeling to concentrate instead on the body part in question. Whenever a human gesture of caring is made, patients feel better. This bond, based on words and gestures that show the physician's concern, are an intrinsic part of the healing process.

> One of the most meaningful things to a patient is to be treated not as an unusual and fascinating case, but as a person. When my daughter, who has beautiful waist-length hair, had to have some of it shaved off when she had her laminectomy she was understandably upset. Her care team didn't think this silly, they cut carefully and then braided it and put it in a bag with her name on it and it was the first thing they gave me post-op. They had done all this while Kirsty was asleep, so she didn't know the difference, but the compassion that went into that little plastic bag with that beautiful lock of hair got to me in a way the horror of all the rest of it hadn't. I cried for a long time, but felt less alone somehow.

Another reason doctors should strive to treat patients with kindness and respect involves their own economic interests. Many studies show that medical malpractice claims are often related more to patient satisfaction with their personal relationship with their doctor than with the quality of their care.

Researchers videotaped patient appointments with both primary care doctors and surgeons to study the communication styles of doctors with and without malpractice claims. They found striking differences between the two groups of doctors. No-claims family practice doctors spent more time with each patient, explained what to expect during the visit more, laughed and used humor more often, asked patients' opinions more, and checked their understanding more. There were no such differences between claims and no-claims surgeons. The researchers discussed whether patients have different expectations of surgeons than primary care doctors. They hypothesized that patients may view surgeons as technical experts and primary care doctors as someone with whom patients desire a warm, connected relationship.[4]

Don't keep people waiting

Patients hate to sit for long periods of time in waiting rooms. People are busy with work and family and resent wasting time. One doctor explains how he handles the problem of keeping his patients waiting.

> *My biggest complaint from my patients, and the one I hear most about other doctors, is that we keep people waiting too long. The deal that I've tried to make explicitly with every single patient is that when they need the time they will get it. Crises happen. When someone comes in for a specific problem, but is really needing major help, I help. So, I tell them that although they have to wait sometimes, when they need extra time, they will get it, too.*

Here's the view of a patient who just refused to wait.

> *I've had to see 30 different doctors during my three-year battle with cancer and I've only had a problem with a few of them. One oncologist at the university hospital canceled three different appointments with me and then on the day I went to see him he made me wait three hours. I told his nurse that I was out of there and I left, only to have him come running after me in the hallway. He was actually mad at me for leaving and said, "You can't leave, we need to go over your treatment." I replied, "I'm finding another doctor" and I walked away.*

> *I found a great doctor at another hospital who had a small office where he saw only a few patients a day. He explained everything to me*

and I never got the all-too-familiar feeling of being rushed through the system. He gave me all the time I needed and my care was handled very competently. We actually became friends.

Most patients don't mind waiting if the doctor explains the reason for the delay and apologizes. It's the all-too-common delay that is never acknowledged that infuriates many patients. They feel that it implies their role is to wait for a doctor whose time is more valuable than theirs.

> *On my first appointment with a new gynecologist, I waited in the examination room for over twenty minutes. She came in profusely apologizing. She said, "Oh, I don't like to start out this way. I try hard to avoid delays, but today's couldn't be helped. I am very sorry." I appreciated the apology, and have not been kept waiting since.*

In some cases, like the following, waiting opens the door for a kind act to occur.

> *After many hospitalizations, I had to bring my husband back in. After three hours, we still were waiting for some faceless lung doctor to install John's chest tube. John's two-time surgeon, Dr. C., stopped in after seeing his name on the board. We told him what we were waiting for and he offered to do it himself right there and then. He's such a skilled and kind surgeon (a rare combo). We were absolutely thrilled. It made John feel so much better about it. Tiny little incision, neat stitches, and minimal pain.*

Provide adequate time to examine, diagnose, and answer questions

Doctors are ethically obligated to provide enough time to examine, diagnose, and answer their patients' questions. In order to "do no harm," physicians need to spend enough time to determine the nature of your illness and answer all of your questions concerning the problem and the suggested treatment. In some busy offices—especially where there is pressure from management and/or plans to strictly limit time spent per patient—this is becoming increasingly difficult. Nevertheless, the doctor has a responsibility to provide the necessary time. It is possible, however, to negotiate the issue of when your questions will be answered. For instance, you could make arrangements to have another appointment or to talk on the phone.

After my radical hysterectomy, I was put on Premarin to lessen the effect of early menopause. It has reduced my hot flashes, which tended to be very uncomfortable at times, but it also has completely eliminated my sex drive, much to the disappointment of my husband. I have tried the patch and break out in a rash. No information was given to me by my doctor about the side effects or effects from long-time use. I have heard about a new natural estrogen available in a pill form, but can't find it anywhere. I asked my doctor about it and he just dismissed the idea, and me, saying, "Now dear, you don't want that, I know what's best for you."

Answering questions takes time, often in short supply in busy medical practices. Diane Komp, M.D., in her book *A Child Shall Lead Them*, discusses being overwhelmed by questions from the parents of a sick child.

I remember the heartbreak of a young mother and father listening to a diagnosis, prognosis, and implications for their future. [But they] moved past their pain, fought back. They armed themselves with a notebook, tape recorder, and telephone...There were times that I was overwhelmed by their questions. But then I remembered that this was indeed war. I had hundreds of patients to care for and they had one surviving child. Let them fight their good fight.[5]

In some cases, doctors are dispensing with physical exams and relying instead on sophisticated tools and tests. You have the right to question your doctor if you feel that insufficient time was spent on a thorough examination.

Using mammography instead of breast examination

Researchers wanted to see if patients who had a mammogram were still receiving breast exams from their doctors (an essential part of a comprehensive screening for breast cancer). They found that three-quarters of the women had comprehensive screening, while the remainder only received a mammogram. Interestingly, female doctors (senior attending physicians and fellows) comprehensively examined 95 percent of the patients, while male attending doctors comprehensively examined only 67 percent, and male residents 61 percent. The study concluded that mammography was replacing examinations for some male doctors, and interventions targeted at them might improve the care given.[6]

If your questions and concerns have been anticipated and answered, your stress and anxiety will most likely decrease. You will more likely comply with prescribed treatment because you understand the condition better and reasons for the treatment. Your trust in your doctor and satisfaction with your medical care will increase. As a result, your relationship with the doctor will be strengthened and your quality of care will be enhanced.

Get informed consent prior to treating

The ethical principle of "respect for autonomy" recognizes the right of patients to be full participants in medical decision-making. Doctors not only have this ethical duty, but they also have a legal obligation to obtain a patient's informed consent prior to treatment. This process has different meanings for different levels of interventions. Naturally, your doctor does not need a signed consent form prior to treating a sore throat. Routine office procedures require only an explanation of the proposed treatment and any common side effects, and your consent. For any treatment requiring surgery and/or anesthesia, a form outlining the proposed procedure and its risks is explained by the doctor and signed by the patient only after all questions have been answered.

> I thought it was a nice touch when my daughter (then 12) was asked to read and sign the consent form prior to her surgery. Obviously, her signature carried no legal significance, but she truly appreciated her participation (as did I).

However, if your doctor is recommending a life-threatening intervention such as an organ transplant or complicated surgery, the informed consent process is lengthy and detailed. In these cases, informed consent is a process, not an event. The doctors, patient, and family should discuss the reasons for the procedure, the procedure itself, the risks and benefits, both common and rare potential side effects, other treatment options, and impact on quality of life. You have a right to have all questions answered, no coercion from the physicians, and time in which to make a decision.

> A bone marrow transplant was not our daughter's only chance for survival, but it was her best shot statistically. Our informed consent process occurred in stages. When we were first in the hospital, a couple of doctors and some medical students sat down with us and went over the informed consent for the protocol. They clearly laid out the choices. They said, "Legally, we have to tell you that you can choose to do nothing. But

the truth is that Adele will die within a month or two without any treat-
ment. However, you do have choices." They outlined the standard treat-
ment for her illness and then they described the clinical trial. They were
honest in telling us that they hoped we'd enroll in the study, but they
didn't tell us what to do. They were clear that we could get out of the
study at any time, for any reason. It was also reassuring when they told
us that the standard treatment had a 70 percent chance of first remission,
but that with the study (which had been going on for some time already)
at their institution, they were getting 85-90 percent remission. Then they
went through the printed forms listing all of the side effects. They told us
which were common (like cardiotoxicity) and which were rare.

Informed consent includes explaining and interpreting complex information so that you thoroughly understand the risks and benefits of any proposed treatment. The information should be given in terms you understand,
should be unbiased, and should include your doctor's recommendation. The
doctor has a responsibility not only to give you the information, but to
ensure that you understand it. The ethical concept of autonomy also obligates your doctor to respect your rights, values, and choices in the decision-
making process. You have a right to know what your medical choices are,
and to accept or reject them.

I learned a long time ago that if I want to be totally responsible for a
decision, I can make it. But, as I get older, I've learned that I don't want
to be totally responsible for decisions for my patients. I involve my
patients to the absolute extent that I can. Often, my job is to explain and
interpret medical information so they can understand it and then they
make the decision. Maybe that's cowardice, but I think my job is educa-
tion and their job is decision-making. But there are situations when it's
more complicated than that. I have a few patients who are incapable of
making decisions because of addictions or mental capacity. I also think
explaining the pros and cons of natural products—such as St. John's
wort—is problematic. There are thirty years of European studies on it—
we know its mechanism of action and that there are rare serious compli-
cations. I have an obligation to inform, but I'm on shaky ground telling
them to take it or not take it. I can look up Prozac in a book and say that
three people in a thousand are going to get seizures from it, but I can't
say that for St. John's wort. So I just tell them what I know and I don't
give an opinion on what they should do.

Doctors not only have an obligation to provide you with all available information prior to treatment, but they must also fully disclose all information pertaining to a diagnosis and treatment options. For example, if you suffered a heart attack and your doctor knew you tended to worry about your health, she might withhold the diagnosis so that you would not be upset. In most cases, withholding information to coerce or deceive violates the ethical concept of disclosure. Many studies show that it is rare for information to worsen a patient's condition, but it is still common for information to be withheld based on the doctor's (or family members') opinions.

A doctor explains how she extends the concept of full disclosure and informed consent to financial arrangements that materially affect patients' care:

> The basis of informed consent is that the physician has the responsibility to tell the patient everything that is pertinent to their care. Patients need all the information so that they direct their own care. I extend that now to financial arrangements and any other conditions in a plan because those materially affect the decisions a person makes. For instance, physicians have a responsibility to tell you where the leading experts are for your condition, even if your insurance won't cover your treatment there. But the patient still has the right to know.

The AMA Council on Ethical and Judicial Affairs (CEJA) supports this position. If you are denied a treatment based on unavailable resources (an organ to transplant) or due to man-made rationing (drug of choice not on managed care organization's approved drug list), you should be told. In 1995, the CEJA published an ethics standard for physicians who find themselves in these situations:

> The nature of the physician-patient relationship entails that physicians of patients competing for a scarce resource must remain advocates for their patients and therefore should not make the actual allocation decisions...Patients must be informed by their physicians of allocation criteria and procedures, as well as their chances of receiving access to scarce resources. This information is in addition to all the customary information regarding the risks, benefits, and alternatives to any medical procedure. Patients denied access to resources have the right to be informed of the reasoning behind the decision.[7]

Discuss health risk behaviors

Doctors need to discuss with their patients the impact of risky behaviors on their health. But most doctors are trained to treat disease—when organs or organ systems malfunction. These abnormal conditions are challenging to diagnose, interesting to treat, and provide opportunities for scientific research. Little time is spent in medical school or residency on health maintenance, disease prevention, or promoting wellness.

Wellness is the sum of everything that makes us healthier. In a wellness model, the doctor's role shifts from that of a mechanic fixing a broken part to a gardener nurturing growth. Smoking, drinking, multiple sex partners, unprotected sex, high fat diets, and other behaviors under patients' control undermine wellness. Doctors have a responsibility to discuss behaviors that enhance or diminish your health.

There is wide variability in the types of health risk behaviors doctors discuss with their patients, as the following study illustrates.

Effect of patient income on discussions of risky behaviors

The Health Institute of New England and the Harvard School of Public Health surveyed almost 11,000 employees of the state of Massachusetts about behaviors that affected their health, such as seat belt use, alcohol consumption, smoking, diet, safe sex, exercise, and stress. They found that low-income persons were more likely to be obese and smoke, and less likely to wear seat belts and exercise. However, as income increased, so did alcohol consumption and stress. Physicians were more likely to discuss diet and exercise with high-income patients than low-income patients. But they discussed smoking with low-income patients much more than with high-income patients. For all health risk behaviors, physicians fell far short of the recommendations of the U.S. Preventative Services Task Force. Only 73 percent of the physicians discussed exercise, 70 percent discussed diet, 61 percent discussed stress, 53 percent discussed smoking, 39 percent discussed alcohol use, 19 percent discussed safe sex, and 16 percent discussed seat belt use.[8]

Most of modern medicine is geared toward treating, rather than preventing, disease. One doctor muses about this tendency:

> *In our culture, people value disease. When you are sick, people are willing to pay a lot of money and do a lot of things to get rid of disease. On the other hand, our society and the individuals in it do not value*

health much. *They just want it fixed when they are ill, but they don't want to prevent illness. They want to smoke for thirty years and not get lung cancer, or if they get it, they just want me to make it better. It just doesn't make sense.*

Keep current with new information

Doctors have a duty to keep current with new medical information. But, with a half a million technical journal articles published yearly, staying up to date is a formidable task. State-of-the-art treatment is usually not essential for minor illnesses or injuries. However, for rare or life-threatening illnesses, learning of the newest treatment advances could save your life. Your doctor has a responsibility to do his best to keep up with the newest information and to obtain a consultation when she needs assistance or upon your request.

> *I believe my doctor is a very good person, who wants me to be successful fighting my disease. At the same time, she has other patients with other diseases. To be honest, I don't think she has the time to research all the journal articles and be completely up to date. Several times, I have brought in abstracts of journal articles when I have questions, and she hasn't yet seen the articles. I think my file is stamped PAIN (in the neck) because every time I go in I have more questions. To give her credit, she will always follow up on my questions, usually within a few days. She said we educate each other. For my own peace of mind, I will continue my independent research, but I do respect her medical opinion, and most times I agree with her.*

Some specialties require periodic recertification in order for the doctor to remain board certified. You may be reassured if you check to see your doctor has recently recertified with her medical specialty board.

Recognize the power of words

Doctors' words have a tremendous impact on patients' minds and hearts. People are extremely vulnerable when ill, and doctors have a responsibility to "do no harm" with their words as well as their deeds. In an article in *Business Week* magazine, reporter Howard Gleckman described how damaging thoughtless words can be when he learned that his father was dying of heart failure: "'Let me put it to you this way: I wouldn't sell him a six-month life insurance policy,' said the cardiologist, who knew everything—and nothing—about the human heart."9

The mother of a young cancer patient describes a similar situation, in which one careless phrase continues to frighten her years after it was spoken.

> One thing that sticks in my mind from our first week in the hospital at the time of the diagnosis is a conversation we had with the oncologist. He told me, "There is no problem curing her leukemia, we just have to pray that we are able to cure what pops up next from the chemotherapy and radiation treatments." I have never been able to get that phrase out of my mind, and it has been three years now! I am sure it was just a poor choice of words, but it is something that is still haunting me.

Often doctors have no idea that they have said something hurtful. You do them a favor to bring it to their attention in a kind way. Not only does it give both of you a chance to repair the damage to your relationship, but it helps the doctor understand a bit better the power of his words. One doctor remarked, a bit ruefully:

> Occasionally, I say things to people that really hurt them, and I have no idea. Sometimes people tell me, or write me a letter, and I really appreciate it. I thank them for telling me and try to learn from it.

Treat the person, not just the body

Doctors have a responsibility to treat the person, and not just the body part that requires immediate attention. Patients often wish that their doctors had been taught to treat them as a whole human being rather than an illness that happens to occupy a body. Illness is not simply a pathological process, but a far-ranging experience that includes how you feel about it, how it impacts your life, your family, your job. As Sir William Osler, one of the most revered doctors in all of history, said in numerous speeches throughout his life, "You must treat the man as well as the disease."[10] Treating the disease or illness, and ignoring the human who is enduring it, is bad medicine. Barbara Webster, in her book *All of a Piece*, describes this phenomenon.

> Another of my doctors believes that my disease [multiple sclerosis] is so benign that it should not be a factor in my life at all. I have often wished that he could spend a day, one of the bad days, in my body...At least for me, it is much harder to come to terms with something if I am the only one who thinks it is important.[11]

On the other hand, there are doctors who involve themselves intimately with their patients. In the following example, a mother describes the magnificent humor, warmth, and caring of her very ill daughter's doctor:

I loved Michelle's first specialist, and I was just sick when he did not make the transfer to the new hospital with all the other doctors. He was funny and upbeat and perceptive. He knew I needed info, so he would copy articles that he thought I would be interested in, that had to do with Michelle's treatment. He knew she was an "I Love Lucy" fiend, so he would never schedule a visit or procedure while that show was on. He resembled Garth on "Wayne's World," and one year for Halloween, he dressed the part (to the hilt, complete with long blond wig) and made rounds that way. Another year he was a punk rocker. He sent little things in the mail to Michelle; cartoon cut-outs from the newspaper were a favorite item. But he could be serious when need be, and he never tried to sugarcoat Michelle's treatment. He was always honest about her treatment, and did his best for her.

You might also consider the differing roles each physician on your team plays in your care. If you expect your hand to be held by a surgeon or anesthesiologist, you are most likely to be disappointed. These specialists are usually not the people who coordinate your care, know you over a long period of time, and grow to value you as a person. They are providing a service that, while valuable, is generally of short duration. You should expect them to treat you with kindness and compassion, but beyond that, your most human and lasting interactions will occur with your primary care doctor.

I think we as doctors have a responsibility to treat the whole person. I think the people that specialize in diseases should be honest and tell their patients that they specialize in diseases. There's nothing wrong with specializing in diseases—it's a great thing. But people need a health care provider who specializes in just them and who coordinates the care of other people who specialize in diseases. People get mixed up about that. And clearly, some doctors do both. But I think that we need to understand which doctors specialize in their patients, and consider the others to be consultants.

Promote hope

Hope affects the body's ability to heal. While your doctor is obligated to fully disclose all information about your condition so that you can work in partnership, how the information is shared is of tremendous importance. According to the *American College of Physician's Ethics Manual* third edition, "Disclosure should never be a mechanical or perfunctory process. Upsetting news and information should be presented to the patient in a way that minimizes distress."[12] Reynolds Price, in *A Whole New Life*, describes how he found out he needed immediate surgery.

> I was lying on a stretcher in a crowded hallway, wearing only one of those backless hip-length gowns designed by the standard medical-warehouse sadist...
>
> My brother, Bill Price, was standing beside me...when we saw my two original doctors bound our way with a chart in hand. The initial internist would show his concern through the years to come, but all I recall the two men saying that instant, then and there in the hallway mob scene, was, "The upper ten or twelve inches of your spinal cord have swelled and are crowding the available space...We recommend immediate surgery."
>
> Then they moved on, leaving me and my brother empty as windsocks, stared at by strangers.
>
> What would those two splendidly trained men have lost if they'd waited to play their trump till I was back in the private room...?...It might have taken the doctors five minutes longer, and minutes are scarce, I understand, in their crowded days. I also know that for doctors who work from dawn to night, in the same drab halls, it all no doubt feels like one room. But any patient can tell them it's not...[13]

In another case, a sister helps her brother overcome the depression that occurred after a doctor told him his days were numbered:

> I believe that doctors should not give false hope. But they should not lead the patient to believe that there is absolutely no hope either. When my brother was told he was terminal and that he had approximately six months to live, all of his hopes and dreams came crashing to the ground. He was paralyzed with fear and extremely depressed. Because he was depressed, his quality of life was greatly diminished and he did absolutely nothing to help his body cope with the disease. He simply decided to lie down and wait for death to come.
>
> Then my sister and I visited him. We put a feminine touch to his cabin, something he hadn't needed before as he spent his entire life outdoors. We turned his shack into a home (he said castle) and we gave him early birthday gifts, gardening tools, and fishing equipment. It was late September. By the time we left, my brother was up and taking mini-hikes

into the woods and over to his neighbor's house. As we parted ways, my
brother smiled broadly and said: "By God, I might just live to see next
year's garden!"

Some patients will see a prognosis of one-in-a-hundred as the ultimate challenge. Most people, however, are completely deflated. Doctors who leave their patients no hope have a total disregard for the serendipity of life. Few situations are one hundred percent predictable. In the following case, a patient had a doctor who framed her illness in a hopeful way, helping her to muster the courage to face difficult treatments.

When I was diagnosed with cancer, it was during a routine opera-
tion. The OB/GYN who did the operation told my sister immediately
because he knew we were very close. I had known this doctor for several
years and we were good friends. Next day, he told me the news in the
presence of my sister.

I knew from his body language that it was bad, but the words he
used were about fighting this illness together and because of my age and
general condition there were a lot of things that could be done. Bless him.
I never for a moment despaired.

When I left the hospital to go to the cancer hospital, I told him I was
going to survive this thing and that I would be back in five years with a
bottle of champagne to celebrate. It was at that point that I realized
things looked bad from the expression on his face. It took a long time
before he could answer, but even then he said he was looking forward to
it.

It's been nearly four years since that day. Every year in April I get a
letter from him telling me how he heard from my present doctor that I'm
doing so well and how happy he is to hear that.

Know limits

Doctors need to know the limits of their own knowledge and freely share this with their patients. They should willingly say, "I don't know the answer to that question, but I will research it and call you with an answer." Doctors should also not hesitate to say something is simply not known or well understood yet. Science has not yet provided all the answers in medicine—scores of mysteries remain. Dr. Jody Heymann, in her book *Equal Partners,* describes an honest answer from a physician who knew the limits of medical knowledge:

Guillain-Barre is a disease of the nervous system and can attack any part of it; in my case it hit the autonomic nervous system, the part that controls blood pressure.

When it was my turn in line for the influenza vaccine, I asked, "Do you advise those who have had Guillain-Barre before to get the flu shot?"

"I don't know," the physician in charge replied honestly, "Not enough patients have been studied to know."[14]

Doctors also have an obligation to consult with one or more other physicians should they require assistance in caring for you or when you request it (see Chapter 8, *Getting a Second Opinion*).

Your doctor also has an ethical obligation to refer you to other professionals who can provide services out of the doctor's areas of expertise. For instance, if surgery affects life skills, a referral to an occupational therapist should occur. If you become depressed during treatment for an injury or illness, a referral to a mental health professional is appropriate. Complex situations may require multiple consultations, but the ultimate responsibility for coordinating your care lies with your primary care doctor.

I was in a serious accident and had many broken bones. The muscles in my arm contracted while it was in a cast, so I went to a physical therapist to learn how to stretch it out again. After the cast came off my leg, my ankle was frozen in position—wouldn't bend at all. I worked on this in physical therapy as well, with minor improvement. When I needed another consult form from my orthopedic surgeon, he refused to sign it, saying, "Your ankle is permanently damaged and it's time for you to accept it." I said, "But I run and ride horses and do karate. I need to flex my ankle for those sports." He said, "Oh, just take up swimming and get on with your life." I said, "You may be right, but I'm not taking your word for it that I'm crippled. It's my time and my money and I'm going to keep working in physical therapy until it's all better or I'm convinced that it's hopeless. So please sign it." He sighed and signed. I struggled through hours of physical therapy every day for three months and regained full range of motion and strength in that ankle. It's been twenty years, and it still works perfectly.

Maintain confidentiality

Doctors have a legal obligation to keep any information you share with them in the course of your treatment confidential. The Code of Ethics of the

World Medical Association states succinctly, "I will respect the secrets which are confided in me, even after the patient has died."[15] Confidentiality respects your privacy, allowing you to feel comfortable candidly discussing your medical problems, and prevents discrimination based on your medical condition. Your doctor should not repeat or release information about you unless required by law (as in child abuse) or if there is a duty to warn others (exposure to syphilis). Prior to breaking confidentiality, your doctor should discuss it with you and try to work out a way to minimize damage to you.

In this electronic age, keeping private information confidential is difficult. For virtually all health plans, the forms you sign to initiate a claim (or to obtain authorization in managed care plans) include an authorization for record access and release. You can specify that only select portions of your records can be released by writing on the form the restrictions you want. For instance, if you tell your doctor about drug use or a mental illness, that information should not be passed on if you clearly exempt it from the release form.

The laws governing medical record confidentiality vary from state to state in the U.S. The general principles are that:

- Hospital charts and records are confidential.

- The patient or guardian can sign a written request transferring records from one treating physician to another, or the patient can deliver the record from one office to another upon request.

- Access to the records for other than current caregivers requires written authorization by the patient or guardian. Records will be released without this authorization only if subpoenaed or by court order.

- There must be no unreasonable delays in granting access to the records if authorized by the patient or guardian.

No abandonment

Doctors have a legal responsibility not to abandon their patients. This essentially means that, once an agreement to treat has been reached, severing the relationship will only occur if:

- The patient withdraws voluntarily.

- Further care is determined to be unnecessary.

- The doctor withdraws after his patient has had the opportunity to find replacement care of equal quality.

Doctors can decide not to treat you anymore, but they must tell you why, provide alternatives (usually the names and phone numbers of three other providers), give an appropriate amount of time to find the other care, and be willing to care for you until you do find other care. Reasons for dismissing a patient include: making unreasonable demands, nonpayment of medical bills, or consistently missing appointments. Many providers have basic rules; for example, if you miss three appointments, you are sent a letter saying that you will no longer be a part of the practice if it happens again.

Severing a medical relationship is a rare occurrence. The *American College of Physicians Ethics Manual*, third edition, states:

> There are occasions when the patient's beliefs—religious, cultural, or otherwise—dictate decisions that run counter to medical advice. The physician is obliged to try to understand clearly the beliefs and viewpoints of the patient. After a serious attempt to resolve differences, if the physician is unable to carry out the patient's wishes, the physician must withdraw and transfer care of the patient...Continuity of care must be assured to the best of the physician's ability. Physician-initiated termination is a serious event and should be undertaken only after genuine attempts to understand and resolve differences.[16]

Be a healer, not just a technician

Doctors should be healers, not just technicians. The space-age technologies of medicine—the MRI scans, laser surgery, gene splicing—have advanced modern medicine but isolated the physician from the patient as a person. The ancient therapeutic arts of listening, laying on of the hands, and empathy are often ignored. As a consequence, the art of healing sometimes takes a back seat to the biology of disease. Sir William Osler said, "The practice of medicine is an art, not a trade; a calling, not a business; a calling in which your heart will be used equally with your head."[17]

> On the night we were told about our son's diagnosis, as we were leaving the dreaded conference room and returning to his room, not knowing if he would ever see again or if he would live through the weekend, I was walking next to the resident, who told us the bad news. My husband was walking somewhere behind, in one of those terrible slow motion moments. Physically speaking, my husband was taking it much harder than I. He was having trouble just moving forward. I was beginning to feel a real break between him and me. I wanted to move forward

to get to what had to be done. (We were both frantic, but in our different ways). The doctor touched my shoulder and whispered in my ear, "Go hold your husband's hand." With that small little reminder, he brought us back together, where we needed to be to be the most help for our boy. A completely nonmedical, human moment.

Another patient who needs follow-up care after a serious illness praises her doctor's caring.

My doctor is very patient. When I was so nervous about stopping the penicillin, he let me wait another month and try again when I was ready. Just being told that it was perfectly normal and understandable for me to be frightened after doing so well for so long on it made all the difference. If I call his office and explain that I'm sick, I get a message given to him promptly. I don't know how he pulls off the amount of work that he does and never seems to be impatient or ruffled by anything. It's unbelievable.

He also doesn't mind my reading. In fact, we actually work together in this context since I do searches and select articles for him. So he knows I read the technical journals, and he points out really good items.

He asks how I'm doing even if he passes me in the hallway just for a minute (I work in the hospital). If something's going on—like a dermatology problem I've been having lately—he offers reassurance and always asks if I'm feeling better the next time we run into each other. The best way I can think of to describe him is that he makes me feel cared for. Like there is nothing else on his mind at that moment other than me and my situation and what can be done about it. That is something I appreciate beyond measure.

He has a phenomenal bedside manner. Even his voice is comforting! When I was sick this summer and we spoke on the phone initially, I honestly felt better after talking to him. When he says it'll be okay, get some rest, come see me in the clinic if you don't feel better, I can honestly trust him and just get some rest. And as crazy as it sounds, I think this is an amazing gift and one of the greatest things you could ever hope for in a doctor. When you have someone who knows their field, knows you, and is reassuring, in my eyes you have the best of all possible worlds. I feel blessed.

This brief summary of the rights and responsibilities of physicians shows that their central duty is to put the patient's best interests first. Physicians have a responsibility not only to care for malfunctioning body parts, but also help maintain the dignity and spirit of each person. Doctors need to do good, not harm.

If I had to guess, I would say that the principal contribution made by my doctor to the taming, and possibly the conquest, of my illness was that he encouraged me to believe I was a respected partner with him in the total undertaking. He fully engaged my subjective energies. He may not have been able to define or diagnose the process through which self-confidence (wild hunches securely believed) was somehow picked up by the body's immunologic mechanisms and translated into antimorbid effects, but he was acting, I believe, in the best tradition of medicine by recognizing that he had to reach out in my case beyond the usual verifiable modalities. In doing so, he was faithful to the first dictum in his medical education: above all, do no harm.[18]

—Norman Cousins
Anatomy of an Illness

CHAPTER 6

Patient Rights and Responsibilities

Patients suffer things to be done to them, thereby becoming the acted upon, the diminished.
We ignore the fact that patients have an intelligence, experience, and will of their own
and can themselves be a resource in restoring the equilibrium we call health.

—Max Lerner
Wrestling with the Angel

INCREASINGLY, PATIENTS WANT TO BE INVOLVED in their own medical care, to learn about their choices, and participate in decision-making. They want their intelligence, common sense, and individuality to be acknowledged and respected. They want a partnership. Creating such an alliance requires commitment from both doctor and patient. Both parties must assume responsibility for effective communication, clarifying expectations, and sharing control.

Patients have many rights. They have a right to be helped and not harmed. They deserve kind and respectful treatment at all times. Disclosure of all information and giving informed consent prior to treatment are both legal and ethical rights. Patients have a right to refuse treatment. They have a right to expect that all information shared with their doctor remains confidential. They have a right to full participation and control over their medical care.

With these rights come responsibilities. Patients are obligated to learn about their illness, participate in decisions, and comply with mutually agreed-upon treatment plans. They need to provide all pertinent information to their doctor to enable her to diagnose accurately and suggest the best treatment approach. They need to speak up on their own behalf, but treat doctors with respect. Patients have a responsibility to help keep medical costs down, to benefit both themselves and society. They need to pay their bills. And a person's ultimate responsibility is to live a healthy life and make choices that increase rather than undermine well-being.

Patient rights

Patients have many legal and ethical rights, including competent medical care, full disclosure of information, and kind treatment.

Receive considerate and respectful care

Patients have a right to be treated with respect, fairness, and without discrimination. Respect means to be treated with special consideration or high regard. Not surprisingly, the first right listed in the American Hospital Association's *A Patient's Bill of Rights* (see Appendix A) is "The patient has the right to considerate and respectful care."

Descriptions by patients of disrespect in medical settings include: poor communication with doctor, feeling rushed or ignored, lack of dignity during examinations, lengthy waiting room delays, inadequate explanations or advice, inadequate time with doctors during routine visits, feeling that complaints were not taken seriously, and feeling that providers are more concerned with holding down medical costs than giving the best medical care.[1]

> When I was a resident in the emergency room at a regional center, we got referrals from a large area. One day a young, vital guy who works with his hands came in. He had been driving with his arm stuck out the window and his car was hit from the side. The car fell over on his arm and skidded. He was treated at the scene by paramedics, taken to the local hospital, then sent to us. I opened the dressing and looked at his arm. It was an awful injury; his arm was just about destroyed. He was a rough-and-tumble guy who was trying to joke and be brave. He looked at it and said, "It looks pretty bad, doesn't it?" and I said, "Yes, it's pretty rough." I started doing some basic testing. I was holding his arm and asking him some questions when I heard sobbing. I looked up and saw tears just running down his cheeks. I said, "Oh gosh, have I hurt you?" and he said, "No, no, that's not it. You're the first person who has touched it. Everyone else just unwraps it, looks at it, and sends me somewhere else." I was the first person who touched his mangled arm. It was poignant.

Obtain complete information on illness and treatment

Full disclosure of all information is based on the ethical concept of autonomy—the right to decide on treatments based on having enough information to be truly informed. In the past, many patients passively sat back and let the doctors make all decisions for them. Indeed, doctors were often insulted if their patients even raised a timid question. Times have changed. You now have a well-defined legal, as well as ethical, right to full disclosure of all information related to your health. This includes accurate, easily understood explanations of diagnosis, prognosis, test results, and treatment options (including no treatment).

> My mom's primary care physician detected a growth in her lung in February '96 and decided to play wait-and-see without telling her of the abnormality. She had gone to see him because of pain and hoarseness. He made this "don't tell" decision, knowing that one of her sons had died of cancer the previous November, and that one of her daughters, myself, had been operated on for cancer three days after her son's death. Because of his decision, my mom's squamous cell cancer was not diagnosed for several months. By then it was the size of a softball.

Full disclosure takes time—in short supply in many busy practices. Time with patients is also shortened by some group practices and managed care organizations to increase efficiency and lower costs. One doctor discusses his dismay with this trend.

> It is extremely dissatisfying to doctors to be shoved into these ten minute fix sessions. You can provide technical fixes to many problems in ten minutes. And of course, it's cost-effective. It makes money. It's the cheapest model for disease care—but for health care it's not a good model at all.

Disclosure also includes obtaining accurate information about your health plan. You should be fully informed about benefits, costs, and procedures to resolve complaints or appeal decisions. The plan should be clear about their certification and accreditation status, and any known results of participants' surveys on customer satisfaction. All questions about access to services such as emergency care or referral to specialists should be answered.

Health professionals are also required to disclose, if asked, their education and board certification, their years of practice, and experience performing specific procedures. They must also tell you if they have a financial interest in any facilities to which they refer you, for example, radiation or laboratory services. If you ask about any financial incentives or punishments (see more in Chapter 3, Getting What You Need from Managed Care), they need to give you an honest answer.

Similarly, health care facilities such as hospitals or outpatient facilities need to disclose experience performing surgeries or other procedures, accreditation status, any known measures of quality or consumer satisfaction, and their methods for handling consumer complaints.[2]

Participate in treatment decisions

You have the legal and ethical right to fully participate in all decisions about your medical care. If you are unable to make these decisions, then you have the right to be represented by parents, guardians, or family members. Full participation includes a thorough discussion of all treatment options (including no treatment) in language that you understand, as well as the risks, benefits, and consequences of treatment. Your doctor should answer all of your questions and ask about your preferences concerning the treatment options.

My mother died of a brain aneurysm when she was thirty-five. On my thirty-fifth birthday several years ago, I got a painful migraine headache that lasted for days. I was convinced it was psychosomatic because of my history with my mother. But, after seven days I knew something was wrong. I went to my family doctor and asked for an MRI. Amazingly, she trusted my intuition and agreed to the MRI (a $1,200 test!). They said I had a mucocele that was pressing against the front left lobe of my brain, and it could burst at any time. It was an area too sensitive for laser surgery. I was very frightened. Later, after a CAT scan, the ENT specialist said the mass was caused by advance sinusitis and he put me on biaxin to try to dissolve it. Usually the drug works within three weeks. After a month, I went for a CAT scan and absolutely nothing had changed.

The ENT specialist called to say he had consulted with several other doctors and they all agreed that I should have brain surgery—a craniotomy. I said, "Let's give the biaxin one more try." He said, "If it was going to work it would have worked in the month you took it." I said, "Well, I want to give it one more try." He said okay and gave me another prescription. When I went for the next CAT scan, the mass was completely gone—not a trace left.

As the patient did in the above story, you need to take an active part in the medical decision-making process. Note that this patient discussed the options, and she and her doctor agreed on a treatment plan. If you choose a treatment that your doctor cannot medically or ethically support, he may explain the possible consequences of your decision or, in serious cases, ask you to find another physician.

Refuse any treatment

If you are an adult of sound mind, you have the right to refuse medical treatment or spurn the services of specific medical caregivers. For example, if you are hospitalized in a teaching facility and encounter numerous groups of medical students and student nurses streaming through your room, you can refuse treatment from any but your own doctor or the senior person on duty. Often patients appreciate the enthusiasm and willingness to talk exhibited by doctors in training. Most patients, if they are feeling well or have considerable goodwill, are willing to let various students examine their bodies to help them learn their trade. Sheer numbers can, however, overwhelm an ill person's meager resources. If, for any reason, you do not want these students to repeat examinations or procedures on you, you have the right to ask them to leave.

> *I had abdominal surgery and I just felt lousy. I was in pain, and really wanted to be left alone. I was in a training hospital, however, and big groups of students seemed to be staring down at me and wanting to look at my incision several times a day. I got tired of it and had my family put a big sign on the door that said, "No Students Allowed—This Means You." Some of the students thought it was funny and some were offended, but I was left in peace.*

The right to refuse treatment has a long and contentious history. One continuing problem is that doctors and patients often disagree about what is the patient's best interest. One example is the rights of Jehovah's Witnesses to refuse blood transfusions on religious grounds. Often Jehovah's Witnesses consent to surgery, but withhold permission to receive blood or blood products. Some surgeons and anesthesiologists adamantly oppose their right to refuse. They feel that they are being put in the untenable position of allowing a patient to die who could be saved.

> *As an anesthesiologist, I have both medical and legal concerns if someone (such as a Jehovah's Witness) wants or needs surgery but refuses all blood products. If it's a minor procedure where the likelihood of needing blood is slim, I usually just make sure that I, the patient, and his family understand what they do and don't want to have used. Larger*

problems arise when the patient needs to have major surgery such as open heart surgery or aortic aneurysm repair, and they may have a high risk of complications or death if they refuse to allow their surgeon and me to give them blood or blood products should they need them.

In this setting, there are surgeons and anesthesiologists who refuse to care for this patient, or don't allow the surgery to take place, especially on an elective (nonemergency) basis. Alternatively, some physicians (myself included) agree to abide by the patient's wishes, but with reservations. In this setting, I go to great lengths to speak with the patient and his family and make sure they understand the risks of their choices. I tell them point-blank that they could or likely will die. I then write this in the patient's chart and have both the patient and a member of the patient's family sign it to document that we have had this discussion. Even with this amount of interaction and communication, I am still taking a risk, as there have been cases where physicians have followed the patient's wishes and the patient had a bad outcome resulting in suits against the physicians. It is a no-win situation and many physicians are unwilling to take that risk.

Refusing treatment at the end of life can be legally accomplished by preparing a living will (also called an advance directive). By statute, health plans and hospitals have an obligation to educate the public about advance directives, and most require patients to fill out living wills upon admission to the hospital. But patients near the end of life sometimes encounter difficulties when they refuse life-extending treatment.

When I was a resident I cared for a little old lady who I became extraordinarily fond of. She was dying, didn't have a family, and I'd spend twenty or thirty minutes with her every day. We had a real friendship, and I came to understand her very profoundly. But I wasn't her doctor, just the resident. At one point she developed pneumonia. I knew her really well and she had told me she was ready to go, she wanted to die. I actually had to be taken off the case because I would not treat her pneumonia. The chief of the service and the attending physician insisted on treating her aggressively. She and I both tried to convince them not to treat her, but they just couldn't, wouldn't agree. It made me very sad.

These end-of-life misunderstandings (or even disagreements) can be avoided by filling out an advance directive, and giving a copy to all of your doctors. You need to discuss your feelings and thoughts on end-of-life care with your primary doctor, and if in the hospital, with all of the caregivers. In case you cannot make these wishes known, legally appoint a health care power-of-attorney to make decisions for you. Your loved ones can then ensure that you get all of the care you want, and no more.

Not be kept waiting

Just as you show respect for your doctor's time by arriving for appointments promptly, you should expect the same degree of respect for your time from the doctor. Doctors should do their best to avoid long delays in seeing their patients. If you do have to wait, the doctor should explain the reason, and if appropriate, apologize.

> *My doctor is a woman my age whom I knew in college, and for whom I have great respect and warm feelings. Yet, when I go in to see her, usually with a list of well-prepared questions in my mind, I find I don't ask them. First, I wait in the waiting room for 15-20 minutes, then I go into the examining room and am weighed, have blood pressure taken, and am told to get undressed and put on that paper gown. Then I sit, uncomfortably on the edge of the examining table, feeling foolish, perhaps shivering, growing more and more impatient. It is sometimes as long as a half hour. When S. comes in, all I can think of is getting out as quickly as possible. I tell her everything is fine, ask politely about her children, and rush to get my clothes on and out to the garage. Surely there must be a better way?*

If lengthy waits are commonplace, you can call before leaving home to ask whether or not the doctor is running on time and whether you will be able to see him at the appointed time. If not, ask how late he is running.

> *After a reasonable wait, I:*
>
> *1. Ask the receptionist what the problem is.*
>
> *2. Tell her I'm feeling sick to my stomach and can't hold out much longer.*
>
> *3. Tell her I have an appointment with the head of patient relations in the hospital/clinic in 15 minutes and will I be able to make it on time?*
>
> *4. Ask her how the doctor/clinic wishes to be charged for my time, which is $x/hour.*

5. When I see the doctor, I ask him if waiting 1.5 hours for an appointment is routine in his office and how can I avoid it next time?

In some cases, patients don't mind occasional waits because they appreciate the time the doctor spends with them. If the doctor treats them in a warm and caring manner, some patients enthuse rather than complain.

Somehow I ended up with the most wonderful doctor. He's very caring and very willing to answer any questions I have. In fact, a couple of my appointments with him were very late because he was taking so much time with another patient. I didn't mind since he takes so much time with me. I live in Seattle and was worried that, if we had one of our occasional snowstorms, I wouldn't be able to get to the clinic for my treatment (eight miles from my house). When I mentioned this to him, he just looked at me and said that he had a 4-wheel drive and that he would come and get me! And I think he meant it, too! During my treatment, he even called me at home once or twice just to see how I was doing. How many doctors will do that?

Maintain confidentiality of records

The legal right to confidentiality of health care information has been upheld by judicial bodies up to and including the U.S. Supreme Court. Clearly, your doctor has the obligation to protect the confidentiality of your health information. The only staff authorized to see your chart are those who are directly involved in your care.

At the same time, current health care systems require the sharing of information. For instance, insurance companies and doctors communicate regularly concerning payment for services. Rapid advances in information technology and changes in health care delivery can jeopardize your health care privacy. Large groups such as provider networks, information management companies, utilization review committees, and quality review committees now request records. If possible, stay aware of the contents of your records through frequent reviews, and give written permission for disclosure only when absolutely necessary. The permission should be very specific as to what can be released and to whom. You should indicate exactly which sections are authorized for release.

I strongly encourage all of my patients to keep diaries and detailed records about all of their interactions with the health care system, including, when possible, a copy of their own medical records. With the frag-

mentation and ever-shifting system, there is little continuity not only with
one's doctors, but among the various places of care. A drug reaction, an
X-ray result, etc., can be easily missed by physicians. But if patients
become their own best information base, some of the problems can be
avoided. Of course, there is the added benefit of having detailed records
should one have to pursue litigation.

The few reasons for disclosure of health care information without written consent are: public health reporting, investigation of health care fraud, and medical or health care research that an institutional review board has determined cannot use anonymous records. In these cases, nonidentifiable information should be used as much as feasible, and no more information than is necessary to fulfill the specific purpose of the disclosure should be allowed.[3]

Get copies of requested records

Medical records are the property of the hospital or the doctor, not the patient. However, most states have laws giving you the right to review, copy, and request amendments to your medical records. One way to get the particulars of your state law is to contact your state legislator's office and ask her to provide the medical record access law for your state.

Here in Kentucky, a law allows any patient who has been hospital-
ized to get one free copy of their entire medical record. I tell all of my
patients to keep a set of records for each hospitalization. They are the one
that holds the thread and keeps continuous and complete records. If you
have a physician who balks at you reading or keeping records, that
should be a red flag and you should be concerned about that.

Provisions that your state law might contain are:

- The patient must submit a written request to review all or part of the medical record.

- The patient has the right to review his/her medical records at a hospital or doctor's office.

- The review may be supervised to ensure that the contents of the records are kept intact. The staff who supervise are not considered qualified to answer questions about the contents of the records themselves.

- During the review, patients can usually indicate which copies they would like. The law might include a time frame for copies to be provided.

- A fee schedule for copies might be specified, including a search fee to locate the chart and a maximum fee per page copied.

- Patients who either cannot, do not want, or are unable to conduct a personal review can usually specify what copies they want (surgical report, pathology report, X-ray reports, discharge summary, etc.) or request the complete medical record.

Patients often encounter extremely varied responses from doctors when they ask to read or copy their chart, as the following two examples show.

> Each night, after my son was sleeping, I would make my way to the nurse's station and read through the day's entries, get his most recent labs, and review medications. The pharmacy book was nearby, so frequently I looked up medications if I hadn't seen them before. Sometimes I asked for old sections of my son's chart (only the current admission is kept at the nurse's station, the rest was in a file room on the floor). We were given a care notebook and told to keep track of my son's counts, so I assumed we were encouraged to grab the charts to get this information, rather than always pestering the nurses. I think most every parent on the floor did this too, and I've never heard of anyone being refused access.

• • • • •

> I tried to read my son's chart when he was in the hospital, and I was told that I can only do that with a doctor present. Then the doctor intimidated me by saying that in 22 years of being a doctor, no one has ever asked to read a chart. Now the only way I can read it is to pay 50 cents a page! One time, a really nice nurse let me read it as we were taking him down to a CT scan. Another nurse actually let me "accidentally" have it in the room when he came back, and didn't take it away until I was done!

If you run into problems getting copies of your records, it sometimes helps to phone or write to the medical records administrator of the hospital or medical group and ask for help. In addition, copies of medical records are usually provided directly to a new health care provider without fee upon receipt of a written authorization. If you are having trouble getting access to your records, you might authorize an M.D., dentist, naturopath, or chiropractor to receive the records and turn them over to you.

> A few years ago, my general practitioner charged $50 for a few sheets of paper and I complained very loudly. A call to some medical complaint organization revealed that his costs weren't excessive so he was entitled. I yelled a bit more and got the cost down a bit, but he still

charged. At that time, all the other medical people I spoke to were appalled that I'd be charged anything at all. Well, recently my wife wanted to get some records of hers and my son's from his birth. The hospital, which is in the same "family" of local hospitals I got all my records from in 1994 for free (including X rays and lab slides), charges a certain fee per page. Our total cost? $138. I think that's excessive.

Right to an advocate

You have the right to bring an advocate to doctor's appointments, procedures, or hospitalizations. Your support person can be a spouse, family member, friend, or anyone you choose. A companion can help you feel at ease, remind you about questions you forgot, and help you remember later what the doctor said. For instance, if you've recently learned that you have a serious disease or illness, it helps to have an advocate along to take notes or ensure that all questions are both asked and answered. If you are hospitalized, your support person will make sure you get the correct treatments and medicines. In some cases, it just helps to have a loved one at your side.

> *When my son was very ill, his physician and I made the medical decisions. My husband did not know what a protocol was, nor did he ever learn the names of the medicines. He came with me to medical conferences, however, and his presence gave me strength.*

Dr. Edward Rosenbaum explains in *A Taste of My Own Medicine* how he used to be embarrassed when his mother parked herself at the bedside of any family member who was in the hospital. He described how she checked the doctor's orders, diets, nursing care, and the patient. His embarrassment transformed into understanding when his father was in the hospital:

> *It was when my dad had a prostatectomy that my attitude changed...My dad had his operation when he was ninety. Although she was eighty-six, my mother insisted on staying the night with him in his room in the hospital. During the night, the nurse changed the numerous tubes and fluid bottles that were connected to dad without even bothering to turn on the lights. As soon as the nurse left the room, my mother examined the apparatus and found that, working in the dark, the nurse had inadvertently disconnected the equipment. It was not functioning. Had the situation gone undetected, my father would not have survived the night. Such situations are not common, but they do occur. Nurses are overworked. Now that hospitals are becoming more profit-oriented and hiring even fewer nurses, such errors will become more common.[4]*

Patient responsibilities

The dictionary defines responsible as meaning answerable or accountable; able to satisfy any reasonable claim; involving important work or trust. In medical relationships, this clearly applies to patients as well as doctors. Shouldn't we be accountable for the type of care we accept? Doesn't our medical care involve both important work and trust? An excellent relationship requires that both parties shoulder some responsibility for the outcome. The following are but a few of the responsibilities that patients must accept to have a satisfying and smoothly functioning relationship with their doctor.

Treat doctors with courtesy and respect

Doctors have a right to courtesy and kindness just as much as patients do. An environment of mutual respect sets the stage for long-term, satisfying medical relationships. Respectful treatment of physicians includes recognizing that they have values, preferences, and needs, too. One anesthesiologist, who has a soft voice and a caring manner, said sadly, "At least twice a month a patient or a family member threatens me. They'll say, 'If it doesn't go well, I'll see you in court.' It makes it seem as if we're adversaries, instead of allies."

Some simple courtesies that should be practiced with doctors are:

- Arrive on time for appointments.

- Use polite language. "Please" and "Thank you" are always appropriate words to use in any interaction. Abusive language or threats should never occur.

- Use a pleasant tone of voice. A demanding or demeaning tone of voice will not improve your relationship.

- Don't interrupt. Listen closely to what she says, without interrupting, then share your views.

- Apologize if you have said or done something inconsiderate.

- Clearly state your needs or concerns.

- Use the telephone appropriately. Give the doctor a reasonable amount of time to return your call—don't repeatedly call unless something urgent happens. You should call your doctor after hours only for true emergencies.

My young daughter was on chemotherapy and had frequent prob-
lems requiring office visits or phone calls. I really tried hard to call during
business hours: if things were getting bad, I called then rather than wait
until evening, or if she got sick during the night I just waited till morning
unless it was a real emergency. One time I brought her in on a Friday
afternoon because she developed a severe, itchy rash. Our pediatrician
told me, "I'm on call this weekend, so give me a call if things get worse." I
said, "I'm not going to call you at home because of a rash." He said, "Sit
down for a minute and let me tell you something. Taking care of your
daughter is my job. Your kid has cancer and you have never called at
night. I average five calls every night I am on call for constipation. The
kids can't go, they are crying and can't sleep, and the parents call me.
This is every time I am on call. So don't worry about calling me if you
need help. That's what I'm here for."

Some doctors get so used to mistreatment from patients that they are pleasantly surprised when things go well. In the following story, an emergency
room doctor describes meeting with a young woman and her mother.

The other day I had a young woman come in to the emergency room
in heroin withdrawal. I went in there loaded for bear because my last
heroin patient had been so abusive. But she was there with her mother
and was fully prepared to go cold turkey. She had already made arrange-
ments with the halfway house to go in after we got her dangerously high
blood pressure under control. She quite happily accepted the blood pres-
sure medication which would also lessen her withdrawal symptoms. Her
mom told me there was some miscommunication with the halfway house
about when she could go back, so I offered to talk to them to try to help.
The mom went out and got them on the phone. I talked to them and we
got it worked out. They had a reasonable expectation, everyone involved
was helpful and pleasant, and it went well.

Clarify expectations

Part of your responsibility as an informed patient is to have a realistic view
of what doctors can and can't do. There are illnesses that are difficult to
diagnose and some for which no effective treatment exists. It's reasonable to
expect your doctor to make an informed effort to determine the problem,
and when he reaches the end of his knowledge, to send you to a specialist

for further input. It is not reasonable, however, to expect doctors to be able to successfully treat all illnesses or never make a mistake. Barbara D. Webster, in her book *All of a Piece*, discusses such unrealistic expectations.

> *Another factor affecting the patient-doctor relationship may result from the explosion in medical research and technology. We have learned to expect that something will be done, that action can be taken, results assured. So much is possible now that was un-thought-of just a few years ago. MS [multiple sclerosis] presents a case where not much can be done or given. Playing it down may be a response to this fact. I think most doctors would like to be able to do something for their patients; in addition, I think that most patients expect that something will be done. There is a tendency to see doctors as very powerful. A disease such as MS with an uncertain course, an uncertain prognosis, no cure, and only palliative treatment available, confounds that relationship.*[5]

Patients sometimes unrealistically expect that doctors know it all or that doctors can instantaneously fix something that has taken weeks, months, or years to develop. Sometimes they want a pill or a treatment that doesn't include personal involvement such as behavior changes. One doctor remarked, "It's become the American way to demand a pill to fix any problem."

Tell the whole story

Partnership with your doctor requires clear communication. When you go for an appointment, be prepared. Plan ahead and make a list of concerns or symptoms that you wish to discuss. Share difficult or embarrassing information first. Tell the doctor how many issues you have to discuss and ask to be heard without interruption. Your doctor also needs to know what prescription drugs and over-the-counter medication you are taking. If you are also using any complementary or alternative therapies (vitamins, herbs, teas), tell your doctor about those, too. The majority of diagnoses depend solely on what you tell your doctor.

A primary care doctor discusses the all-too-common problem of not hearing the full story.

> *I start out by asking people, "What brought you into my office today?" If they've had an ongoing problem for six months, something brought them in today. I'd estimate that 50 percent of the time there are some underlying issues that are not their presenting complaints. I have*

patients who come in and give me little itsy bits at a time. Each time they come in they tell me another symptom that I don't know about. It's really difficult.

The situation is quite different in busy emergency rooms. Doctors in emergency rooms only want to hear about the emergency and nothing else. Chronic or non-acute problems should not be brought up in your emergency room story; such complaints only waste time and confuse the issue.

We have a different problem in the emergency room than the primary care doctors do. We just want the one problem that brought them in—not a whole litany of complaints. One of my pet peeves is people who come in with a shopping list of unrelated complaints. It's not unusual to have someone who arrives with a work-related ankle injury say, "You know, my shoulder is a little sore, and my other ankle is bothering me—could you shoot an X ray of them while I'm here?" They know it's on the boss's ticket. Patients need to realize that if you have more than one chief complaint in an emergency room the doctor starts to wonder. If we hear several problems, we keep trying in our minds to relate it to the main injury or illness.

Telling the whole story has benefits other than just getting the right diagnosis. Researchers at the Primary Care Outcomes Research Institute conducted four separate controlled trials on patients with ulcers, hypertension, diabetes, and breast cancer to see if there was a relationship between patient assertiveness and health outcomes. The researchers coached the patients prior to appointments on questions to ask, negotiation skills, and methods to overcome embarrassment and anxiety. In all four trials, subsequent testing showed that the coaching increased the patient's communication and involvement during appointments, and they subsequently felt better and had measurably better health (for example, lower blood pressure).[6, 7]

Speak up

Passive patients get plenty of medical advice, but not always the best health outcomes. Part of effective communication with your doctor is speaking up about your concerns, thoughts, and values, and asking questions until you understand exactly what you have and what the proposed treatment is. Your doctor cannot factor into the treatment equation your perspective if you do not share it. The following study shows the degree of reluctance some patients still have when making the most basic of requests.

End-of-life decisions also require clear communication. One study from the Center for Evaluative Clinical Sciences showed how poorly patients and doctors communicate about whether the patient would like to be resuscitated by CPR should their heart stop. Of 2,636 pairs of doctors and patients, up to one-half of the doctors did not know or did not agree with the patient's preferences. These misunderstandings not only lead to a course of care at odds with the patients' wishes, but, in the case of patients who do not wish resuscitation, consume large amounts of hospital resources unnecessarily.[9]

Learn about condition and treatment

Partnerships with medical professionals are based on patients taking an active role in learning about their illness and the options for its treatment. Ways to learn about your illness are:

- Ask your doctor questions and make sure you understand the answers.

- Get a second opinion if necessary (see Chapter 8, *Getting a Second Opinion*).

- Research your illness and treatment options (see Chapter 13, *Researching the Medical Literature*).

- Express wishes and concerns clearly.

    I have a connective tissue disorder called Marfan syndrome. This condition affects, among other things, the heart, lungs, skeleton, blood vessels, and eyes—basically everything—since everything is made up of connective tissue. Among the doctors on my health team are a general internist, cardiologist, orthopedic surgeon, ophthalmologist, allergist/ asthma specialist, and endocrinologist.

Most recently, I discovered that people with Marfan syndrome are at risk of having very poor bone density at a very young age (I made this finding when, during a bad bout with a cold, I fractured a rib while coughing). I'd been to a local Marfan chapter meeting about a year before this episode, and vaguely recalled hearing about bone density issues, but in general, it was not well documented with regard to the Marfan syndrome.

So I set out to find out as much as possible and brought all my findings to my newest specialist (the endocrinologist). I knew I liked this new doctor when she so eagerly accepted (and pored over) my documentation, and was very open to hearing about my experiences and overall input on the Marfan syndrome, specifically as it related to bone density. Since Marfan is a fairly rare disorder, most doctors either don't know anything about it or only know basic details—it's really up to the patient to stay abreast of all the latest advances in treatment, and keep yourself and your doctor informed.

Patients' needs for information differ. You may want just basic information and your doctor's recommendation, while others may pursue in-depth research on their condition. Your feelings may also shift as your situation changes.

Share responsibility for decisions

You do not need to blindly follow what your doctor recommends. In the best of all worlds, your doctor would ask how you felt about his proposal and if there are any potential problems with his recommendation. But even if he doesn't ask, speak up and say what you would like to do and why. For instance, you may have a problem with the pill schedule, or you may not be able to have elective surgery next week due to family problems. The doctor will not know your feelings or life situation unless you tell him. This allows the doctor to explain more fully the proposed treatment or to make an alternate proposal based on your input. Your doctor may simply view the risks and benefits of a course of action differently than you do. After you have shared the full story with your doctor, and spoken up about your own feelings and concerns, it's time to jointly decide on your treatment.

I know that there are doctors out there that treat people like cogs in a machine. Those are the ones I run from and I run fast. If I ever feel the least bit uncomfortable, or am given that "pat on the head," I speak up. This is only my opinion, but I believe you have to have trust and a good working relationship with your doctor. You must also be informed yourself so that you understand all that is going on. Together you will be making some major decisions about your life.

I trust that my doctor will give me the information to make an informed decision about my treatment. I trust that when my doctor does not have all the answers, she will tell me, and together we will find them. I trust that my doctor considers me a person, not just a patient. I trust that my doctor has enough trust in me to allow me to seek alternatives.

I trust that my doctor will always explain to me what she is doing and why, whether it be a change in treatment or medication. I trust my doctor to keep the lines of communication completely open. Because of this trust, we have had heavy discussions, arguments and differing opinions regarding my treatment plans. Because of this trust, we have cried together and shaken our heads together in disbelief. Because of this trust, I feel I am getting the best treatment possible.

Yes, I trust my doctor. But it is a two-way street.

One treatment option worth discussing is to do nothing. Watchful waiting has fallen out of vogue since technology has boomed and malpractice suits have increased. Doing nothing is no longer popular. However, many maladies are self-correcting. Keep in mind that for many illnesses, doing nothing is sometimes a viable (and inexpensive) option.

When my young daughter had a seizure in church many years ago, our doctor was out of town. The doctor taking his place told me that she needed an EEG and complicated work-up to determine the cause of the seizure. When Dr. M. came back to town, he said, "I hate to put a child through all those tests unless we really need to. What do you think about just waiting to see if she has another?" I thought it was an excellent idea. It's been thirty-five years, and she never had another seizure.

Comply with a mutually acceptable treatment plan

You have the ethical and legal right to fully participate in all treatment decisions. Once the decisions are made, you then have a responsibility to make a good faith effort to comply with the treatment. It is frustrating to doctors when patients do not follow the agreed-upon plan, or even worse, say they did when they didn't. In a partnership, both patient and doctor are responsible. So, once you've agreed, follow the plan or call the doctor to tell him why you can't.

I have patients who've walked around with something for four or five years, and they come to me expecting it to be better in a week or two and it just doesn't happen. High blood pressure, for example, requires lifestyle changes. I try to see them frequently for three or four months to make sure they stick to the new program. It's their responsibility to do the best they can, and I try not to make them feel guilty if they don't. It's hard.

Patients need to be informed of the consequences of noncompliance. If you forget to take an aspirin, it probably won't matter; but if you use your asthma inhalers improperly, you could end up in an emergency room in crisis. Doctors and pharmacists should inform patients of the risks associated with not complying with the agreed-upon plan. In addition, numerous studies show that better health results from compliance.

Following doctors' advice affects outcomes

The Medical Outcomes Study analyzed information from 1,751 patients with diabetes, hypertension, and heart disease to determine if remembering and following physician's recommendations affected the level of their disease. Among patients in all three disease groups, more than 90 percent recalled recommendations about medication, while far fewer recalled advice on diet, exercise, and other self-care activities. Following the doctor's advice varied considerably according to the nature of the recommendations; for example, 91 percent of diabetics took prescribed medications but only 69 percent followed a diabetic's diet and 19 percent engaged in regular exercise. Those who followed all the doctor's recommendations had better health: diabetics had lower serum glucose and patients with hypertension had lower blood pressure. The study concluded, "The majority of chronically ill patients failed to recall elements of potentially important medical advice and did not always adhere to advice that was recalled."[10]

In the above study, most of the chronically ill patients took their medication faithfully, but had problems making lifestyle changes. The following study shows that many elderly patients have trouble managing their many medications, resulting in hospitalizations.

Medication noncompliance in the elderly

Researchers in Massachusetts interviewed 315 elderly patients admitted to the hospital to determine how many of the patients entered the hospital due to complications from noncompliance in taking medications. They found that 33 percent of the patients were not taking their medications correctly. Some of the reasons for the noncompliance were forgetfulness, confusion from seeing different physicians, numerous prescriptions, and concerns over medication expense. Of the 315 elderly patients admitted, 89 went to the hospital because of an adverse drug reaction. The study concluded that several preventative measures could be taken, including a simpler schedule with fewer pills to take each day, reducing the costs of medications, better communication between doctor and patient on side effects and drug effectiveness.[11]

In some cases where noncompliance puts others at risk, patients and doctors have legal obligations to fulfill. A doctor tells about methods used in a tuberculosis clinic to ensure compliance.

Compliance takes on a whole new dimension when we talk about infectious diseases like AIDS or tuberculosis. I used to work in a pediatric TB clinic and there we tried to enforce compliance. We required them to come in for observed therapy (taking the medicines in the clinic) or we sent public health nurses out for home visits. My public health orientation clearly differentiates between infectious and noninfectious diseases. If someone doesn't manage their diabetes, it doesn't hurt anyone else. But, if they are infecting others, it's a whole different situation.

Help keep costs down

Health care costs have dramatically increased over the last two decades. Patients have a responsibility not only to their individual insurance company or managed care plan to help keep costs down, but also to society as a whole. Health care is a limited resource, and the dollars you use for your care are dollars not available to another patient. In addition, profligate use of resources increases the cost for everyone. Health care consumers have a responsibility to use only the resources they truly need.

In my area, most of my patients are issued a prescription card by their insurance company which allows the patients to get medication for free or for a small fee (typically $10). I've found that this results in

*patients immediately not caring about the cost of the medication. They
routinely ask for the most expensive one. The classic example is the two
medications used to treat sinus infections—the old, effective standby costs
$8, while the new, effective wonder drug costs $180. I always start with
the $8 one, and if the patient is allergic or it doesn't work, then we try the
next one. But the people with the cards often demand the expensive drug.
I try to explain to them that their insurance will be more expensive
because they are not willing to actively help me to help keep costs down
by figuring out the least expensive way to treat the illness.*

Discuss money and pay all bills

Patients are obligated to pay for the service their doctor provides in a reasonable amount of time. Timely payment allows the doctor to pay employees, benefits, rent, utilities, and other costs. Patients who are tardy cause an
accounts receivable problem for doctors, causing the doctor's practice to
owe more money than is coming in.

If you have a problem paying for your medical care, talk to your doctor and
the bookkeeper about it. Often, a payment schedule can be set up to allow
you to pay a smaller amount for a longer period of time. Many physicians
donate a portion of their services to patients who don't have insurance and
cannot afford their care. Rather than just not paying the bill, try to work out
a mutually satisfying solution.

*The first time my daughter was released from the hospital after a
chemotherapy round, I stopped at the hospital pharmacy to fill a prescription for antinausea drugs. My insurance plan at the time required
prepayment for prescriptions. I would then have to submit forms for 80
percent reimbursement which took weeks to receive and was always less
than expected. When the pharmacist asked for $1,200 for the prescrip-
tion (only four days' worth), I just stood there shell-shocked and trying
desperately not to cry. The woman, bless her, recognized my poorly
hidden distress and just gave me the medicine!*

*The next day, I happened to mention my inability to prepay to the
hospital social worker. He immediately set up the billing so all outpatient
prescriptions were charged as inpatient (fully covered) costs. I was surprised at how easy it was when I just asked.*

Complain constructively

You have a responsibility to complain constructively to your doctor. A laundry list of grievances or an argumentative tone undermine your partnership. Try to focus on just one problem, present it in a positive manner, and conclude with a suggestion on how to fix it. Chapter 7, *Problem Solving*, contains numerous suggestions for positive problem solving.

And remember, doctors deal with ill or injured patients all day long, every working day. They deal with people at their worst who may not be so easy to get along with at their best. Not all patients are patient or even polite with their M.D.s. It is an emotionally and physically draining job.

Unless you speak up, your doctor won't know that something she said or did offended you. It also helps to keep in mind that it's hard to know what one person might find offensive. Each patient is different.

> It must be very difficult for doctors to gauge when to say what. Just because some kinds of comments would irritate me now doesn't mean they would evoke the same reaction from others. A comment that I find condescending may actually be comforting for some other women. That same must be true for comments about prognosis, statistics, etc. I always want to know the truth, even if it's painful, but others need to keep hope alive, and they don't want to hear any grim statistics. A skilled and compassionate doctor or nurse can adjust his or her manner to suit each patient, but it's not surprising to me that many medical professionals fail dismally in this regard. They're only human, after all.

Understand that patient and doctor have different perspectives

Satisfying relationships require recognition that each person has a unique perspective. Differences between patients and doctors can be vast. Just recognizing that the other person has a valuable and crucial viewpoint can build bridges and forge bonds. Recognition that the other view has value allows you to listen quietly without anger or judgment. And from the quiet listening sometimes comes understanding.

Dr. Joseph E. Harding wrote of this phenomenon in an essay contained in *A Piece of My Mind*. He described an incident during his residency when he interviewed a man and diagnosed the rare illness myasthenia gravis. He was thrilled with his discovery, but his patient was sad and quiet. It was then that the patient's world was suddenly illuminated:

> Mr. Thomas told me he knew he had myasthenia gravis. I was put out. "Why didn't you tell me? Why did you let me go through the history and give you Tensilon when you knew all the time what was wrong with you?" "I am sorry," he said. "I was hoping if I told you my symptoms, you might diagnose something else—a disease you could cure. I take my medicine, but my case is difficult to control. I am not doing well. I am afraid."
>
> I was embarrassed and disappointed, but most of all I felt sorry for him. I had been so euphoric about diagnosing my first case of myasthenia gravis that I had forgotten about my concern for Mr. Thomas.
>
> From that day to this, I guard against thinking of patients as interesting. Diseases are interesting. Patients are sick.[12]

Barbara Webster discusses the differences between her doctor's view of her multiple sclerosis and her own in her book *All of a Piece*:

> Akin to this is something that I feel very strongly about every time that I see my neurologist. I have a benign form of this disease. He deals every day with acutely and grievously ill people. In his world, I am clearly one of the lucky ones. Seen through his eyes, I am quite well. In my world—especially compared to the way I used to be—I am not OK at all. I try to remember that. It is, in part, a question of perspectives. For me, it is of major importance that many days I must struggle to walk. In his world, I walk very well.
>
> I think of a day when I was walking along and suddenly felt something very strange or, rather, I felt nothing at all and wondered if my shoe had broken. Well, my shoe was fine. My ankle had collapsed and there was no sensation attached to that event. There was suddenly no support there. I reported this to my doctor and he said, "Oh, yes, that was an ankle collapse." For him, it was another transient symptom; for me, it was much more...[13]

Maintain a healthy lifestyle

If doctors could wave a magic wand and get a wish about their patients granted, it most likely would be that they eat well, exercise, and avoid stress, alcohol, and cigarettes. More than 875,000 deaths in the U.S. in 1990 were caused by behaviors that undermine health—totaling over 40 percent of all deaths. The costs to society are staggering—$179 million from cigarette and alcohol use alone. The old adage "an ounce of prevention is worth a pound of cure" is simple common sense.

However, most Americans prefer to eat loads of fat and sit in front of a TV or computer screen rather than go for a brisk walk or bicycle ride. We'd rather not hear about prevention; we like magic bullet drugs that fix it quick. Millions of dollars are poured into ever more elaborate technology, while preventative actions like hand washing, good nutrition, and prenatal care get short shrift.

Perils of smoking

Smoking, the leading preventable cause of death in the U.S., causes more than 400,000 deaths a year. In 1994, 48 million Americans 18 and over smoked. Half of all lifetime smokers die of a smoking-related disease. Quitting smoking reduces the risk of premature death by as much as 50 percent. The total economic cost of smoking (including lost productivity) has been estimated to be about $100 billion, with direct medical costs accounting for more than 75 percent of all national medical expenditures.[14]

Wellness isn't simply the absence of sickness, rather, it's a way of living that emphasizes healthy living. Our responsibility as patients extends to decisions we make every day—eating less fat and more vegetables, buckling up the seat belt for all car rides, practicing safe sex, quitting smoking, drinking alcohol only in moderation, eliminating all but essential drug use (both prescription and over-the-counter), and exercising regularly.

One of my teenaged patients came in with her tongue pierced. It was badly infected—all red and swollen. I explained that some people could tolerate this type of piercing and others couldn't and I didn't think she was cut out to have this thing in her tongue. She really wanted to keep it and demanded an antibiotic. I made a deal with her—I'd give her four days of keflex, and if the infection was cleared up completely by then, great. Either way, I wanted her to come see me in four days. She said she wanted to consult her piercer, but I explained how our perspectives would probably be quite different. I wrote on her chart that I advised she immediately remove the object in her tongue. She never came back.

Navigating the health care system and becoming a full partner in treatment decisions requires time, effort, and commitment. Understanding both your rights and responsibilities helps you to maximize your chances for a rewarding relationship with your doctor.

I have learned that it is necessary to stay on top of things, be sure all essential tasks are done by doctors, their staffs, and other clinical practitioners and that I make sure I know what the alternatives are (and there are always alternatives).

Vigilance is essential, and it requires that I keep myself as well informed as I possibly can. Even so, I will make mistakes, too. But caution, an eye out for problems, frequent questions, and follow-ups to make sure things are getting done are what is required. Such patients are sometimes not loved by their doctors, but we're not here to be loved by our doctors. We are here to get the best medical care we can. And it's hard to be a good manager of one's own medical situation. Things have changed from the old days. Knowledge is now a far more basic need.

CHAPTER 7

Problem Solving

Don't find fault, find a remedy.

—Henry Ford

IN THESE TIMES OF SPACE-AGE MEDICINE, some of us still yearn for Marcus Welby—with his comforting manner, shy smile, and complete knowledge. When the expectation for perfection in our doctors collides with reality, friction results. And it's not surprising that when life, health, or comfort are on the line, problems can quickly escalate into crises. Identifying and fixing disagreements quickly will help preserve, and sometimes strengthen, your relationship with your doctor.

The first half of this chapter outlines many common problems that patients face in their sometimes prickly relationships with their doctors, and the remainder discusses methods for recognizing and dealing with them.

Common problems

Patients and doctors have different temperaments, life experiences, and expectations. As in any relationship, disagreements are inevitable. This section examines several common problems encountered in medical relationships.

Differences of opinion

Active patients disagree with their doctors on occasion, especially if they have to see them frequently due to a chronic or serious illness. Medical relationships are similar to any other interpersonal relationships—with frequent interaction, friction is inevitable. It is usually far better to work through it than to give up.

In the following situation, a mother feels that her son is getting inadequate pain medication, but the doctor disagrees.

I usually use the "honey" approach first. I've found that asking nicely works wonders. But, on one occasion when my son was in the PICU (pediatric intensive care unit) after a bike accident that fractured his skull, I really worked up a head of steam. They had my son sedated, but were giving him, I thought, inadequate pain medication. He was unconscious, but still crying. The nurse called the doctor to ask if she could give the same amount of drugs on a different schedule to try to make Nick more comfortable, but the doctor said no. The nurse was very upset.

I asked her to put a note in the chart stating, "Parent demands to meet with doctor first thing in the morning to discuss pain management." I also called and left messages with his trauma surgeon and his pediatrician to get reinforcements. I just wasn't going to let Nick suffer. It turns out that the doctor from the night before went on vacation, so another doctor, whom I had never met, walked in and said, "Hello, my name is Dr. S. I have rewritten the orders to eliminate the sedation and increase his pain meds." Problem solved.

No shared decision-making

You have a legal and ethical right to fully participate in your medical treatment. If you have spent time researching and studying your illness and treatment options, only to be told by your doctor that he is in charge of the decision-making, conflict is guaranteed.

I lost my first oncologist by asking too many questions. From my reading, I thought I should have one type of chemotherapy, she chose another. I thought she probably had a reason, and wanted to know what it was. She told me that she couldn't give me a medical school course. She was very insulted and suggested I would probably be happier with another oncologist.

I was devastated when this happened because I was not being hostile when I asked the questions. It actually worked out better for me because I next had an oncologist who loved to talk and would answer any question. I always knew I would have to wait for her because she took too long with every patient, but it was worth it.

Not being given the full story

Doctors sometimes tell only part of the story. Some of the reasons for such selective presentations are: saves time, prevents questions, sways patient to accept recommendations, and protects patients from upsetting information.

Regardless of the reason, a biased explanation is totally unacceptable. Withholding knowledge of all the facts strips patients of the information they need to make informed decisions.

I was scheduled for a routine hysterectomy necessitated by constant right-sided abdominal pain. I was told the surgery was fully elective and I could decide against it if I wanted, "after all it's not like you have cancer or something." The morning after the surgery I was informed that I had an ovarian cyst, but not to be concerned as these are always benign. Upon leaving the hospital I was told that the pathology would be ready in a day or two and I left expecting a call. Two weeks passed and no call, so I called the doctor. He said, "I have good and bad news. You had cancer—the cyst was malignant, but I consulted with two gynecological oncologists and both agreed that it was not so bad, and most patients survive this type of cancer."

I was, to say the least, stunned by his abruptness and his total lack of concern or compassion. He did mention the pathologist's name which I was too shocked to remember. In fact, I did not even remember what description was given to the malignant cyst. A return call got me the name of the pathologist and the tumor description. It was a mucinous cystadenocarcinoma of the left ovary.

I called my husband (a veterinary pathologist) and he immediately made an appointment with the head of pathology at the hospital. Our discussion with the pathologist, who was forthright and honest, led to a much different picture of my possible future. The tumor had penetrated the capsule and had released mucinous contents into my pelvis, and so things were not so simple. I had pseudomyxoma peritonei which is generally a recurrent problem and additionally these tumors in the ovary are frequently accompanied by tumors in the appendix and omentum. He thought I should consider additional surgery to rule these out.

I did in fact have another malignancy in my appendix that was diagnosed months later. Again I was accused of faking symptoms. Again it required a trip to the emergency room and this time a threat of a lawsuit if the diagnosed hernia, which I agreed to give permission to repair, proved not to be a hernia. Fortunately this resulted in my being seen by a very skilled senior surgeon. He admitted me immediately after palpating a mass. He looked at the resident and said, "This lady ain't fakin'." Surgery revealed that the mass was a malignancy in my appendix.

Not being believed

As medicine tilts more and more toward the bells and whistles of complex machinery, the human voice is sometimes ignored. Many patients complain that their doctors and nurses believe the machines, rather than them.

> I had liver surgery and was in great pain. The nurses were short-staffed, and when I rang the bell for help, it took the nurse one half hour to come. I told her that I was in bad pain, but she checked the morphine machine and said that the right rate of morphine was going through the epidural (needle in the back) and that I was fine. I kept calling all night long and she kept saying I was fine. She finally called the pain team— three doctors. They couldn't find anything wrong either. But I was in agony.
>
> By the next morning, I was in such extreme pain that I could not move and could barely talk. An orderly came in to get me up to exercise and I said I couldn't move. He said, "Oh, come on, you can do it," and pulled me up. I started to scream. Luckily, my mom and dad walked in at that moment, and my father took over. The pain team came back, and when they took off the tape to check the epidural, they found the needle hanging free—it was not even in my back.

Lack of sympathy

Doctors can sometimes treat patients as merely problems to fix, rather than complex human beings with needs other than just medical. Most patients recognize that the doctor's expertise is not in emotional support, but it is also clear that people need to feel cared for and heard in order to heal.

> When our son was going through his three-year protocol for leukemia, we often consulted his hematologist about various side effects he was experiencing. The doctor (a very experienced and well regarded doctor) often said, "No, that's not related to the treatment. Never heard of that before." At first I thought she was deliberately minimizing in an effort to keep us from getting upset. Then I noticed that the nurse was standing right behind her and was nodding big time about the things we were experiencing. In the hall she would later tell us, "That happens with a lot of kids."
>
> The fact remains, one of the things we really needed more of as we went through this with our son was validation of our feelings. We weren't complaining to the doctor about the drugs. We just needed to know that

others experienced what we experienced and yes, it can be a bitch. No more, no less. Few of the medical staff were able to do this. It wouldn't have taken long, but a little would have gone a long way.

Excessive waiting

Doctors are busy people; so are patients. But patients sometimes find themselves waiting two months to get an appointment, then waiting an hour in the waiting room, and perhaps enduring two weeks of worry while waiting for test results. Waiting heightens emotions such as fear or anger, and may result in a frustrating visit.

Three days after my tonsillectomy (I was 38), I went to the surgeon's office for a follow-up appointment. I was feeling ill, and my mother had to drive me there. I was scheduled to see his assistant first—she asks questions and takes blood pressure and temperature. I waited thirty minutes, then asked the receptionist when I would be seen. She said, "As soon as the assistant gets back from lunch." I waited 15 more minutes, feeling sicker and more angry by the minute. The assistant arrived, very happy and cheerful.

When the surgeon came in, I said, "I don't appreciate sitting here for 45 minutes waiting for your assistant to return from lunch when I'm feeling so ill." He raved about her, saying, "She's very competent and a great employee." I told him that I thought he was an excellent surgeon, but his office management left a lot to be desired. Then I told my allergist (who had recommended him) what happened. She picked up the phone, called him, and told him if she ever heard another story about mistreatment of her patients, she would never refer another one to him. A few days later the assistant called me and apologized.

Billing problems

If you keep good records of your office visits and tests, errors will probably be easy to identify. Hospital errors are more common, and sometimes harder to prove.

The following patient resolved her problem with a review of her hospital chart and a letter.

My specialist charged $125 for an appointment. The only problem was that he charged for hospital visits that he did not make. For instance, he'd poke his head in the door, notice that I was on the phone, wave, and disappear. Then I'd get a bill for $125.

I called his office and was told that his bills are always correct. So I copied my hospital chart and made a list of the dates in which he had made a notation in it. These visits did not match his bills. I wrote him a letter noting the discrepancies between his visits and his billed visits (he billed me for 10 phantom visits). I attached a copy of the pertinent pages from my chart and sent a copy of the letter to my insurance company. The bill was adjusted.

Problems during procedures

Patients often aren't aware of their legal right to stop a procedure or refuse treatment. In most states, unless they are a danger to themselves or others, adults have the right to refuse medical care. If a procedure is not going well, you have the right to tell them to stop.

I was having a full body skeletal survey done, and I wasn't feeling well. The X-ray technician was very tentative, and he was doing things in a different way than I was used to. He also seemed to be taking way too many X rays. Usually, they take them standing up because it is just diffi-cult for me to lie down on a hard table due to multiple back fractures and harrington rods. He insisted that I lie down, so I did. Then I was able to see the name tag hooked to the bottom of his shirt. It identified him as a student and there was no supervisor present. I said, "Get me off this table!" He said, "You're not done yet." I responded, "Yes, I am." I wrote to my orthopedist (who had referred me there for X rays), the hospital administrator, and the head of radiology. My orthopedist was aghast, the head of radiology apologized, and now I get only senior technicians.

Conflict resolution

The previous section contained just a sampling of the myriad problems that result in conflict between patients and physicians. How can you resolve these vexing problems? The following methods will outline ways to identify and fix misunderstandings and disagreements with your medical caregivers. Patients share many stories of how they persevered until the problems were resolved and what they did if the problem simply couldn't be fixed.

Plan the meeting

Your problem will probably get worse, not better, if you explode at the doctor or staff when you are very angry. Usually, it is better to leave if you are very upset, and wait for your emotions to cool before taking action. Planning a strategy may help you resolve the problem. The following are ideas on what to consider during your planning process:

- Understand the problem. Think about and clarify the nature of the problem.

- Decide to whom you need to talk. You may need to talk with the billing supervisor for bill problems, the doctor about treatment disagreements, or the nurse for rude behavior.

- Get expert information. You can skip this if the problem is about your relationship, e.g., wanting the doctor to not interrupt you so often. If, however, the disagreement is of a technical nature, for instance, choosing between two treatment plans, arm yourself with expert opinions.

- Decide on a strategy for the meeting.

- Consider obstacles.

- Have a positive attitude and expect to succeed.

- Carry out the plan. Set deadlines and goals for yourself, then gather appropriate information and make the appointment.

A couple of months ago I complained to my doctor about wearing the paper vest, and then I wrote about it to the computer discussion group. So many responded that I compiled the best comments and took them to my doctor on my next visit. He agreed with it, and had a nurse check into getting cloth gowns. But the hospital refused to provide gowns and his partners said it would be impractical and expensive to change things.

So, at my next appointment, I took a stand. I wore a big, loose blouse without a bra instead of a paper vest. My doctor came in and said, "I like your new vest." It worked just fine, and I felt like a human being again with my clothes on. It made a huge difference to me. So that was that. I will never wear the paper thing again.

Make an appointment to talk

Combining your conflict resolution talk with an examination may backfire. First, you may not have enough time to fully discuss the issue. You also will be at a bargaining disadvantage if you are lying on a gurney looking up at the doctor. If the doctor is not expecting the discussion, you may start off on the wrong foot. Too often patients irritate doctors by bringing up an unexpected subject late in an appointment, throwing the doctor's schedule off and making it less likely that he will hear your problem with compassion. Lastly, it is common courtesy to forewarn the doctor that you have specific issues to discuss, so that he has time to think about and prepare for the discussion as well.

One doctor remarks on the ability of some doctors to hear what patients are saying.

> Some doctors have such a strong ego that they can't even hear a patient's constructive complaint. You have to be very comfortable with yourself to be a good doctor and there are a lot of doctors out there who are not. If they feel that they are being challenged, it affects their sense of self. Many of them cannot be objective about the situation and really hear what's being said. Sometimes they become defensive or belligerent.

When you call for your appointment, tell the receptionist that you need to talk to the doctor and it may take a while. This should ensure that you are given more than a ten-minute slot for your discussion. If the doctor knows she has time for a discussion, she might be less likely to interrupt or rush you. Knowing you have a chunk of time may help you relax, as well.

> I was extremely concerned about some of the side effects of the treatment my young daughter was experiencing. I called the pediatrician's office and told the receptionist that I needed a lengthy appointment to discuss the problems. I wrote down the side effects that I was concerned about (so that I wouldn't forget any in the heat of the moment), looked into some other treatment options, and went to the appointment with my notebook and articles.
>
> When I went in, he took me to his office rather than an examining room, and we both sat down. He looked exhausted and I felt teary. He apologized at not giving me his full attention and explained that he had been rerouted due to snow the night before and ended up driving all night to get back into town (a mountain pass had been closed). We decided to discuss it another time when we both felt better. And we did.

Get an advocate

If you feel intimidated or overwhelmed, it may help to have an advocate at your side during your appointment with the doctor. Even if you feel strong, another person to take notes or listen to explanations can help you keep focused on questions you're asking. If you feel intimidated, an advocate may help equalize the power equation with your doctor.

> We have an elderly client with breast cancer whose doctor (a female surgeon, I might add) treats her like she is senile. The patient is 80 years old and quite disabled, but mentally sharp as a tack. She is, in fact, a highly educated and sophisticated woman. But the surgeon keeps treating her like a child. She was trying to ask questions and discuss treatment options with the physician, and the physician would have none of it. We have spent a lot of time with the patient pointing out that she did have some treatment options, and getting her to speak with physicians within her plan who could fill in the picture with absolutely necessary data. In the end, one of the patient's friends, who happens to be a psychologist, went with her to one of the appointments. All she did is sit in the corner and listen and take notes. However, the physician treated the patient completely differently when someone else was present taking notes.

Send paperwork early

If you need to bolster your position with documentation, fax or deliver it several days before the appointment. You may, for instance, be discussing a difference of opinion on your treatment plan. If you have researched the illness, you probably have recent articles or treatment guidelines to share with the doctor. If he has time to read, think about, and verify the information (perhaps even research rebuttal papers), you will more than likely have a fruitful discussion. It isn't fair to try to discuss articles that the doctor has not had a chance to read. It frustrates him and may be a waste of time for both of you. Or you may just want to discuss how much information you need to feel comfortable, as the following woman does.

> In two weeks I'm going to start chemotherapy for breast cancer, and I'm very frustrated and confused. I don't think my doctor is communicating with me in the way that I need for my emotional well-being.

> I've written him the following note:

> Dr. G. and Staff:

> These are just a few of the questions that have been running through mymind as I sit here trying to plan my life for this next year.

I want to know:

- *What is the current treatment plan for me?*

- *Where will it be administered?*

- *How long will it take?*

- *Will I need someone to drive me home?*

- *To what type of facilities will I have access while being infused?*

- *How should I dress?*

- *Is there anything I could or should bring with me?*

- *What can I expect afterward, i.e., nausea, weakness, etc.?*

- *What precautions will I need to take?*

- *How long and what kind of follow-up can I expect after the initial treatment?*

I am a planner! I am the kind of person who needs to know what is going to happen to me. I feel most comfortable when I know what's coming.

Knowledge is power! I am an intelligent person and know myself better than anyone else. My expectation is that we will be partners in fighting this disease. However, I can't take part in my own life if I'm left out of the planning. I know that there will be unforeseen obstacles. But I will be better prepared to deal with them and better able to be coopera- tive if I start out with some kind of a plan.

I need to feel I'm not alone! I feel as if I'm hanging out here in the wind all by myself without support from your office. I have been given no information at all.

Sincerely,

[my name]

In the above heartfelt yet clear note, the patient tells the doctor and staff what she needs to feel more prepared and comfortable. She explains the type of relationship she hopes will develop, and she asks specific questions. The tone is not accusatory. She's asking for help. Sending a letter such as this ahead of time vastly increases your chances of getting the information you need and preventing a problem from escalating.

Watch your body language

A large amount of what you communicate during a discussion is done non-verbally by body position, eye contact, and distance between you and your doctor. Give some thought to how to use body language to your advantage. For instance, don't try to discuss something important if you are lying down and the doctor is standing at your bedside. If you are confined to a hospital bed, crank up the head and ask the doctor to sit down so you are looking eye-to-eye. Similarly, don't try to talk over something important if you are in an examining room sitting on a table in a short gown. Make arrangements to talk with your clothes on, preferably in the doctor's office. Practice your tone of voice before the meeting. You should strive to sound like a colleague, neither adversarial nor submissive.

State the problem

A clear description of the problem in a nonaccusatory voice sets the stage for resolution. Use concrete terms to describe the problem, and try to limit yourself to one problem per meeting—a long laundry list will create more conflict, not resolve any. In the following case, a businessman states his complaint and offers a solution in terms that made sense to the hospital staff.

> I asked to get my transfusions after 5:30 P.M. so that I could stop losing all of my vacation and sick time. I was spending four hours a day between 9 and 5 at the hospital attached to a bag. Transfusions can remove hours and hours of work time, but it need not be so!

> I pointed out that my insurance was paying close to $250,000 for my bone marrow transplant. In my world of industrial sales a $250,000 customer was treated like a king! I asked that they see me as a customer of that hospital and that their office hours for transfusions were not convenient for this big time customer. I needed to get transfusions after work or lose my job and the big insurance.

> When I put my request in money and customer service terms, they had no valid objections except that it had never been done. I was warm and pleasant at all times, but very insistent that they find a way. They did.

> Here is my point. We should help the medical profession learn good customer service skills. They will never know if we don't speak out.

It also helps to be concise. You might write out or outline what you plan to say, and practice in front of a mirror. When talking to the doctor, make your description of the problem short and to the point. The longer you talk, the more likely it is that you will be interrupted. If you are interrupted, say, "I would like to finish my thought. It will only take another minute or two. Then I'll be very interested in hearing your ideas."

You may be more comfortable writing than talking face-to-face. If this is the case, try to use the same positive tone in your letter. One woman encountered numerous difficulties during her husband's long illness. She explains her approach:

> I've written several truly nasty letters myself. Then I tear them up and write a more polite, brief note detailing the problem. Since I have a vegematic tongue (it slices, it dices...) the nasty notes should never be seen by anyone but myself. But writing them really helps clear out my system.
>
> I also make it a point to write thank-you letters to doctors and health care people who have gone out of their way for John.

Explain how you feel about the problem

One excellent way to prevent more confrontation is to use "I" messages. If you state the problem in terms of how you are feeling, it is less likely to sound blaming and more likely to be heard. For instance, you could say, "When you told me the diagnosis and then turned and walked out of the room, I felt terrified and abandoned. I would have felt much better if you had expressed concern or had held my hand." This kind of description is easier to hear rather than a blaming one like, "You treated me like a lump of meat rather than a person."

Clarify what you would like to see happen

After you describe the problem, consider offering a potential solution. This lifts you out of the "complainer" category and into a partnership attempting to work out a constructive solution. Complaining frequently ends in circular discussions of accusation and response, rather than working toward a solution. Setting a clear goal will more likely result in you getting what you want.

My son was in a burn unit for second and third degree burns. The staff there was a group of dedicated and wonderful people. One of the things that they had to do every day was remove the old skin. They applied softening cream, removed the bandages, sprayed the wounds with water, and scrubbed the area to get the skin off. Sometimes they used tweezers on tough pieces. It was painful, but had to be done. I wanted to be in there with my son, but there was a rule against it. I was nice but persistent. I just kept bugging them. I asked his doctor to write a note giving me permission, then I approached the head nurse and asked for permission. They finally just had me scrub and gown, and in I went every day.

Listen

After you have stated the problem and what you would like to see happen, stop. It is your turn to listen without interrupting. Make eye contact and lean forward to indicate your interest. Avoid body language that indicates a closed mind, such as crossed arms and legs, turning away, or moving about.

Restate what you heard

After the doctor stops talking, restate briefly what you heard. For example, if you told the doctor that you wanted to change blood pressure medications because of unexpected side effects, and he explained several other drugs that you could try, respond, "I hear you say that x, y, and z drugs are all possible replacements. Which would you recommend and why?" If, however, the doctor gives a long reply that says there are no alternatives to treat your problem, you could say, "Are you saying that in your judgment there are no other methods to treat my problem?" Then listen for the answer.

Negotiate

Once you and the doctor have each clearly stated your positions, talk over the options. You have a right to vigorously negotiate for what you want. In *Going for the Cure*, Francesca Thompson, M.D., needed two catheters surgically implanted in her chest, but knew how to clearly state the problem and her wishes:

Chip Moore, my surgeon...comes by to discuss the surgery he will be doing tomorrow, placing the two Hickman catheters, one on each side of my chest. I ask him where the incisions will be, and how big? Less than an inch, about three inches down from the top of the shoulder, in line with the bra strap. It won't be too noticeable. I tell him I don't want the exit on the front of my chest, because I scar very badly, and I don't want to give up v-neck styles. I insist on this...Can you tunnel down to my abdomen? I don't wear two-piece bathing suits. Chip gauges the distance. No, our tunneler isn't that long. But the distance to just below my armpit is about right. And the exit scars will be hidden in my bra line. I sign the consent...[1]

Agree on a plan

Your negotiations should end in agreeing upon a plan of action. Make sure that you are comfortable with the solution.

> We had a problem with the pediatrician's office not calling the specialist's office with the results of my son's blood work. This would result in worry for me and delay in changing his medications. I told the pediatrician's nurse that I knew how busy they were and how I hated having to keep calling them to get the results. I asked if it was possible for them to give the lab authorization to call me with the results. They thought it was a great idea and it worked well. The lab would fax the doctor the results, but call me. I would call the specialist and find out if I needed to change his meds. The specialist would fax the med dose change to the pediatrician's office. It was a win/win situation: the doctor's office wasn't interrupted, they got copies of everything in writing, and I was worry-free.

Agree to disagree

Assertive patients sometimes find that, after a thorough discussion, they simply disagree with their doctor. If you've calmly explained your decision, listened to her side, and still have a different opinion, then it's time to agree to disagree. In rare cases, if your doctor feels that your decision is life-threatening or unconscionable for some other reason, she might remove herself from your case. Usually, however, you will just move on.

> Our pediatrician and I rarely disagree, but when it happens it is resolved in a healthy and graceful way. One instance that comes to mind was over occupational therapy. I thought my child would benefit from a particular type of therapy. The doctor didn't. I brought him in bibliographies of articles from the last two decades. He wasn't impressed. We discussed it and ended up just disagreeing. He didn't feel comfortable writing a referral for a therapy he thought was not helpful, so I didn't ask him to.

I just told him it was refreshing to hear his point of view and I wished I could change his mind. Then we both laughed. I worked with my insurance company and got the therapy covered, and I still have a great relationship with the doctor.

Whatever you decide, try not to leave the office dissatisfied. If you can't reach agreement, tell your doctor what you are going to do. For instance, you may say, "I'll have to think about what you've said and decide what to do later." Or you could say, "I feel that this is an important issue. Could we make another appointment to talk some more?" You could end the discussion by stating the obvious: "I think we're beating a dead horse. We just disagree. I respect your position, and I hope you do mine. Here's what I've decided to do…"

Problems in the hospital

You sometimes don't have time for deliberation when a problem arises in the hospital. Your best bets are to ask a nurse for help, talk to the social worker or chaplain, talk to the hospital's patient advocate, or get a family member to try to resolve the dispute. It's hard to talk tough when you're flat on your back.

I'm an ICU nurse in a teaching hospital. If someone is having trouble in the hospital, I advise them to find a talkative and friendly nurse and ask for advice. There is no better source of information. If I think a resident is in over his head, I try to talk him into calling the attending doctor. If he doesn't, I call the doctor myself. Sometimes the residents get mad, but the patients get the experienced help they need.

If the problem has not been resolved by talking with the doctor, nurse, or social worker, find out about the hospital's process for addressing ethical issues. Hospitals are required by the Joint Commission on Accreditation of Healthcare Organizations to have a method of dealing with ethical problems. Many hospitals, and even some health plans, have ethics committees. How you access this committee varies from hospital to hospital. One doctor describes the system at the teaching hospital where she works.

In our hospital, a patient can pick up the phone, call the hospital operator, and ask to speak to whoever is on call for the ethics committee. We also put a brochure in the admissions material that describes the committee and what it does. It serves anybody—patient, doctor, nurse, social worker. It is a neutral entity. Usually, issues come forward from the patient representative, social worker, nurse, or chaplain. Any issues are addressed, such as organ donation, end-of-life issues (turning off ventilators, hydration, feeding), and balancing economic issues with patient care. Another area is resolving ethnic/religious issues of the patients that are not understood or respected by members of the care team. They basically mediate between people with problems.

Mending fences

If you feel that some damage was done to your relationship in the discussions, you might consider mending fences. This doesn't mean capitulation; rather, it means putting the dispute in context. For instance, if you have had a satisfying and long relationship with your doctor, you might want to write a letter to tell him the things you appreciate about his care. Or you may need to simply clear the air.

> *This summer, I let a backhanded, insensitive comment by one of my son Nicholas's doctors send me into a downward spiral. I then felt myself losing confidence in several of the health professionals caring for Nick— some things justified, others not so justified. It took an almost two-hour meeting with the primary physician to restore my faith in our medical team…it was a difficult meeting, but well worth it. My husband and I prepared a list of items that had been bugging us for months. We asked our questions, listened carefully, jointly made decisions, and then took the opportunity to verbally evaluate the services we'd received at the clinic during the past year. By the way, we didn't simply complain, we recommended solutions and offered assistance. At the end of the meeting, all parties were "singing from the same song sheet again."*

The following are some suggestions for things that help with problem solving in medical situations, and things that tend to make things worse.

Do	Don't
Deal with one problem at a time	Bring in a long list of problems
Speak respectfully	Speak critically
Focus on your goal	Digress
Offer clear information	Challenge what he knows
Ask questions to clarify	Make assumptions
Anticipate disruptions	Allow intimidation or interruptions

Problems that can't be fixed

Some disputes can't be resolved, and some relationships break beyond repair. If you find yourself enmeshed in one of these situations, finding a new doctor may be your best recourse. Chapter 9, *Changing Doctors*, discusses when and how to change doctors.

More serious problems—impaired physicians, serious medical errors, violations of confidentiality—require outside help. For an overview of your options in these situations, refer to Chapter 11, *Taking Action if You Have Been Wronged*.

Whenever I have a disagreement with my doctor, I simply point out, as nicely but firmly as possible, that she is certainly the expert on the clinical aspects of my treatment (diagnosing, assessing risks, evaluating and providing tests and treatment options), but I am the expert on my values. My personal needs and concerns need to be considered in making decisions. Only I can bring these to the equation and speak to them.

I think it is very important that doctors realize the limits of their knowledge just as patients must recognize their own limits. Doctors aren't objective, fully informed people even when they think they are. They bring their own biases to their practice, the limits to their knowledge, and their human ability to make mistakes and misjudgments. I think patients have a responsibility to check up on and watch for the all-too-common failures and mistakes that plague medicine no less than any other area of human knowledge and action.

CHAPTER 8

Getting a Second Opinion

Even when two doctors of equal ability have the opportunity to investigate a patient's complaint and prescribe treatment, their opinions may differ. Medicine is still an art, with vast territories open to legitimate debate and dispute.

—Lewis Miller
The Life You Save

IT'S REASONABLE TO EXPECT DOCTORS to be knowledgeable and caring, but unfair to expect them to be perfect. Doctors are human, and they sometimes make mistakes. Moreover, the amount of medical information is exploding, and there is simply too much for one person to master. Indeed, the best treatment for your illness may even be one of the unknowns—the mysteries—of modern medicine.

Where facts leave off, opinions begin. In these gray areas, experience and judgment are as important as knowledge. Conscientious doctors welcome consultations and encourage second opinions. In fact, many insurance companies require one before they authorize payment for surgery or treatment.

Even if you are devoted to your doctor or fearful about antagonizing him, you owe it to yourself and your family to seek another opinion if there is any question about a diagnosis, proposed treatment, or intervention that may drastically change your life. As William Howard Taft once said, "Trust your mother, but cut the cards." This chapter discusses when to get another viewpoint, how to pick the best doctor to provide it, and how to use the information once you have it.

When you need a second opinion

Doctors usually have several choices for treating various illnesses. The doctor's recommendation may be based on what he thinks is best for you, or it might be mandated by your insurance because it is cheaper. You need to know all of the options and discuss them freely with your doctor before you agree to medical treatment. Unfortunately, your doctor may not share this vital information with you if he is rushed, is pressured by his employer to keep costs down, or feels that it is his job to make decisions for you.

If, at any time, you are uneasy about any part of your care, you should not hesitate to get another opinion. The Principles of Medical Ethics of the American Medical Association clearly support seeking additional opinions: "A physician shall...obtain consultation, and use the talents of other health professionals when indicated."[1]

You should not worry about hurting your doctor's feelings. Especially for complex cases, most doctors welcome confirmation of their diagnoses. And most, if they truly care for their patients, prefer to hear if they are wrong before misdiagnosis causes possible harm. Often, it is not a matter of correct or incorrect diagnosis; rather, it may be an honest difference of opinion on the diagnosis and/or treatment by two competent doctors based on identical facts. In these cases, you should learn all you can about the background and reasoning of each doctor, and make the final treatment decisions yourself.

Following are seven specific situations in which it would be wise to get another medical opinion.

If your primary care physician suggests one

If your primary care doctor suggests that you see a specialist to help diagnose or devise an appropriate treatment plan, go get the second opinion. Competent primary care doctors know when expert advice is needed. Your doctor will probably recommend a physician, and may even make the appointment for you.

> When my seven-year-old daughter began to show signs of premature puberty, I brought her to our pediatrician. He said that we could wait and watch, or we could go to a pediatric endocrinologist in a large city quite a distance away. I asked what he thought would be the most prudent course of action, and he said, "If she were my daughter, I'd go and have it checked out by the expert." We took his advice.

If your insurance company requires one

Insurance companies are in business to make profits. Many now require a second opinion prior to any but emergency surgery. Their cost analysis shows that the small cost of the second opinion is offset by the savings from preventing unnecessary surgeries. If your insurance company requires one, go get it, from the best specialist you can find.

If surgery or a major procedure has been recommended

Standards for determining when surgery is necessary fluctuate from region to region, from hospital to hospital, and from doctor to doctor. Controversies over medical and surgical treatments rage in medical journals and in doctors' offices across the land. However, when a doctor's opinion is given to the patient, it often is presented as compulsory, not optional. Unless you are in imminent danger of dying—in an emergency room with a life-threatening illness or injury—don't be swayed by a doctor pressuring you to "get this done immediately."

Any surgery not necessary to preserve life or function is called "elective." Cosmetic surgery is elective, but so is gall bladder surgery, open heart surgery, and most other surgeries. Whether elective surgery is necessary is a matter of opinion, and opinions sometimes vary wildly. For example, the rate of tonsillectomies is going down, but the number of cesarean sections is at an all-time high. As you can see from the following study, doctors frequently disagree.

Results of a mandatory second-opinion program

In Massachusetts, more than 2,500 Medicaid patients were referred for second opinions prior to elective surgery. Of these, 14.5 percent of the doctors giving second opinions disagreed with the first physician's view that surgery was necessary. About a quarter of the second opinions for hysterectomies, knee operations, and back operations deemed the surgery unnecessary. Patient decisions on whether to have the surgery were greatly affected by the second opinion: 85.5 percent of those patients whose second opinion confirmed the first agreed to the surgery, whereas only 31 percent of the patients whose doctors disagreed were operated on. In the year after the program was implemented, there was a 20 percent reduction in Medicaid surgeries.[2]

It is always a good idea to get a second opinion prior to elective surgery or an invasive procedure because only you can make the ultimate decision on whether the potential benefits outweigh the risks and costs (see Chapter 10, *Questions to Ask About Tests, Drugs, and Surgery*).

I had a cardiac stress test during a routine physical. My doctor was concerned about the blood flow in my heart, so he scheduled a arteriogram. This showed narrowing in two of my coronary arteries. However, I

had never had any pain or other symptoms from this problem. He sched-
uled an angioplasty (a procedure where they put a catheter with a
balloon tip into the coronary arteries to enlarge the vessels) without even
discussing the pros and cons with me. I went for a second opinion because
I was uncomfortable taking those risks when I didn't even have any
symptoms.

Don't stop at just getting a surgical second opinion. Doctors also base their suggestions on results from X rays, blood work, and pathology (microscopic examination of tissues). If a major intervention is proposed, take the slides to an independent pathologist for a second opinion. Get a second reading of the X rays by a different radiologist, and have the blood work repeated (lab errors are common). For instance, of 535 men referred to Johns Hopkins Hospital for removal of a cancerous prostate, seven were found not to have cancer at all after a review of their biopsy results by another pathologist.[3] While this is a low percentage of errors (1.3 percent), for the seven men who were spared the risks of major surgery, as well as possible lifelong impotence and incontinence, it was a second opinion well worth having.

Jody Heymann, M.D., described her operation for a brain tumor and the aftermath in her book *Equal Partners*. Three days after the traumatic ten-hour surgery, her surgeon admitted that they had operated on the wrong part of her brain because they did not repeat the MRI done at another hospital. He explained that the MRI was done from a different angle than he expected, and the tumor could not be reached from the part of her skull that was removed. He wanted to operate again to remove the tumor. Not surprisingly, she went to another doctor for a second opinion.

If diagnosis is uncertain

Some doctors find it hard to say, "I don't know." If you sense that your doctor is stumped, or if there seems to be no clear reason for the suggested treatment plan, get a second opinion. It may uncover a totally unexpected problem or it may be identical to your first doctor's opinion. Either way, you will have more information on which to base a decision than you did before the second opinion.

I had been taking Stephanie to our pediatrician for a cough that
would not go away. She had the cough on and off for months and kept
running fevers for no reason. She also developed bruises on her legs and
complained that her legs hurt. But I did not think of saying anything to

him about that because the most severe thing was the cough. The week before she was diagnosed, he saw Stephanie (for the fourth or fifth time) and it was the day he was leaving on vacation. He told me that he heard a heart murmur and she was wheezing. He diagnosed her as having a childhood heart murmur and severe asthma. I thought that the diagnosis was dead wrong, so I told his associate that I wanted her to see a cardiologist. The cardiologist found a massive tumor in her chest that was crushing her aorta and trachea.

If symptoms persist after a reasonable length of time on treatment

Whether a disease or injury is acute or chronic, a proper diagnosis and appropriate treatment should alleviate some of the symptoms. Even in diseases that are not well understood and are notoriously hard to treat—such as lupus and rheumatoid arthritis—there are therapies that can provide noticeable relief, although not a cure. If a few months have gone by and you do not feel better, you should talk to the doctor about alternative approaches. If he seems unsure of the diagnosis, or unwilling to discuss other methods of treatment, it's probably time to seek a second opinion.

Soon after birth my son started having problems with chronic ear infections, a persistent groin rash, and scalp rash. His pediatrician treated him with multiple antibiotics and topical steroids without success. The problem would get worse, subside, then reappear. After about six months, we went to a different pediatrician for a second opinion. His only suggestion was stronger steroids and antibiotics. We went to an ear/nose/ throat specialist who recommended tubes in his ears—they didn't help. We took him to an older, experienced pediatrician, who said it could be histiocytosis (a rare immune system disorder) and he ordered a skin biopsy. It came back negative.

Our son continued to deteriorate. We also saw a Chinese herbalist and several naturopathic doctors, but unfortunately, they were as baffled by the root cause as everyone else. They did provide invaluable health support for his ear and skin infections. We then tried an allergist—who put him on several different diets without success. The dermatologist had nothing to offer other than the steroid creams. We took him to the dermatology clinic at the large regional children's hospital. They brought in an entire team and we walked away with 10 prescriptions for antibiotics and steroids. Nothing helped, and he continued to get worse. We thought that each doctor was seeing only one piece of our son, not the whole. We were desperate. Finally, when he was almost two years old, they did another skin biopsy, and it showed histiocytosis. They went back and found the one from a year and a half before, and discovered that it had shown the disease but had been misread. He was put on chemotherapy, had radiation, and is now a healthy 11 year old.

As parents, you have a huge responsibility as advocates and caregivers to your child. Our advice is to find a doctor you are comfortable working with. Ask questions until you understand what the doctor is recommending and trust your heart—it's a reliable barometer.

When deciding on treatment for a life-threatening or disabling illness

You have nothing to lose, and your life to gain, if you seek another opinion after a diagnosis of a potentially fatal or disabling disease. Doctors are not infallible, and there is always the chance that the diagnosis is wrong. In addition, the doctor who diagnosed you may not be aware of the newest or most effective therapy for your type and stage of disease. You will always learn something from a second opinion: a deeper understanding of the illness or, perhaps, a better grasp of the treatments available. Or you may be reassured that the original doctor's diagnosis is correct and the suggested treatment is state-of-the-art. Trusting that you are getting the best that medicine has to offer is, after all, an important part of healing.

When I was diagnosed with cancer, it was a relatively high priority for me to be treated locally. I was a single parent with two teenagers, one of them acting out in anger and one of them hovering around me. I was under stress and I did most of my own caretaking.

The idea of looking for experts and driving around for consultations did not appeal to me at all. However, I felt I owed it to myself to search out a second opinion before making a decision on my chemotherapy treatment after surgery. My own oncologist (who said that if he had cancer, he'd get several second opinions) gave me the name of a doctor at the University of California at San Francisco and arranged the consult.

This specialist (who is widely respected in northern California) basically told me that I had "garden variety" breast cancer and either the treatment my oncologist had recommended or another common regime was the best treatment for my diagnosis. Even though he didn't tell me to do anything different, it was very reassuring to me. He respected my doctor and knew he had worked with clinical trials at the National Institutes of Health. I ended up being much more sure that I was making a rational choice, with very little extra effort.

And I could satisfy myself—and those well-meaning advice-givers that every cancer patient runs into—by saying that yes, my doctor knew what he was talking about.

• • • • •

I went to my family doctor for a physical. I mentioned some swelling that didn't hurt. He decided to meet with an oncologist who reviewed my biopsy slides and two bone marrow biopsies. This oncologist's premature conclusion was that I had high grade lymphoma and needed to start chemotherapy immediately and plan on having a bone marrow transplant. After the shock and accepting the diagnosis, I was preparing myself for the catheter surgery and the treatment to follow. While at the radiology department getting tests, I asked myself why I needed such treatment at a time when I felt so good.

I called my family doctor again to get his opinion and to ask for a referral for a second opinion by a different oncologist. After reviewing the information available, we agreed to postpone immediate treatment and schedule a second opinion.

The second opinion doctor reviewed all of the same information and suggested that I monitor my blood and other vitals for a period of time to track the progress of the disease (marginal zone lymphoma). He explained all of the information to my satisfaction (something doctor #1 wouldn't do) and encouraged me to look at my whole lifestyle to determine the best healing approach. He did say that I may need some treatment in the future, but there is no reason to start now when I feel great and the disease is apparently idle.

Between this second oncologist and my family doctor, I have learned a valuable lesson about taking my health into my own hands. I have to make the decisions—the doctors are just resources with experience to help provide me options.

Whenever you are uncomfortable with how your care is being managed

You need to have confidence in the doctor to get the maximum benefit from your treatment. If your pediatrician says your baby has a heart murmur but it's nothing to worry about, ask him why you shouldn't worry. If your asthma is not responding well to treatment and your doctor says there is nothing else that can be done, ask more questions. If you are not reassured by the answers, get a second opinion.

Once my mom started treatment, she started having very high blood pressure after the chemotherapy. She was worried, and we were terrified. What we couldn't understand is why this doctor and his staff weren't even checking my mom's blood pressure before and after treatment, particularly after the problem of dangerously high blood pressure occurred after the first treatment. She had to ask them to do it! I flew out to see them, and we arranged for her to get a second opinion with the university medical oncology department. The doctor and his nurse together spent about two and a half hours with us, answering all those pent-up questions that my parents, my sister, and I all had. Afterwards, my mother decided to switch to the university's program and she is very glad that we suggested that she look around for more information.

• • • • •

I am in my early forties and have problems with extremely heavy menstrual flow and severe cramps. It really impacts my life. My OB/GYN told me that I was premenopausal and there was nothing that could be done. I was not comfortable with that diagnosis, so I asked around among my female professional colleagues and got the names of several gynecologists with good reputations.

At the start of the first appointment with the new doctor, I pulled out a list and said, "I hope you don't mind, but I have a list of concerns and questions." She said that it was wonderful that I was prepared and she often suggested to her patients that they do that very thing. When I explained my symptoms and after she had examined me, she said, "I hate to second-guess another doctor, but your symptoms are just the opposite of a woman entering menopause." She went on to outline a several-step process. The first steps were all lifestyle changes. She wants me to make some diet changes, exercise daily, and take calcium for three months. If I am not feeling better, then we move on to step two. I finally feel like someone is paying attention and cares. I also like trying to change my lifestyle to relieve the symptoms, rather than just start taking medicine for it.

You need to trust your intuition. If you feel uncomfortable with the treatment proposed, or just sense that something is not quite right, get a second opinion to gather more information. Even if you only find out that the proposed treatment is the standard of care for your condition, the second opinion will ease your mind and increase your trust. On the other hand, your intuition may be sending loud signals because something is truly wrong, as the following college student found out:

A friend of mine once told me: "Mike, if an allergist ever tells you, 'You're cured,' walk in the other direction and take your wallet with you."

About fifteen years ago I got to test his advice after being told that my adolescent acne condition may have been the result of a food allergy. I still remember his name: Dr. Z. He was very well respected in his field, from what I heard.

He gave me two tests. In one, they make numerous tiny pin pricks on your arm and apply a small drop of solution onto each to see if various substances caused a rash on contact. The next test was just plain silly. I was supposed to sit alone in a room, be still, relax, breathe evenly and concentrate, drink a small cup of liquid solution, wait, try to sense whether I felt anything different as a result (like a hot flash or a nervous feeling), wait a few minutes, then go on to the next cup of liquid—all this repeated for over two hours. Well, of course after not very long I started to go into sensory deprivation out of sheer boredom. None of the liquids made me feel any different as far as I could tell, and toward the end I even started to imagine I felt different because I wanted to have something to report. Frankly, I was hallucinating.

After all that, he said that based on the tests, his conclusion was that I was allergic to milk, beef, and cocoa. He would write up a note so that I could present it as a special dietary request to my college food service. He said, "As far as I'm concerned, YOU'RE CURED." He sent me on my way.

Bells should have gone off in my head, but I endured an entire semester eating stuff like tofu pasta sauce and supplementing my protein needs with salad-bar chickpeas. What did I do when there was no change in my condition? I cut more things out of my diet, including nuts and all animal products. Nothing changed while I was on these diets, or off them for that matter. Eventually my skin problem receded dramatically, at the same point in my life that it receded for my dad, who after all gave it to me.

How to get a second opinion

Seeking a second opinion should not be done in secret. Going behind your doctor's back can create antagonism and undermine your relationship. It also prevents the specialist giving the second opinion from having access to relevant medical records and test results from your current doctor. If your physician suggested the consultation, you have no problem. If, on the other hand, you initiate the request, you could receive a variety of responses. To present the request in the best light, and to minimize potential for resistance from your doctor, try one of the following approaches:

- **Give advance warning.** "You know, Dr. J., I think you have given me wonderful care for years, and I both like and respect you. But I am concerned about my increasing chest pain and our plan for treating it. I think I'd feel reassured if I saw a cardiologist to get his view on my options."

- **Be honest.** If you use "I" statements such as "I feel" or "I hope" or "I think," it is less likely to create conflict. For instance, you might say, "I understand that you think surgery is the next step to take in treating this illness, and I have great respect for your opinion, but I just feel that it isn't the time for that yet. Perhaps if I talked to another doctor, I'd gain a bit more perspective on my options."

- **Ask questions.** To find out if there are different approaches to your problem, you could say, "I really respect your opinion on this matter. Do you think other doctors would all agree that this treatment is the only one for my condition? Or are there different approaches that are considered state-of-the-art? Talking to another doctor with a different viewpoint might help me sort out my options."

- **Invoke your family.** You might say, "I value your thoughts on this, but I think I owe it to myself and my family to get another opinion before proceeding. I never make decisions without considering all of my options."

Any negotiation is more likely to succeed if praise is included. Notice in each of the above examples, praise is given to minimize the chance of the doctor responding poorly. After all, you probably want to return for further care, or you would have simply changed doctors. Diplomacy acts as a lubricant in all relationships, including medical ones.

If your doctor resists your suggestion for a second opinion, consider changing. Any doctor worth his salt should be willing to have his judgment reviewed. You also have a right to a second opinion, and that right should be respected by your caregivers. Conscientious doctors like to have their opinions confirmed, or their mistakes uncovered, before any harm results. Second opinions help you make better, more informed decisions. One doctor, when asked why some doctors discourage their patients from getting a second opinion, stated succinctly, "Ego and money."

Our son was born with a birth defect called hypospadias. This meant that the opening through which urine passes was not located at the tip of the penis, but on the shaft. When my infant urinated, he sprayed urine out; it did not come out in a straight stream. Had he been an older boy standing at the toilet, he would have urinated on his shoes.

I asked our pediatrician for a referral to a good urologist and was sent to someone he trusted. Everyone in the urologist's waiting room was quite elderly. We asked and were told that a couple of hypospadias repairs were done here yearly. After examining our son, the urologist said there was nothing he or anyone else could do to fix this problem without seriously jeopardizing my son's urinary tract. He also said there was a fifty percent chance our son would need additional surgeries due to scar tissue build-up.

I went back to our pediatrician and asked for a referral to the regional children's hospital for a second opinion. This request was met with great resistance and assurances that the local urologist was an expert, that managed care wouldn't pay for the surgery out of our designated area, etc.

We took our son to the children's hospital. The doctor walked in, examined our baby, and said, "Oh, quite a mild case." I asked what the chance of a second operation was. "Maybe a three percent chance that we'll need to go back to remove scar tissue." We then asked how many times he had performed this operation. "About five or six times a week." The moral of our tale: go to someone with lots of experience. Our son is doing great!

Once you've informed your current doctor, you must find the best consultant possible. Go to a doctor independent from the first—preferably at a different institution—rather than someone recommended by your primary doctor. Doctors often trade referrals and are loathe to criticize someone they may know socially and on whom they depend for referrals (hence income). Your primary doctor is also most likely to send you to someone who shares her philosophy. So, where do you go?

- Call a national organization for your illness or condition, if one exists. Refer to Appendix C for the numbers for dozens of such organizations. For cancer, call 1-800-4-CANCER. For rare diseases, call 1-800-999-6673. Ask whomever answers the phone to send you literature on the organization and any available lists of physicians who specialize in the disease. Call members of the scientific advisory committee listed on the organization's literature. Briefly tell them that you are searching for a second opinion from a physician skilled in treating your illness. Often, these specialists obtain information on your prior history and all lab results from your physician, and may consult either on the phone or in person.

- Ask other doctors or professionals (nurses, dentists) whom you know personally for recommendations. Also, ask the local medical society for two or three names of physicians who specialize in your area of concern. If you assemble several short lists, the best doctors' names will tend to appear often.

- Call the nearest medical school and ask if anyone on the staff specializes in your condition or if they could recommend two reputable physicians in the field.

- Use the information in Chapter 13, *Researching the Medical Literature*, to locate and read the current research on your condition. Call one or more of the authors of the journal articles to ask for the name of a clinician specializing in your illness.

- Go to the Internet site for Mediconsult at *http://www.mediconsult.com/home/service/* to get a second opinion for specific conditions from experts.

Remember that physicians who share the same specialty generally share the same biases for their treatment; surgeons most often recommend surgery, and internists generally try medication as a first step. If surgery has been recommended, get a second opinion from a different type of doctor. If an orthopedic surgeon recommended a knee replacement, see a rheumatologist—a specialist in joints. If heart surgery has been recommended, see a cardiologist. At the very least you will get a different viewpoint, which will add to your understanding of the choices.

After you have chosen the physician and made an appointment, arrange to have your records sent ahead, or pick them up and hand-carry them to your appointment. Ask ahead of time if test and blood results will suffice, or if the new doctor is going to require some or all of the tests to be redone. Also, ask about fees and check to see if your insurance will cover the charges.

Make sure to bring a written list of any questions that you wish to ask during your appointment. The second opinion should include a thorough record review, physical examination, and discussion. Have the doctor explain, in detail, his findings and opinions, and ask to have the report (and any additional test results) sent to your primary care doctor, and a copy sent to you.

How to best use the information gained

If the second opinion differs from the original, ask both doctors to explain how they arrived at their conclusions. Inquire about the scientific studies on which their recommendations were based, what test results they looked at, and their reasoning. You will learn a lot from these discussions. It may be that one doctor is more current than the other. For instance, if you have migraine headaches and one doctor shows you recent guidelines from the American Academy of Neurology that outline the newest and most effective treatments, that's compelling evidence. On the other hand, there may be no best treatment, and the two doctors may recommend different but equally effective treatments. Or the doctors may simply disagree over whether you need a surgical procedure, for example, a hysterectomy, and explain by citing their own training.

An important point to keep in mind is that doctors tend to feel uncomfortable criticizing their colleagues. Jody Heymann, M.D., describes this tendency in her book *Equal Partners*:

> *Tim and I called Dr. Manson for another opinion...Was the fact that the surgeons missed the tumor the first time so unreasonable that we should not go back to the same group?...There are, in general, two approaches doctors take to this type of question. There are doctors who will never comment on another physician's work to the physician's*

patients. Then there are doctors who give their honest opinion to patients because they recognize it is important to the patient's future care for them to know the truth. We realized that only a minority of physicians would break the unspoken but binding vows of loyalty to other physicians..., but we hoped we would be able to learn the truth as members of the brethren ourselves.[4]

To avoid problems of this sort, make sure to tell the doctor that you are not interested in a critique of the other doctor, but merely an unbiased second opinion. For example, if the second doctor indicates any reservations about the proposed treatment, such as, "It's unusual to..." or "Some doctors don't consider that the first treatment of choice," make sure to press for more detailed information. Ask for a diagnosis, alternative treatments, the risks and benefits of each, and his recommendation.

> On Friday I got a second opinion for what to do about my gall bladder cancer. I saw a doctor who is a chief of gastrointestinal oncology and a professor at the medical school. I went in with my list of questions and we talked for a long time. The main issue is whether I should have radiation and chemotherapy. He said—and this phrase really sticks in my mind—"If you get five oncologists together to consider your case, you'll get six different opinions." Basically, he thinks it comes down to philosophy. Radiation and chemotherapy don't have a good track record against gall bladder cancer. It's unclear whether they help at all. An aggressive oncologist who wants to try anything that might work would recommend doing treatment. An oncologist more concerned about the detrimental effects treatment can have would recommend against it. He added that he prefers to undertreat rather than overtreat, and so recommends against the radiation and chemotherapy, but can well see how a different doctor would reach a different conclusion. I feel like I'm at a crossroads in the woods, and I don't know which way to turn.

Once you have all of this information, go back to your primary doctor and discuss it. If the opinions differ, a third opinion may be necessary. Many insurance companies pay for third opinions in cases like these. If you feel yourself leaning strongly toward a specific treatment, choose that one.

> When my daughter was first diagnosed with bone cancer and I was still in shock, family connections brought me phone calls from the chief attending physicians at a very highly regarded cancer institution in another state. They wanted to see my daughter and have her treated at their hospital. As I probed for additional information, I discovered that

they were not in favor of or performing the limb salvage surgery which the local surgical specialist said was the recommended treatment. The Boston hospital tried to convince me that I was making a terrible mistake using an Ohio doctor (said with much disdain), but I did not have the energy to travel so far from home and felt comfortable with my decision, especially after researching the medical literature.

Remember that just because opinions differ, it doesn't necessarily mean that one is right and one is wrong. Experts disagree because medicine is an art as well as a science and because definitive information covering all aspects of the situation is sometimes simply not available. For example, it could be reasonable and effective to treat a condition with surgery or with drugs, or even with two different surgical techniques. Or the best treatment may simply not be known. Ultimately, you must gather the information, talk it over with your doctor, and decide.

I'd probably be dead if I hadn't received a fifth opinion for my multiple myeloma (a type of cancer). At the age of 37, I fractured my back. My orthopedist treated the fracture, but never asked the important question, "Why does a healthy young woman with no history of trauma have a broken back?" I went to get another opinion, and this doctor noticed multiple cancerous lesions on my X rays, which had been overlooked by the orthopedist. This doctor told me that I had cancer, but it was 85 percent curable. (This is not, in fact, the case. There has never been a documented cure, although more of us are living for many years after the diagnosis.) He wanted me to have a bone marrow transplant (BMT) immediately. He didn't give me much information or discuss options, so I went to get a third opinion. This oncologist wanted me to start on chemotherapy right away. I declined.

A friend did research for me at the medical school library, and for the first time, I began asking questions. The current doctor wouldn't answer questions, and repeatedly told me that I was going to die if I didn't start chemotherapy immediately. I went to a major cancer center for yet another opinion, and they recommended that I have more tests to pin down the type and stage of my cancer before deciding on treatments. We did this. After reviewing the results, they recommended that I not have a BMT or take chemotherapy, but instead do nothing unless the cancer advanced. Meanwhile, I continued learning about my disease, and contacted an international expert across the country. He has been my telephone consultant since, and together we make all of my treatment decisions. Through a combination of selected chemotherapy, nutrition, acupuncture, physical therapy, and herbs, I have had a good quality of life for almost five years. All due to persistence, and that fifth opinion.

CHAPTER 9

Changing Doctors

We do not know our own souls, let alone the souls of others.
Human beings do not go hand in hand each stretch of the way.

—Virginia Woolf

DOCTORS AND PATIENTS SHARE A UNIQUE INTIMACY that is quite different from other professional-client relationships. Your doctor is entrusted with personal information about your body, health, and lifestyle that requires delicacy and confidentiality. If you have a healthy partnership, you are more likely to follow her recommendations, feel confident about your treatment, and, perhaps, heal faster. If that trust is irreparably broken, changing doctors may be necessary.

You have probably put time and effort into establishing a relationship with your doctor and may dread starting all over. While changing doctors is disruptive, it can be a great relief if the relationship has deteriorated beyond repair. If you have used the information in the chapters on communication and problem solving without resolution of the problems, the time has come to seek another caregiver.

This chapter helps you identify the reasons why it may be necessary to terminate a medical relationship, and looks at some reasons why you may not wish to do so. It shows you how to notify the doctor you are leaving and how to make a smooth transition to the new doctor's practice. Many patients share deeply personal stories about why, when, and how they changed doctors.

Reasons not to change

Changing doctors, especially during serious illness, is a disruptive and upsetting business. It entails shopping for a new doctor, worrying about the old doctor's feelings, filling out forms to transfer records, and making sure that there is no lapse in care. For these reasons, if the situation is salvageable, try using the techniques in Chapter 7, *Problem Solving*.

The following sections contain some examples of situations that can be salvaged.

Misunderstandings

Life is full of misunderstandings. During a brief doctor's visit, when fatigue, worry, or illness (the patient's or the doctor's) clouds understanding, confusion can grow. A few questions or a follow-up phone call can sometimes resolve the problem.

> *I had a very stormy time with my son's doctor when I asked to read the protocol (document that explains in detail a clinical trial). Dr. L. had seen me talking to parents of another ill child. I had known this couple for 10 years and our children were in school together. The father was a physician.*
>
> *Dr. L. refused to let me read the protocol. In fact, he was so upset he wrote me a three-page letter saying that the other parent/doctor was trying to interfere with his treatment of my son. He wrote of the many years that he had devoted to medical school and the financial sacrifices he had made to do research on childhood cancer. He insisted that I trust his knowledge and treatment plan. It was a very angry letter. He basically said that he wanted exclusive rights to advising me about my son's medical care.*
>
> *I wrote a letter back explaining that I was talking to the other doctor as a parent, not a doctor. I was not going behind Dr. L.'s back. I pointed out that Dr. L. had already arranged several consults for us, and if I had a problem or needed another opinion I would ask him about it as I had in the past.*
>
> *Then we had several phone calls trying to resolve the matter. He ended up giving me the protocol to read in the hospital and told me that I was not allowed to photocopy it or take it out of the hospital. He added that he wanted to have a conference with me after I finished reading it.*
>
> *When we had the conference, I asked several questions and explained to him how much better I felt now that I understood the evolution of the research on the drugs being used. It was a comfort to read it. He told me that he was surprised that I had understood so much and was amazed that I found comfort in it. I think it changed his mind a bit on how parents use knowledge.*

Unrealistic expectations

Evaluate your expectations before changing doctors. What is reasonable to expect from a doctor is warmth, expertise, ability to listen, willingness to answer questions, awareness of limitations, and willingness to consult with other experts. Patients should not expect house calls, nonemergency after-hours calls or appointments, free care, lengthy visits dealing with nonmedical issues, or miracles.

> *Most people don't recognize how often their expectations exceed what the doctor can do. Take acute back pain. There are very few serious problems that cause acute back pain in young people (under fifty). We usually don't know what the hell causes it. X rays are useless for non-traumatic back pain. Yes, you can move on to incredibly expensive modalities like CT scans and MRIs, which might give you an answer, but they will not affect treatment for the short term. We say, "It could be a disk problem or a pulled muscle." They say, "Well, what is it? I want to know." I try to educate them and explain that the initial, short-term treatment is the same, regardless of the cause. They need to rest a couple of days, get postural advice, and take anti-inflammatories. And wait. But most people want a quick fix. Unless you're getting numbness, tingling, bowel and bladder changes, or fever, that's all you should do for the first couple of weeks. It's very frustrating for everybody: they want something done, and they want answers and we don't have them.*

Isolated human error

Doctors are human and make mistakes. Often the mistakes are caught by nurses, technicians, or the patient himself. Sometimes, they slip through and cause physical or emotional distress, or, in rare cases, injury or death. If there is a clear pattern of sloppiness or errors, change doctors. If, on the other hand, your doctor makes one mistake, think about the error in the context of your entire relationship and see how you feel. You may be holding him up to a standard that no mere mortal can meet.

> *When my son was very ill, the doctor sent medication home to give for the next several days. I checked the dosage and they had made a math error, giving me ten times the correct dose (they moved the decimal point one place over). I called and told them and they were horrified. Both the nurse and doctor apologized, and the nurse left the office to*

*drive to the house with replacement medications. She apologized again. I
told her that it was OK, they were only human. I was just glad that I had
checked.*

Reasons to change

Few healthy adults change doctors. If you only see your doctor once a year
for a checkup or a minor ailment, differences in philosophy have little
impact, and a lack of warmth is easier to overlook. However, living with a
serious or chronic illness can be one of life's great struggles. If you have a
physician whom you trust, can rely on for state-of-the-art medical treatment, and can count on for advice and support, the struggle is greatly eased.
If, on the other hand, your doctor adds to your discomfort rather than
reducing it, change.

The following sections contain stories from many patients who explain how
they made the difficult decision to change doctors.

Scheduling problems

If the doctor has office hours that make it difficult for you to get to appointments, you may wish to change to someone with business hours more
aligned with your schedule. Changing doctors for this reason is relatively
stress-free. After you have located a new doctor (see Chapter 2, *Finding the
Right Doctor*), simply tell your old doctor the reason for the change and sign
the necessary form to have your records sent to the new practice.

In other cases, the conflict arises not from office hours, but rather the doctor's requirement for frequent checkups that create time and expense problems.

> *My doctor gave me a prescription for migraine headache medication.
> She would only give me a month's worth, and required me to come
> monthly to the office for a checkup. I had to take off work, drive a half
> hour, wait in her office for a half hour or more, then have a cursory exam
> in which my blood pressure was taken and I was asked if I was having
> any problems. I explained to her when I received the prescription that I
> worked at a large government facility that had a clinic with a nurse
> available every day. I told her it would be much more convenient if I had
> my BP taken there. She refused and insisted that I keep traipsing down to
> her office. I resented it.*

I asked to be seen by her partner (who had been the person that I was initially referred to, but I ended up with his partner because his schedule was full). He gave me a three-month prescription (which he refills when I call his office), and told me to call anytime I had a side effect or any questions. He was very nice and I still go to him.

Not the best person for your illness

Some patients simply do not receive state-of-the-art care from their current physician. Consider the following story, in which a man with several different medical problems was overwhelmed with unpleasant side effects from numerous medications. A change to a group with a different perspective and a willingness to eliminate some medicines made life much brighter.

In the last year I shifted all of my medical (even dental) care to Johns Hopkins, and using the same procedures, same medicines, and same protocols, the difference in my medical care and health is like the difference between night and day.

The medical insights are superior, the invasiveness is now far less frequent, and the far greater openness, honesty, and frankness are refreshing. I now take a minimum of medication for my colon and cardiovascular conditions. I have lost 35 pounds in the past year (good), I am no longer wrapped in a "dulled sensorium" (beta blockers), I am no longer protected from reacting to adrenaline flows (calcium channel blockers), I am now completely weaned from systemic cortisone (bad for my heart and other long-term negatives).

I'm much healthier—with far less intervention! My IBD (irritable bowel disease) hasn't been this well-behaved in 20 years!

You'd almost think I was now getting medical care in a different country, if not on a different planet, yet the other doctors are no more than ten miles away!

If you have a good relationship with your primary care physician (general practitioner or family practice doctor) but you require specialized care, consider keeping your primary care doctor as your medical quarterback—the person with the big picture of your health care. Presumably, your doctor referred you to the specialist in the first place and has received reports back on your progress. If you have developed a chronic illness requiring frequent visits to the specialist, however, you might decide to use the specialist as your primary physician.

When our daughter was diagnosed with cancer, we were fairly new to the area. Our pediatrician was nice, but we had only seen him a few times. Since treatment for the cancer would be lengthy (over two years), and travel distance was the same, we decided to just use the oncologist as our primary doctor. That way there would be no need to communicate with different offices that would just add to our stress. It worked out fine. Now that she's finished with her treatment, we go to the pediatrician again, and there have been no hard feelings.

In this case, simply tell your primary care doctor that you think it makes more sense to use the specialist as your primary doctor due to the frequency of your appointments.

Loss of trust

Confidentiality is the cornerstone of patient care. Except for legally defined exclusions (such as child abuse, which has to be reported to authorities) what you say to your doctor should go no farther. If the doctor violates your trust, and word is spread about an illness or injury that you expected to be kept secret, the results could be minor (embarrassment) to catastrophic (loss of job when your employer learns you have AIDS). A breach of doctor-patient confidentiality that causes damages to you is grounds for taking action. (See Chapter 11, *Taking Action if You Have Been Wronged.*) If the only damage that occurs is to your trust, change doctors.

I had severe back pain that went down my leg. I could barely walk and had to hire someone to care for my horse for me. My internist diagnosed a bruised tailbone and a pulled muscle. He wanted me to take muscle relaxers, but I told him they made me nauseous. He told me to do whatever I normally did for exercise, which was walking every day. The pain steadily increased and I would cry as I walked. I kept going back to the doctor and he would say that I wasn't "meeting him halfway" because I wouldn't take muscle relaxers. I ended up in bed, sobbing with pain. I had an electrical throbbing sensation down my leg. It felt like my leg was pulsing with electricity. If I stood up, it would feel prickly, then go numb. I called the doctor's office in tears, said I was in terrible pain and asked to speak to the nurse. The receptionist told me she was too busy to talk to me. I told her I was going to the emergency room. The receptionist replied, "If you had taken the muscle relaxers like the doctor told you to last month, you wouldn't be in this situation right now." Not only did the doctor or nurse violate my confidence, but I had the doctor, nurse, and receptionist all blaming me for my own pain. It turned out I had a ruptured disk.

Serious errors made

Mistakes are more common than you might think. A Harvard study estimated that more than 80,000 deaths are caused each year by medical mistakes.[1] If a serious error has happened during your medical care, your confidence and trust—both crucial components in healing—may have been undermined. Some patients forgive, hoping it will never happen again, while others change to someone whose expertise they trust.

When I was first diagnosed with diabetes (I was 43) the doctor prescribed oral medication. I was with an HMO then (no more!) and hadn't really needed a doctor before, so it was the first time I saw him. Looking back with what I now know about the disease, he gave me precious little information. He was nice enough, but said nothing about scheduling me for any kind of educational follow-up.

The day after I started taking the medication, I became violently ill. When I called to say I needed to speak to my doctor, the nurse could tell I was in trouble and advised me to come to the emergency room right away, offering to send an ambulance if there wasn't anyone who could bring me.

After I was properly hooked up to an insulin IV, I overheard the emergency room doctor talking to another doctor. He was furious that my doctor had prescribed oral medication instead of putting me on insulin. He said that he should have known from my tests that oral meds would not be appropriate. Later, when I was out of danger, one of the nurses told me I could have died if I hadn't come in when I did.

I stayed in the intensive care unit for about 24 hours. The nurses were extremely kind to me—supportive, helpful, and patient. I was then transferred to a regular room for another couple of days. I was given lots of information, visited several times by a diabetic advisor, saw a dietitian—the works.

I don't expect every doctor to know everything about every condition, but I do expect them to be conscientious about their lack of knowledge/ experience in an area, and to take the time to consult with a more knowledgeable colleague before deciding on a course of action.

Lack of empathy

Some doctors are so out of touch with patients' feelings that it may not be worth your time to problem-solve. The only solution is to walk away, or in the following case, fly away:

While I was a college student at a large private university with a prestigious medical school, I found a single, small pimple-like lump in my labia. There was no itching or pain, but I thought it odd. I went to the student health center. There I had to sit in my paper gown in a hallway with several other women, also basically naked. This was quite uncomfortable. Eventually I saw the doctor, who immediately was saying, "tsk, tsk" and "uh oh," but wouldn't say why. He said he'd have to do some STD (sexually transmitted disease) tests and started asking very detailed questions about my sex life, which had been monogamous for at least 6 months. I demanded to know what it might be. He said, "I've never seen anything like this that wasn't herpes. But don't worry, your sex life won't be ruined. You'll just always have to use condoms for the rest of your life, and childbirth will be tricky." I was stunned and asked how it could have happened. He said, "Well, usually there are symptoms within two weeks, but it can be up to two years after exposure that there are any problems." He gave me an ointment to use while I waited for the test results.

I immediately went to the library and started researching herpes. The photos were horrible. The tests were due back in two days. On that day, I got a call saying the sample had been left out overnight and that I needed to retake the test. Then, when I went in, they didn't know what I was talking about and denied there was any problem. I called the next day, and the next, and the next for results (they wouldn't call me). They still weren't ready.

Finally, about a week later, the results were in and I was told I had to pick them up in person. I went in to the same doctor and he said that all my STD tests were negative and that I didn't have herpes. Stunned, I said, "Well, then what is it?" "Nothing, I guess. Just a little pimple," he said casually. After using the ointment for another week or so, it simply went away. My disgust with the process and the disregard for my feelings did not. That was the last time I visited the student health center. Finding out I had a pimple took three trips and a week of anguish. Everything about my experiences there made it clear that they weren't interested in keeping me as a client, they didn't respect my feelings, and they weren't interested in maintaining a high quality, well-organized operation.

After that, I flew home to Boston to visit my family doctor if I had a problem.

Communication breakdown

Some doctors are just poor communicators. It may be caused by a basically shy temperament, lack of time, lack of interest, paternalistic philosophy, or simply not having adequate interpersonal skills. In some cases, you might be willing to accept poor communication if the doctor has superior technical skills or other qualities that you prize. However, poor communication and lack of warmth often are the reasons patients take their business elsewhere.

The following reasons are commonly given for changing doctors:

- She won't answer questions.

  I am a small woman, and my doctor was even smaller. Once when I was in the hospital, I asked a specific question about my blood work results and she reached up to pat my head and said, "Now, don't you worry about such things, that's our job." I was stunned, but did manage to reply, "I think it's a reasonable question. Are you going to give me an answer?" She mumbled a very simplistic answer, so I went and found an attending doctor to give me a thorough answer which really reduced my anxiety.

- He's paternalistic.

  While I was in college, a male doctor at the student health center asked me the name of my birth control pill so that he could give me a prescription for another month's worth. I'd been on several brands, having to change due to migraines, so I had to double-check to make sure I told him the correct brand name. I'd brought my pack with me and pulled it out of my purse to check the name. The doctor, actually an intern, exclaimed, "You don't know the name of your pill? Now, what if you were in an accident and had to know?" Before I could explain, he said in a voice generally reserved for speaking to kindergartners, "OK, today's lesson is to memorize the name of our pill. Can you do that?" He then quizzed me on it! I walked out feeling completely humiliated and embarrassed. It was the classic talking down to patients that doctors are so chided for doing. As a smart young woman, who was being responsible about birth control, I was deeply offended. I still regret that because I was pressed for time, I didn't go complain to the head of the staff.

- She just doesn't listen.

  I was taking propranonol for severe migraine headaches. I started taking it in the winter, and I soon started getting swollen, white fingers whenever it was cold. No matter how many gloves I wore, it happened and it was painful. I was also getting light-headed occasionally. I told my doctor about the side effects, and she replied, "That's not a problem." I said, "It's a problem to me." She told me not to worry about it. I then asked if these were common side effects from the drug and she said, "No." She just had an attitude that she knew better and that I was bothering her with minor complaints.

  My sister looked propranonol up in the PDR (physicians' desk reference) and found out that these indeed were possible side effects. I brought this info to my next appointment and she categorically stated that the info was false. She did call me later, after looking it up, and said that these were possible side effects, but only in combination with other medications. I changed doctors.

- He takes away hope.

  One member of our cancer support group tells the same story at each meeting about her general practitioner telling her to get the "pine box" ready when he visited her in the hospital after her surgery. Her surgeon arrived shortly after and was able to calm her down and offer her encouragement. Now eight years later she is happy to be alive and well, but still expresses her anger at her GP's thoughtless and hurtful words.

- He won't tell me side effects of treatment.

  My dad has prostate cancer and what he needs is honesty with hope. He is 82 years old, primarily self-educated, but extremely intelligent. His urologist prescribed hormone therapy without explaining any of the female side effects he would develop. My dad was tired, stressed by treatment, and felt that the doctor wouldn't answer his questions and he wasn't going to beg. He began to physically, emotionally, and spiritually suffer. So I got on MedLink, found out all about the common side effects and told him he was not imagining things or going crazy (something he feared), but was experiencing expected and very common side effects to hormones. He turned to his radiologist, who talks to him and listens, for support. His spirit has returned, the cancer was successfully combated, and he's doing much better—he's now 83!

Philosophic disagreements

Severe differences in philosophy warrant changing doctors. You, for instance, might have a terminal illness and wish to stop treatment to go home to die among family and friends. If your doctor is on the aggressive end of the spectrum and wants to exhaust all possible treatments, conflict will result. The reverse situation also occurs, when the patient wants to continue trying new treatments, but the doctor says nothing more can be done.

Another common conflict occurs if doctor or patient wants to use pills, while the other party wants to try lifestyle changes or adopt a wait-and-see approach. Differences about alternative or adjunctive treatments can also rupture relationships.

Incompetence

Some patients just get bad care. If your doctor is not well versed in the newest treatments for your illness or injury, you might get better care if you find someone more experienced.

I have Marfan syndrome and have been taking medications for a heart problem since I was fourteen years old. When my beloved cardiologist moved across the country while I was a teen, she wrote me an open-ended prescription for the drug, which I took for the next five years without ever visiting a doctor. In college, I began to have dizzy spells and heart palpitations so I went to see a cardiologist. I was young and quiet and didn't know that I could interview him to see if he had any experience treating patients with Marfan. He told me that I would need open heart surgery when my aorta grew to six centimeters wide, or by the time I turned twenty-six years old, whichever came first. I went into an emotional tailspin. Later, I discovered at a National Marfan Foundation meeting that age has nothing to do with when you need the corrective aortic or mitral valve surgeries, which, at age thirty-six, I have yet to have.

When I began researching my condition, he wasn't at all interested in hearing about the latest studies or learning from me (his only patient with Marfan, I later learned). I asked him about the possibility of having an MRI instead of cardiac catheterizations every other year which were emotionally and physically difficult for me. He completely dismissed the MRI as being in the research stage. He was irritated at me asking and had the attitude that I shouldn't be questioning such tests and treatments. But I was completely involved—it was my body.

My brother began having heart palpitations and he went to the same doctor. When my brother mentioned that I went to him (me, his only patient with Marfan syndrome) the doctor said "Just remind me—how long ago did she pass away?" I changed doctors.

You move to a new location

Moving is the most common reason for changing doctors as well as one of the easiest with which to deal. Whether you moved across the state or jumped from one coast to the other, you will have to find a new doctor. The easiest method for handling the transition is to ask your current doctor for a recommendation. Follow the steps outlined in Chapter 2, *Finding the Right Doctor*, to identify and interview candidates. After you have made your decision and feel comfortable with your choice of doctor, request in writing that your records be sent to the new office.

Doctor retires or dies

If your doctor retires, he will have provided information and a transition to a new physician. After a period of adjustment, make a conscious decision about whether to stay with the new doctor or search out another with whom you might have a more satisfying relationship.

We went to the same family doctor for twenty years. The stress of a large solo practice became too much, and he took a job in the local teaching hospital's emergency room. He recommended a replacement and we both saw Dr. G. for twenty years. He is retiring this year, and he recently employed two young doctors in the practice. He was gradually phasing out, so we saw both the new doctors several times. Neither my husband nor I felt able to communicate well with them, so we are looking for a new family doctor for the first time in decades.

If your doctor dies, you may suddenly find yourself scrambling during an illness to locate a new doctor. Refer to Chapter 2 to learn how to find a new doctor who meets your needs.

When a doctor sells her practice or leaves a group practice

Most sales of medical practices happen because the selling doctor is moving to another geographical area, chooses to retire, or changes jobs (such as from an HMO to a private practice). When a practice is sold to another doctor, the new doctor should make an effort to notify the patients that they will have a new doctor when they return to the office. This not only warns the patients, but also gives them an independent opportunity to change doctors. If the notification process breaks down, you might learn in an unprofessional and upsetting way that your doctor has left a practice.

> *My doctor belongs to a group of eight family practice doctors.*
> *Several years ago, I went in for an appointment, and someone I'd never*
> *seen walked in. I said, "You must be in the wrong room, I'm Dr. S.'s*
> *patient." He said, "No, he moved back to his home state so his children*
> *would be closer to their grandparents." I hadn't been notified. The next*
> *time I went in, the second doctor had also left and I was not notified. I*
> *left the practice after that.*

How to change doctors

Once the decision to seek a new doctor has been made, consider taking the following steps to ensure a smooth transition:

- **To ensure continuity of care, find another doctor before you leave the old one.** Try to learn from the past problems and choose your new doctor carefully to prevent the trauma and disruption of another failed relationship.

- **Be candid with your old doctor.** An explanation for the change should be given either verbally or in writing. It's only fair to let the doctor know that he has a problem staff person or a manner that you find abrasive, as it may spare other patients the trouble that you have experienced. An example of what you might say is, "We do not seem able to resolve our differences, so I have made arrangements to see Dr. So and So in the future." If you decide to write a note, the following example might help.

> *Dear Dr. Smith,*
>
> *I am leaving your practice because _____ (we cannot agree on*
> *treatment plans; you are continually two hours late for appointments;*

you refuse to answer my questions; you made a serious medical error,
etc.) Please send all of my records to the office of Dr. So and So at _____
(include address) by _____ *(include date).*

Thank you for your prompt attention to this matter.

Sincerely,
[your name]

- **Have your medical records forwarded.** You can either write a note as in the above example, or go to the old doctor's office and sign a medical records transfer form. Physicians are required by law to transfer all records upon written request.

> *You don't have to be polite or impolite, but be direct. I have changed twice, and one doctor I had seen for fifteen years! I picked the new doctor I wanted, made an appointment, then asked the office of doctor #1 to forward the records to doctor #2. Then I wrote a letter to the doctor I was leaving to explain why. The first one called me the same day he got my letter to discuss it. I told him I would always come to him for a second opinion, but I wanted a doctor who would give me more time, and with whom I could talk.*

> *The second doctor did not care why I changed, but since we disagreed on everything, I think he knew why. Both times it was a huge relief—don't wait, just do it.*

CHAPTER 10

Questions to Ask About Tests, Drugs, and Surgery

The main problem plaguing too many patients is that they are so respectful toward—or intimidated by—their doctors that they don't realize they have a right and an obligation to be assertive in gathering facts about their situation...Once you know the kinds of questions that should be raised, you'll be in a much stronger position to prevent errors that could threaten your health and even your life.

—Richard M. Poddell, M.D.
When Your Doctor Doesn't Know Best

TESTS, SURGERY, AND TAKING MEDICATIONS are often necessary in order to diagnose and treat injury or illness. As an involved patient, you need to understand the nature and the purpose of all proposed medical procedures as well as the possible risks and side effects. It is vital that you have all pertinent information in advance in order to make knowledgeable decisions. As Norman Cousins wrote, "Living in the second half of the twentieth century, I realized, confers no automatic protection against unwise or even dangerous drugs and methods."[1]

This chapter will clarify the questions you need to ask to be truly informed and equipped to make decisions about your medical care. It describes when tests might be unnecessary or even harmful, questions to ask about tests and procedures before consenting, and easing the uncertainty of waiting for test results. Methods to evaluate what medicines to take are explored. Questions to ask about surgery and how to determine when surgery may be unnecessary are outlined.

Medical tests

The days of doctors making diagnoses based on history and physical examination alone are long gone. Instead, most patients are subjected to one or more tests, some with the potential for serious complications. In addition to being risky, tests can be uncomfortable, time consuming, privacy invading, and expensive. Doctors may prescribe tests to help make a diagnosis, to establish a baseline prior to treatment, or to monitor the effects of treatments.

Unfortunately, a few doctors may also order unnecessary tests out of habit, a desire to increase income, or to protect themselves from possible litigation. Dr. Edward Rosenbaum, in *A Taste of My Own Medicine*, explains his mixed feelings about testing:

> I have a dilemma. If I complain, I will have tests. If I don't complain—no tests, but possibly a missed diagnosis. Unfortunately, unlike the usual patient, I happen to know that tests are not necessarily innocuous. Doctors love to do them; it makes medicine seem more scientific. In recent years, because a missed diagnosis may mean a malpractice suit, physicians have had a tendency to overtest; it's called defensive medicine.[2]

In contrast, some doctors are pressured by managed care organizations to decrease the number of tests to cut costs rather than being allowed to use their clinical judgment about what tests are necessary. Understanding some basic principles of effective medical testing and asking the questions listed in this chapter will help you make choices about the appropriateness of prescribed tests.

Routine, but unnecessary

Many tests, once given routinely, have been shown to be unnecessary or even harmful. One recent study found that $30 billion is spent on pre-operative tests in the U.S. each year, 60 percent of which are unnecessary. In addition, injury can result from the further evaluation and treatment of false-positive results.[3] The annual or pre-hospital-admission chest X ray is a good example.

Routine chest X rays

An article in *American Surgery* cited many studies which concluded that routine pre-operative chest X rays continue to be widely used despite high cost and low yield. To analyze the usefulness of routine pre-operative chest X rays, 403 patients undergoing operations were studied. The study examined the number of abnormalities detected during pre-operative chest X rays and how often results of the chest X ray resulted in postponement or cancellation of the surgery. Only 2 of the 403 surgeries were canceled due to abnormalities discovered by the X ray. The article projected the cost of needless pre-operative chest X rays in the U.S. to be more than $1 billion per year.[4]

If you don't have symptoms involving your chest and are not having chest surgery, you can politely refuse a chest X ray. Simply ask what the purpose of the X ray is, and what the risk is of discovering an unknown problem in your chest or lungs. If you are in good health and without symptoms, the risk that you have a serious problem is probably extremely low.

Science is a study in probabilities. If the likelihood of missing a chest abnormality is one in five hundred, you might feel safe in refusing the X ray. Once you are fully informed, the decision should be based on your values and tolerance for risk, not the doctor's habits or comfort. Given identical information, two people often make opposite decisions. If you decide to refuse a procedure, the doctor should outline the possible consequences of your decision and the likelihood of their occurrence.

Making decisions on tests for your children is even more difficult. When parents hear, "Your child is very sick. He needs some diagnostic tests," they often respond, "Where do I sign?" Parents feel pressured to give their children the very best modern medicine has to offer. It is usually far easier to refuse for yourself than for your child. That said, consider how much more important your decisions are when made for another. Don't our children have the right for us to fully explore the reasons for all proposed procedures and tests? Aren't suggestions based on hunch or habit as common for children as for adults? Consider again the common chest X ray:

Routine chest X rays for children

The prestigious medical journal *Pediatrics* conducted a retrospective study to assess the value of pre-operative chest X rays for children. The study compared children admitted to two hospitals, one that required pre-operative chest X rays, and one that did not. The purpose was to study the number of unknown chest abnormalities discovered by routine X rays and to see if patients who had received a chest X ray experienced fewer anesthetic or post-operative complications than those children who were not x-rayed. In all, 1,924 cases were studied; in 749 a chest X ray was taken. Nine clinically significant chest abnormalities were discovered, with only three (0.4 percent) resulting in cancellation of surgery. There were no differences in anesthetic or complication rates between the two groups. The study concluded that routine pre-operative chest X rays on healthy children should be discontinued.[5]

Defensive medicine

In addition to the number of tests that are administered out of habit—such as routine pre-operative chest X rays—doctors are prescribing many more tests to reduce the risk of being sued for malpractice. Many doctors are justifiably worried about lawsuits. There have been some well-publicized multi-million dollar lawsuits, and malpractice insurance has skyrocketed in recent years. In response, doctors are changing the way they practice. "Wait and see" has been replaced with ordering tests "just in case." In one study at Pennsylvania State University, researchers surveyed physicians to measure defensive medical practices and found "in all of the scenarios, many physicians chose aggressive patient management styles even though conservative management was considered medically acceptable by the expert panels that developed the scenarios."[6] In *M.D.: Doctors Talk About Themselves*, one doctor describes changes in attitudes as well as test ordering:

> *The physicians sued most often are those most highly trained, but they have the shortest and least intimate contact with patients and their families. They often meet the family in a crisis situation. It may be that they are highly paid and they are arrogant, but that is not what causes them to be sued. They're sued when something doesn't turn out the way people want it to turn out, even though it may be completely out of the doctor's control...*
>
> *Doctors will talk about the cost of defensive medicine that has been made necessary by malpractice suits, and the money wasted on needless tests, and that sort of thing. All that's true. But the real cost is a change in attitude, a loss of enthusiasm. That is immeasurable. It's the price the American public is paying and will continue to pay—the loss of the physician as their advocate.*[7]

Ironically, according to a Harvard study, doctors dramatically overestimate their risk of being sued—their estimates were three times the actual rate. This inflated perception of risk increased test ordering and caused a reduction in practice scope.[8]

Patient demands

Many patients desire—and sometimes demand—that the doctor do something, whether it is medically justified or not. If, after a thorough discussion about the treatment plan, you feel that your doctor is not doing enough, a second opinion might clarify the situation for you (see Chapter 8, *Getting a Second Opinion*).

Conversely, you may need to demand necessary tests in some managed care situations. More and more, patients are facing situations in which they find that critical tests, labs, and X rays are not being ordered for them, especially in capitated systems. Your doctor may be in the ethically uncomfortable position of facing financial penalties for ordering more than the allotted number of tests or procedures for his patients. If you are facing this situation, strategies for coping are found in Chapter 3, *Getting What You Need from Managed Care*.

> *The problem these days is whether your doctor is doing what needs to be done. I always tell my patients and consumer groups that they need to be more aware of their own needs, their bodies. If things aren't getting better, you need to be assertive and ask lots of questions. Networking with other people with the illness and researching will help you discover if crucial tests or treatments have not been recommended. It's also worth paying out-of-pocket for a second opinion on your own from somebody who is not going to be influenced by your insurance plan.*

Questions to ask about tests and procedures

If your doctor has proposed a test or procedure, the following are questions that you should consider asking before consenting to the test:

- What is the purpose of the test?
- How will it contribute to diagnosis or treatment?
- Are there simpler or less risky ways to get this information?
- If so, what are your reasons for not choosing those methods?
- What are the risks associated with this test?
- Do I have any particular risk factors for this test?
- What are the possible side effects and how often do they occur?
- How reliable is the test?
- How reliable is the testing facility?

The skill and experience of the technician giving the test and the quality of the equipment being used are an often overlooked aspect of testing. For instance, if you are going for a mammogram, the center should be accredited by the American College of Radiology (ACR). Many facilities fail when they seek accreditation. To find out if your center is accredited, call the American Cancer Society (1-800-ACS-2345) or the National Cancer Institute's information service (1-800-4-CANCER). Make sure that the technicians are registered and state licensed. Go to the same center for every mammogram to ensure that your past films can be reviewed by the radiologist. As with many other procedures, quality tends to improve with volume and experience. The ACR requires that the radiologist be board certified and reads at least 480 mammograms a year; however, busy centers do thousands of examinations a year.

- Who will do the test?

If your primary care doctor offers to perform a specialized procedure, make sure he or she is qualified—and experienced. For instance, if you are over 50, have blood in your stool, or have a family history of colon cancer, you may need a yearly sigmoidoscopy—a procedure in which a two-foot-long flexible scope is inserted into the colon to check for cancer or polyps. An unskilled physician could perforate the colon—a life-threatening complication. For best results, go to a gastroenterologist who has performed several hundred of the procedures with a low rate of complications.

When I was a resident, patients often asked me how many times I had done a procedure. I usually spoke around it, for instance, I'd say, "Yes, I've done many of these with so-and-so," because I don't really think it's fair to tell somebody that it's my first time on my own. They have the right to ask to have an attending doctor present, and, frankly, the resident should have a right—but they don't always get it—to have a supervisor there as well. I felt out on a limb many times, especially in obstetrics, when I was on my own with little experience. When training doctors, they put a high premium on self-reliance and independence.

- When will I have the test done?
- How long will it take?
- Will it require hospitalization?
- Please explain in detail exactly what will be done during this test.

- Can I expect any unusual feelings, pain, or sensations during this test or procedure?

- Should I bring someone to drive me home?

- Are there special instructions to follow before or after this test?

- Are there any symptoms that may occur that I should call you about (pain, bleeding, fatigue)?

- Will I need to be seen after the test is done?

- What does this test cost?

- Will my insurance cover it?

- When will I get the results?

- How will you inform me?

- How can I get a copy of the results for my personal records?

- What is your plan if this test or procedure does not result in a diagnosis?

Tests can be simple and quick—drawing a vial of blood for a blood cell count—or painful and risky. Getting answers to the above questions, in terms that you understand, will provide you with the information you need to consent to or refuse the procedure. You will also know what to expect and thus will avoid any nasty surprises.

If the answers are confusing or incomplete, stop the doctor with a phrase such as "Could you repeat that, please?" or "I'm not familiar with those terms. Could you explain it using different words?" If he is talking very quickly, it is perfectly acceptable to ask him to slow down. It is also very helpful to bring either a tape recorder or a note pad to make sure that you don't overlook or miss any crucial information. Patients frequently bring spouses or friends with them so that four ears hear the doctor, rather than just two. In some cases, you might be too sick or medicated to hear and comprehend clearly. Stress also affects hearing and memory in many people, so having an advocate present is a great help. Others feel more comfortable dealing one-on-one with their doctors.

> *I need someone with me when I visit the doctor. Even with another set of ears listening, it's sometimes hard to understand because there is so much information to absorb. I sometimes bring a tape recorder with me, so I can listen again at home. That way I don't miss anything important.*

If the test requires you to sign a consent form, ask for it in advance. More often than not, the form is given to you just before the test is about to start, so that if you take the time to read it carefully, you are holding up the show. It's very uncomfortable to read the fine print when everyone is waiting for you to sign, and even worse if you need to ask questions or get something clarified. So prepare ahead and ask to take home any written consent form.

Learning all that you can about tests will make you an informed and involved partner in your health care. If you would like to read more on this topic, two excellent books that explain most tests and procedures in plain English are: *The People's Book of Medical Tests,* by David Sobel, M.D., and Tom Ferguson, M.D., New York: Summit Books, 1985, and *Everything You Need to Know About Medical Tests,* written by 70 doctors and medical experts, Springhouse, PA.: Springhouse Corporation, 1996.

Additional questions for children's procedures

If a procedure is recommended for your child, ask all of the questions listed earlier, as well as the following:

- Why does my child need this procedure now? What are the risks or benefits of waiting until a later date?

- Does the facility that will do the procedure have a social worker, child life therapist, or nurse who will work with my child ahead of time to prepare her for the procedure?

- Is sedation for the procedure available?

- Describe the test in detail so that I can prepare my child. Are there any pamphlets or videos my child can read or watch that will explain the procedure?

- Does the hospital give children tours to help prepare them for the procedure or hospitalization?

Waiting for results

If you are worried, waiting for test results can be excruciating. You can lessen or prevent this agony by making prior arrangements with your doctor to get the results at a specific time. You could say, "I find it hard to wait for results. What arrangements can be made so that I will hear as soon as possible?" The doctor then might tell you that he will schedule the test early in the week to avoid a delay in reporting over the weekend. You might also learn from this question that the doctor will be in the office only on certain days; the test can therefore be scheduled to coincide with his schedule, ensuring that he can call you with the results. Make sure that you have an appointment to discuss the results if the doctor does not want to phone you.

When I have a test such as a bone scan, I am not willing to wait to get the results from the referring doctor. I want those results as soon as they are available. The stress associated with these tests is not from the tests themselves, but from the wait to get the results.

When my oncologist orders a test such as a bone scan, I ask him to have his nurse make my appointment at a time when the radiologist will be present to read the film and to request that the radiologist discuss his findings with me immediately following the bone scan.

I arrive for the scan with all of my previous films and reports and a written note that says something to the effect of "Dear Dr. Radiologist, This is a request that you explain your findings to me before I leave the premises today." I give the note to the technician and ask him to take it to the radiologist and get his reply prior to starting the bone scan. In every instance, the radiologist has pleasantly explained his findings to me within twenty minutes after the end of the test. In fact, the radiologists have thanked me for the information that I have provided them concern-ing my complicated case and have asked additional questions. I am able to explain much more of my history than is written in the records they receive. If you bring in the old films yourself, you will not have to wait for the radiologist to locate them to make comparisons and complete his report. I have recommended the same procedure to many other patients in my community, and it has worked every time with many different radiologists.

The key things are to get the oncologist's approval and to let the radiologist know before the test is done that you are expecting an imme-diate oral report. If the radiologist is not willing to discuss his findings with you, then take your business elsewhere.

Another patient, who requires periodic bone and CAT scans, pestered her surgeon so often for results that he gave her a phone number to call to get the results herself. When she tried the number, it turned out to be the tape dictated by the radiologist who interpreted the scans.

It is extremely common for test results not to be transmitted to patients in a timely fashion, if at all. Consider the following study from southeastern Michigan.

Delays in reporting test results

A survey was conducted of 161 attending physicians and 101 residents in family practice and internal medicine in southeastern Michigan. The study investigated how physicians handled patients' test results from the time the test was ordered until the time any required follow-up was completed. Thirty-two percent of the doctors had no reliable method to make sure that the results of all tests ordered were received. One-third of the physicians did not always notify patients of abnormal results because, the physicians said, the results were trivial or the patient was expected in the clinic soon. Residents were far less likely to notify patients of abnormal results. Only twenty-three percent of physicians reported having a reliable method for identifying patients overdue for follow-up. The study concluded that the lack of a system to get results, dependence on follow-up to tell patients the results, and failing to know when patients were overdue for follow-up could result in poor care and increase the risk of malpractice suits.[9]

When you are having trouble getting the results of your tests, it is often easier to just ask someone else in the office or clinic. One mother describes her successful method of working around a difficult physician:

> On my daughter's last day of treatment for leukemia, I asked the fellow when we would get the results of the bone marrow aspiration. It was important—no cancer meant celebration, while cancer cells meant that the arduous treatment was unsuccessful. She said that end-of-treatment bone marrow aspirations were at the bottom of the pathologist's priority list and that the written results would not be available for days. Instead of fighting, I just waited until the fellow left, then I found the director of the clinic and asked her very politely if she would go down to the pathology lab sometime that afternoon to check on the bone marrow results. She said, "Absolutely," and she called me three hours later.

Understanding the test results

Once you have obtained the test results, how do you interpret them? Ideally, if your doctor is a good communicator, she will have explained the results of the history, physical exam, and all test and procedure results. Clearly, part of the discussion should cover not only what the diagnosis is or isn't, but also what treatment is recommended. The discussion should also include the prognosis, as well as back-up plans should the recommended treatment not be successful. If the doctor has volunteered all of the information that you want and need, you will walk out of the office secure in your understanding of diagnosis, prognosis, and treatment. If, on the other hand, you have questions whirling around in your head, or you feel confused or fearful, it's time to make a follow-up appointment for further discussion.

When you call to make a follow-up appointment, tell the receptionist that you need an appointment for discussion of your diagnosis and treatment. By doing this, you should get sufficient time for questions and discussion. Go to the meeting with a friend or relative, a tape recorder, or pad of paper so that you can review the information at your leisure at home. The following sections suggest questions that you might ask your doctor during this appointment.

Diagnosis

Tell your doctor that you want a complete explanation of what your illness or condition is. Some possible questions are:

- What do I have?
- Do I have a mild or severe case?
- What caused it?
- How did I get it?
- What is the usual course of this illness?
- Will it affect other parts of my body?
- Is it contagious?
- Are there any organizations that can provide more information about my illness or help with the problems that result from my illness?
- Is it possible that this diagnosis is wrong?

Treatment

You'll want to know if there is more than one treatment option, and what the benefits and drawbacks of each treatment are. Ask your doctor:

- What treatment do you suggest?
- How does this treatment work?

- Is this an experimental or investigational treatment?

- Is this treatment considered the standard of care for this illness?

- Are there other treatments available for this illness?

- How long does this treatment last?

- What are the common and rare short-term and long-term side effects?

- Are there diet changes or other measures that I can take to lessen the effects of the disease or the treatment?

- If the treatment doesn't work, what next?

- What would happen if I didn't treat my illness (or disease)?

Before agreeing to any treatment for a serious illness or disease, find out if there are treatment guidelines available. These guidelines, put together by panels of super-specialists in each specialty, outline the state-of-the-art treatments and any controversies in the field. For instance, the American Heart Association has published guidelines—called a multi-disciplinary consensus statement—on the use of carotid endarterectomy (surgery to clean out the carotid arteries in the neck). This document explains surgical risk using four categories: proven, acceptable but not proven, uncertain, proven inappropriate. Since this major surgery involves substantial risk of stroke, knowing what the experts in the country would suggest given your situation might dramatically increase the information you have about your options.

Many specialty boards publish guidelines for a variety of conditions. For example, the National Heart, Lung, and Blood Institute issued new guidelines in 1997 on the prevention and treatment of high blood pressure. The American Academy of Neurology has published guidelines on treatment for concussions, and the American Academy of Otolaryngology (ear, nose, and throat doctors) has guidelines that clarify appropriate treatment of the adenoids and tonsils.

To find out if any guidelines exist for your illness or condition, contact the American Board of Medical Specialties at 1-800-776-CERT or find the address for the particular specialty in Appendix B, and either call or write asking for the most recent guidelines. For cancer, the National Cancer Institutes have patient and physician guidelines written by experts that outline the state-of-the-art care for each specific type of cancer. These guides, called PDQ (Physician Data Query), are available free of charge by calling the NCI information line at 1-800-4-CANCER or visiting their web site at *http://cancernet.nci.nih.gov/.*

If the suggested treatment is medication and/or surgery, ask the questions listed later in this chapter. If the treatment is experimental or investigational, refer to Chapter 12, *Clinical Trials*.

Prognosis

The biggest question on your mind will probably be "What's going to happen to me because of this illness?" Getting thorough answers to all your concerns will help you feel more in control and better prepared to deal with the illness.

- What do you expect to happen in the future with my illness (or disease)?

- How long will I have it?

- What is the chance of recurrence?

- Is there anything that I can do to prevent recurrence?

- Does the illness (or disease) tend to have long-term side effects?

- Will the disease affect my lifestyle (hobbies, sports, travel)?

It is likely that your doctor will not be able to answer all of these questions in one visit. Let him know at the beginning of each appointment that you have questions and ask the most important ones first. Recognize that he may have patients waiting and, after the first few questions are answered, ask if you should make another appointment or phone call to cover the rest. You won't get thorough answers if your doctor is feeling pressured by time, but make him realize that you do need the answers in order to increase your understanding and lessen your worry.

Medications

Many patients view taking a drug as a cure for whatever ails them. However, of the thousands of drugs currently in use, most do not cure conditions; rather they relieve symptoms, alter mood, or delay progression of disease. Moreover, there is always a trade-off in using drugs; they may help one problem but create or exacerbate another. For instance, many patients who use antibiotics develop diarrhea and/or yeast infections. While these risks may be worth taking if the alternative is an unchecked pneumonia, they are not worth risking for an upper respiratory viral infection, for which antibiotics are useless anyway.

Benefits may not outweigh risks

Prescribed medications are not always necessary. At least part of the blame for over-prescribing rests with patients. Patients often want a doctor to prescribe something for every medical complaint. Prime-time TV and glossy magazine ads—relatively recent phenomena—add to patient demands for the latest popular drugs. Some patients do not want to hear the doctor's objections. Sometimes, unknown or dangerous side effects occur, and the drugs are taken off the market after being widely used.

> *I have had patients who feel I haven't done anything unless they leave with a prescription. It is not unusual for patients to come in "knowing" what's wrong with them and what they need to "fix" the problem, and I'm just a means to get it. For example, I've had patients come in with a cold and say, "I've got a cold, I'm going on a trip and I want some amoxicillin (an antibiotic)." I then have ten minutes to explain to them that their cold symptoms are due to a viral illness and that antibiotics are ineffective against viruses. I also explain that they will have the cold symptoms for seven days if I give them an antibiotic or a week if I don't. They still insist on a prescription.*

> *The problem with this scenario is that the patients end up being inappropriately given antibiotics for an illness for which the antibiotic will not have any beneficial effect. The most frightening part, which can and has occurred, is this in turn may lead to development of bacteria that are resistant to many if not all of the antibiotics available to treat bacterial infections. This can lead to life-threatening, untreatable infections, especially in hospitalized patients. The difficulty is in getting the patient to understand these principles without creating an argumentative, confrontational, and inefficient patient interaction. It is a real and common problem.*

To be able to derive maximal benefit from medications while minimizing the risk, you must be very practical and persistent in your approach. After you learn the potential benefits, risks, strengths, limitations, interactions with other drugs, and unknowns about each medication prescribed, you will be able to make educated choices about which drugs to take.

Weight loss drugs cause heart and lung problems

The FDA took two enormously popular diet drugs off the market in the fall of 1997, after learning that they can cause heart valve abnormalities and life-threatening lung disorders. The two drugs, Redux and fenfluramine (the fen in fen/phen), were originally approved for obese patients (those more than twenty percent above their healthy body weight) in conjunction with exercise and a low-calorie diet. However, they were widely prescribed to anyone wanting to shed a few pounds. In addition, after a 1992 study showed that fenfluramine and phentermine (commonly called fen/phen) worked more effectively when combined, their use skyrocketed despite lack of FDA approval for the combination and warnings from the manufacturer. In 1996, an estimated 6.6 million prescriptions for fen/phen were written. One study showed that 30 percent of the users of fen/phen had damaged heart valves.[10]

Questions to ask about medications

The following are questions to ask your doctor about any medication she has recommended.

- What types of drugs are used for my illness and how do they work?

- Why are you prescribing this particular drug for me?

- Is this drug approved by the FDA for this particular use? (Once the FDA approves a drug, any doctor can legally prescribe it for any use.)

- Is there anything I can do that might eliminate the need for taking this drug?

  Many cases of mild hypertension (high blood pressure) can be successfully treated by using low-salt, low-fat foods; regular exercise; reducing alcohol intake; and reducing stress. Many doctors would rather write a prescription than work with patients on lifestyle changes, and many patients would rather take a pill to "fix" the problem than try to prevent it. However, if you learn all of the potential side effects of many common medications for high blood pressure—sexual problems for men and women, shortness of breath, fatigue, hives, headache, dizziness, slow heart rate, to name just a few—you might be interested in trying the alternatives first.

- Will this drug cure my illness? If not, what effects on my symptoms should I expect?

- What would be the consequences of failing to take the drug?

- How long do I take the medication?

- How often do I take the drug? Is there a certain time of day that I should take it?

- Are there any special instructions for taking the drug (with food, with lots of water, etc.)?

- Does the drug interact with food, sunlight, alcohol, other drugs?

  An often overlooked drug interaction occurs in women who use birth control pills. Some antibiotics—penicillin, tetracycline, rifampin—decrease the effectiveness of birth control pills. You may get rid of your bronchitis, but end up pregnant! Barbiturates and hydantoins (e.g., Dilantin) also make birth control pills less reliable. Make sure to tell your doctor about *any* prescription or over-the-counter drug or vitamin that you take, before taking the new prescription.

  I have a neuromuscular disease and many drugs, including some vitamins, are toxic to me. I have a list that my pharmacy and doctor have, but the latest problem was a result of injections: cortisone, aristi-cort, and of all things, Novocain. The first two were administered by my regular doctor and the Novocain by my dentist within three days of each other. What a reaction! I looked like a raspberry for several days.

- Are there any dangerous side effects? Am I at special risk for any of the side effects? Remind the doctor of any chronic conditions you have, such as diabetes, asthma, or hypertension.

- What are the short-term and long-term side effects of the drug and how often do they occur?

  Most doctors have not personally experienced the problems involved with each different chemotherapy regime. Other than a published list from the drug company, the patient does not have access to much information. My doctor, for example, outlined only the most serious known problems involved with the various chemotherapeutic agents and steroids I was on. Then, too, some problems, like my inability to concentrate, were dismissed as being age related. I'm happy to announce that, since my chemotherapy ended, I have gotten much younger!

- What should I do if I experience any side effects?

- If I forget a dose, what should I do?

- If I take too much, what should I do?
- Is a generic substitute equally effective?
- Should the drug be stored in special places such as the refrigerator or in the dark?
- Will this drug cause a problem if I become pregnant or breastfeed?
- Will the drug affect my sex life?

    Many of the drugs used to treat high blood pressure—especially the diuretics such as Clonidine, Minipress, Reserpine—can cause sexual problems in both men and women. Don't stop taking the drug or change the dosage on your own if you experience distressing symptoms. Discuss them with your doctor. She should work with you to change the medicine or dosage schedule until the problem is resolved. If she is unresponsive or embarrassed, refer to Chapter 7, *Problem Solving*.

- What is your plan if this medication doesn't work?
- Do you know of any way to reduce the expense of taking this drug?

Additional questions for children's medications

Whenever your doctor writes a prescription for your child, ask the questions above that are appropriate for children, as well as the following:

- Has this drug been studied in large groups of children? If so, what was the outcome? If not, what are the risks in giving it to my child? Many drugs given to children have been studied only in adults, so the short- and long-term effects on children are unknown.
- Will this drug affect my child's appetite, growth, temperament?
- Will this drug have any impact on my child's ability to learn?

    Almost every one of the many seizure drugs that my son has taken has caused a decrease in his ability to focus and concentrate on school-work (or anything else) and they have also slowed down his processing speed. It just takes him longer to understand or figure things out. It's important for parents to anticipate these side effects so that they can work with the teacher. Parents also need to be prepared to identify these side effects, get appropriate help, and explain to their child that the changes are due to the drug, not anything else.

- If it is a drug given for a chronic condition, ask, how will this affect my child over time?

When my son was being seen at a large children's hospital, they didn't volunteer loads of information, but if you asked a question you got an honest answer. When we began seeing a neurologist for my son's seizure disorder, he prescribed a new seizure drug and said, "Oh, this will stop these seizures." I really never expected to see another seizure. Six weeks later, he had a big one, and I called them feeling frantic; I thought something must be dreadfully wrong. The nurse just said in a cheerful voice, "I guess the honeymoon season is over." Why didn't they tell me? Why wasn't I forewarned? I guess I wanted so to believe that the seizures were gone. But I think it's better to know the truth, no matter how hard it is to hear.

Precautions after a drug is prescribed

Before you take the first dose of any prescribed medication, consider consulting the *United States Pharmacopoeia Drug Information for the Consumer*, a book published yearly, which contains a tremendous amount of information in lay language about thousands of medications. This book will tell you how the drug works, describe the common and rare side effects, and warn about interactions with other drugs. It will also tell you the standard dosages and for what illnesses or conditions the drug is prescribed. This book is located in the reference section of most libraries.

For those interested in thorough, technical information, locate *The Physician's Desk Reference* (PDR) in the U.S. or the *Compendium of Pharmaceuticals and Specialties* (CPS) in Canada. These contain the drug company's description and formula for each drug, contraindications (situations when the drug should not be used), precautions, usual dosages, reported adverse reactions and their frequency, and treatment for overdoses. The reference sections of most libraries, hospital libraries, medical school libraries, and nursing stations in hospitals usually contain these books.

There are a few precautions that should be taken when using the PDR or CPS. They use technical language—a medical dictionary is helpful if you are not familiar with the jargon—and they also list every side effect or adverse reaction ever reported. These can be overwhelming to read. Since the potential benefit from using the drug should far outweigh the potential risks, the information needs to be considered in that light. On the other hand, reading the possible side effects may help you to clarify your own thoughts concerning the need for the drug.

It is also extremely common for a drug to be used for several purposes other than those listed in the indications section because the only listings allowed are those for which there is government approval. Also, the dosages recommended for you may differ from those listed in the PDR or CPS because of various reasons, including newer information available in the medical literature, or your particular situation. It's also possible the doctor or pharmacist made a mistake. When questioned, your doctor should be able to clearly explain why your dosage schedule is different from that recommended, or why the drug is being used for a purpose different from those indicated. It is far better to closely question your doctor and pharmacist and run the risk of being viewed as a problem than to blindly trust and regret it later.

The information from the PDR can also be found on the drug package insert contained in the box your drugs come in. Ask your pharmacist for this insert for each of your medications and check the section for drug interactions. Before taking a new medication, it is wise to tell your pharmacist all of the prescription and over-the-counter medications that you are taking, and he will check them all on their computerized drug interaction list prior to giving you the new prescription.

I kept a file of all the package inserts for each chemotherapy drug that my daughter took and I'm glad that I did. Once, early in treatment, her muscles just stopped working: she couldn't walk, swallow, lift her head, even open her eyelids. I went through all of the inserts again carefully, reading about interactions. I learned that the manufacturers of vincristine warned against giving the drug L-asparaginase within 24 hours of getting vincristine. It said that the L-asparaginase slowed the excretion of the vincristine by the kidneys, thereby increasing the vincristine's toxicity. One of the side effects of vincristine is muscle weakness.

I highlighted the section and showed it to the doctor and asked to have the two drugs given on different days, rather than at the same time as the protocol required. She said that we were supposed to follow the protocol (my daughter was enrolled in a clinical trial). I replied that my daughter was having a severe reaction and we needed to be flexible. I added that I was willing to withdraw from the study if they didn't adjust the dosing schedule to comply with the manufacturer's recommendations. We changed the dosing schedule and my daughter was back up on her feet with eyes open in no time.

When you pick up your medication from the pharmacy, check the label to make sure that it says your name, the correct drug and dosage, and any contraindications—such as, take only with milk or avoid sunlight. Ask the pharmacist if any additional literature is available on the drug. Often, pharmacies give out preprinted sheets with easy-to-understand descriptions of the drug, its uses, dosing schedule, and possible side effects.

> When I went in to pick up my daughter's dilantin, I noticed a problem right away. Usually I get a bottle of 100 pills, and they are given to me in the manufacturer's white container. This time, they were in a regular, round, brown pharmacy bottle. So I removed the cotton and looked at the pills; they were white tablets instead of yellow triangles. I said, "These aren't dilantin." The woman said, "Yes, they are, we just gave you the generic version." I said that I didn't want them. She went to get the pharmacist, and he looked and his face went white. He said "These are depacote." The mistake could have had severe consequences.

If you are hospitalized, check the label for each drug before you let them give it to you. Make sure that your name is on it, that it is the correct drug, and that the dosage is correct. If you are feeling too ill to perform these essential tasks, make sure that you have a relative or friend stay with you to be your advocate. Mistakes in giving medications are shockingly common in hospitals, as the following study illustrates:

Medical mistakes

Harvard researchers studied the hospital records from the state of New York and discovered that in a one-year period more than 13,000 New Yorkers were killed and 2,500 were permanently disabled due to medical care. Over half of the deaths were due to negligence. When the numbers are extrapolated to the entire U.S., they estimate that 400,000 patients nationwide are the victims of negligent mistakes or misdiagnoses each year. Of these, they estimate that 80,000 result in death.[11]

Not only do hospitals make mistakes—your neighborhood pharmacy is fallible, too. Consider the following study.

To prevent such mistakes, before taking any drug or letting someone in the hospital give a drug to you, know the correct name and exact dosage for the prescribed medication. The following are common sources of errors:

- **Confusion over drug names.** Many medications sound and are spelled similarly. For example, vincristine and vinblastine sound similar, but have different actions and dosages. Other examples of frequently confused drugs are cisplatin and carboplatin, Amiodarone and Amrinone, Covera HS and Provera, Leukeran and Leucovorin, Norvasc and Navane, Norvir and Retrovir. If the orders are scribbled or simply misunderstood by the pharmacist, you could be given the wrong medication.

- **Confusion over drug name abbreviations.** Drugs can have the same abbreviation, for example, methotrexate and mitoxantrone are both sometimes referred to as MTX.

- **Ambiguous orders.** Handwritten prescriptions are sometimes unreadable. If the pharmacist appears to have difficulty reading the prescription, ask that he call the doctor to verify the order. Ambiguity also results if clinical trial protocols are not written with precise language.

- **Medicine given incorrectly.** Some drugs are taken by mouth, some by intravenous line in a vein, some by injection into a muscle, and some by injection into the cerebrospinal fluid in the backbone. Some drugs are given quickly (called IV push), while others need to be given slowly to prevent problems. Make sure that you (or your advocate if you are in the hospital) know which drugs, in what doses, are to be given at what time. You should also learn the proper way each drug should be given.

A free pamphlet advising consumers on how to use medicines safely is available from the FDA. Special sections inform patients about possible problems with medications during their hospital stay. Also covered are: protections against tampering, how/where to get medication counseling, and some tips for giving medicine to children. To order *FDA Tips for Taking Medicines: How to Get the Most Benefit with the Fewest Risks*, send a letter with the publication number, FDA 96-3221, to this address:

FDA
5600 Fishers Lane
Rockville, MD 20857
Attn: HFE-88 (for single copy)
Attn: HFI-40 (for 2 to 25 copies)
or fax your order to (301) 443-9057

Many medications are very expensive and, in some cases, are not covered by insurance plans. If cost is a hardship for you, ask your doctor if he knows of any assistance programs. Many drug companies have programs to provide free medicines to needy patients. Eligibility requirements vary, but most are available to those not covered by private or public insurance programs. Ask your physician to request, on letterhead, a free copy of the *Directory of Prescription Drug Patient Assistance Programs* from:

Pharmaceutical Research and Manufacturers of America
1100 15th Street NW
Washington, DC 20005
1-800-PMA-INFO

Surgery

Rather obviously, every surgery carries with it risks. The risks from the procedure itself include trauma, infection, problems from anesthesia, unexpected results, and even death. There are also costs in time away from work and family, pain during recovery, and out-of-pocket cost for the procedure. Emotional costs can be fear, pain, anxiety, and worry. As with tests and medications, before consenting to surgery, you want to make sure that benefits outweigh risks.

Surgery is one area when procedures that begin as innovations sometimes evolve into common practice with little, if any, close scientific scrutiny as to their effectiveness. Tonsillectomies, for example, were routinely performed on thousands of children afflicted with sore throats or repeated respiratory infections. Even today, inappropriate tonsillectomies are performed despite substantial scientific evidence showing that the tonsils play an important role in the immune system. Tremendous variation in surgical procedures occurs in different geographic areas, as the following study shows.

Variation in the rate of spinal surgery in Washington state

There is a lack of consensus on how to treat neck pain, and wide variations in spine surgery rates exist. Researchers evaluated the rate of spine surgery in Washington state from 1986-1989. Excluding cases involving trauma, infection, or malignancy, 5,173 surgical cases were analyzed. They found a sevenfold variation among counties for cervical spine surgeries (fourfold to thirteenfold for specific procedures). Data showed that spine surgery is increasingly common with wide geographic variation.[13]

A reasonable question to ask when surgery is first proposed is, "What is the scientific evidence that supports the use of this surgery for my problem?" The following patient asked that very question when her gynecologist recommended a hysterectomy:

After the birth of my second child, I developed a very uncomfortable prolapse of the bladder and rectum which made even walking painful. I tried every nonsurgical intervention available without success. Without question, I needed surgery.

When my gynecologist was discussing the surgery with me, I was surprised that she added, "And I routinely take out the uterus during this surgery." I asked why and she said that the uterus would probably prolapse soon anyway and we might as well take care of the entire problem with one surgery. I asked her if there were studies which compared groups of women who kept their uteruses compared to those who had them removed during the prolapse surgery. She said, "No." I said, "Would you call removal of the uterus during this surgery the standard of care throughout the nation?" She said, "You know, without any studies, all I can say is that we tend to do as we were trained. At Duke, we took the uterus; at other centers, they don't. There are definitely two schools of thought." I declined the hysterectomy and have had several years without problems.

As you can see, just because an authoritative source of information presents something as fact does not make it the only option. Selective questioning, in a respectful, inquisitive tone, can yield valuable information.

Questions to ask about surgery

If you have been referred to a surgeon, ask the doctor referring you the following questions.

- Why are you referring me to this particular surgeon?

- Is she affiliated with the institution with the most experience doing this surgery?

- If insurance coverage were not an issue, what would be your recommended treatment?

- Is this the person you would recommend if your mother or father needed this procedure?

When you go to the surgeon for your initial visit, ask the following questions.

- What training do you have for performing this procedure?

- How many cases do you do annually?

  The number of surgeries the doctor does each year is important for several reasons. First, it takes experience to get and maintain the technical expertise necessary to be skilled at any particular procedure or surgery. Additionally, if a doctor is performing a high volume of procedures, it means he is respected by colleagues who are referring numerous patients to him. Lastly, it takes practice to maintain a high level of expertise in any given procedure, so you need someone with recent, frequent experience. It is reasonable to expect a surgeon to have performed at least forty of the procedures that you need in the previous year.

- How many patients with my illness do you treat?

  If you have a rare disease, don't go to a doctor who has never treated your disease. It is surprising how common it is for patients to stay with their hometown doctor for treatment of complicated illnesses. One study published in the *Journal of the American Medical Association* determined the differences in survival of women with breast cancer based on the type of hospital in which they were treated. The highest survival rates occurred at large hospitals and large community hospitals. Small community hospitals had lower survival rates, and HMO hospitals had the lowest rates of all.[14]

- What is your success rate? How do you define success?

If your surgeon defines a successful coronary bypass operation as one in which the patient's chest pain is reduced by one half and you think you will be pain-free, this discrepancy in expectations needs to be resolved ahead of time.

- What is the rate of complications?

Question your primary doctor or do some research to make sure that the surgery proposed is the most likely to alleviate your problem while minimizing complications. For example, several years ago, the standard of care for prostate cancer involved major surgery that often resulted in permanent impotence and sometimes incontinence. Now there are new techniques for removing the prostate that prevent impotence. Radiation is also used in many cases. And often, no treatment is given for this slow-growing cancer. If you have prostate cancer, see an oncologist who treats a large number of men who have this cancer to help you sort out your options.

- Is the procedure done on an outpatient basis? If not, how long is the average hospitalization?

In some managed care environments, doctors are under increasing pressure to get patients out of the hospital quickly after major surgery. For example, many hospitals are performing mastectomies on an outpatient basis. They give general anesthesia, remove the breast, and send women home with pain pills and chest drains that need to be cleaned, cared for, and monitored for infection. While some independent women with good support at home desire this surgery outpatient, most do not.

Every time that I hear about outpatient modified radical mastectomy (MRM), my blood just boils. If a woman really wants to go home on the same day as a MRM, that is fine, she should go home. But I think that the majority of women really need to stay in the hospital and should have that option. I had a really tough time when they sent me home the same day after my lumpectomy. I had a headache, nausea, and vomiting in the car, and could have benefited from an overnight stay. But I could not even imagine coming home the same day as my MRM. I couldn't even move until the next day. And I was nauseous. And the pain from the lymph node dissection was excruciating. And I was scared—scared of hurting myself, of caring for the wounds and drains, and of getting sick, which I did several times. Even when I did go home, I had my sister-in-law (who is a nurse) stay for four days. I didn't even have the strength to cut a bagel! And I was in good shape when I went into this!

Two ways to remain in the hospital are complaining of severe pain and/or nausea. Make sure the nursing staff documents in writing your request to remain hospitalized. Often, this will give the doctor a basis for ordering additional days in the hospital.

- What are the usual risks of this surgery? Do any of my medical problems put me at increased risk?

- How many follow-up visits will be required?

- What is the normal period of recuperation?

Specify that you want to know the length of time until you return to your normal activities, and tell the doctor what your normal activities are. There may be quite a difference between the time it takes to start walking out to the mailbox again and when you can resume running marathons.

- Who will be my anesthesiologist? What are her qualifications?

    When I went to have a hysterectomy, I asked my gynecologist which anesthesiologist she felt most comfortable working with. She gave me three names with #1 being her top choice. She said that hospital policy forbade her from scheduling her surgery according to the anesthesiologist working, but that patients could do so. So I called and received the anesthesia schedule, and we set the date for my surgery accordingly.

- Who will be performing the actual surgery?

This is vital information. Often, at teaching hospitals, residents perform virtually all surgeries while supervised by senior physicians. You may feel comfortable having your surgeon supervise, but if you don't, make sure that you verbally make your wishes known to your doctor. You will also have to cross out the sections on the consent form giving blanket permission and clearly specify, in writing, that you are consenting only to having your surgery performed by one specific person, and name him.

Additional questions for children's surgeries

If your child's doctor has recommended surgery, ask all of the questions listed earlier in the chapter. You might also want to determine why the surgery is needed at this particular time. Some other questions to ask are:

- How often have you performed this surgery on a child the age of my child?

- Could you provide me with articles that explain the scientific basis for the necessity of this surgery for children?

- Is there a nurse or child life worker on staff who takes the child on a tour of the facility and explains the entire surgery to the child beforehand?

- If my child has to stay overnight in the hospital, what is the policy on parents staying in the room? Are there roll-away cots or pull-out couches to sleep on?

- What are the possible short-term and long-term consequences from this surgery on children?

- Will the anesthesia be done by an anesthesiologist with extensive experience treating children?

The surgeon recommended [my wife] have the lesion removed and biopsied immediately to determine if it was malignant. If so, he explained, she had a number of options—ranging from mastectomy to lumpectomy…However, he made it clear that he was not convinced that lumpectomy had proved "as good" as mastectomy—and if she chose that option, she would have to get another surgeon to operate…

After talking it over, my wife and I decided that the first step was to get a second opinion. An oncologist…examined her and ordered a mammogram X ray of her breasts.

After seeing the report, he assured her that with such a small tumor…there would be no increased risk to her in waiting a few days, thinking it over, and having a lumpectomy rather than a partial mastectomy…

Because of a urinary tract infection, she was put on antibiotics for a week preceding surgery. By the fourth day of medication, the "lump" had disappeared. The biopsy was no longer needed. The new surgeon's best guess was that the antibiotics had cleared up what must have been a localized infected breast cyst.

Close calls like that make you appreciate the value of accurate diagnosis, of knowing the treatment options, of second opinions from specialists who are totally independent of one another, of a little time, and, yes, of good luck.[15]

—Thomas Scully, M.D.
Playing God: The New World of Medical Choices

CHAPTER 11

Taking Action if You Have Been Wronged

Before the names of just and unjust can have place, there must be some coercive power to compel men equally to the performance of their covenants.

—Thomas Hobbes
Leviathan

MOST DOCTORS ARE HARD-WORKING, dedicated men and women who care deeply about their patients and spend most of their waking hours trying to help them get well. Unfortunately, a small number of doctors injure or kill people through gross negligence, out-of-date training, impairment due to alcohol or drugs, and other causes.

This chapter explains a range of actions that you can take if you have been injured by illegal or substandard medical treatment. Actions can include: forgiving the wrong, writing a letter to the doctor to let him know how his treatment has affected you, complaining to various licensing and review boards, suing for medical malpractice, and filing criminal charges.

Will taking action do any good?

Many patients just shrug their shoulders and say, "It wouldn't do any good to complain, nothing will happen anyway." Historically, doctors have closed ranks around their weaker colleagues and have been unwilling to take steps to censure them when appropriate. In the past, testifying against a fellow doctor frequently resulted in fewer referrals—a type of shunning. Times are changing, however. In some recent cases, if a doctor covers up for a colleague or fails to report a serious problem, he can be found equally liable. Now, more than ever before, you are likely to spark a positive response if you complain about wrongdoing.

Several positive outcomes can result if you take action when wronged. Among these are:

• You may be compensated for your injuries.

- You may contribute to the effort to remove the bad doctors, protecting other patients from similar harm.

- You may ensure that wrongdoing is justly punished, and the punishment may function as a possible deterrent to others.

- You may cause personal change in the targeted doctor. For instance, if the licensing organization discovers impairment due to alcohol or drugs, they may require the doctor to participate in a treatment program in order to practice.

> *A local family practice doctor was sanctioned by the state for sexually abusing two female patients and making inappropriate remarks to three others. His license is restricted so that he cannot see patients without a chaperone in the room, he must remain in mental counseling, and pay an $11,000 fine.*

When contemplating whether or not to take action, think about what you want to accomplish and how best to achieve that goal. For instance, if you want the physician to lose his license to prevent an identical injury from happening to other patients, a malpractice suit will not be the appropriate path to choose. Instead, you'd need to pressure the hospital to revoke the doctor's admitting privileges or the state to lift his license. If your wish is that the nurse, physician, or dentist get into a treatment program for drug or alcohol abuse, the local medical society or state licensing board are most likely to require these actions. Perhaps you have been incapacitated by a horrible medical error and are no longer able to work—a cash settlement from a malpractice suit may be what you need to survive. Many medical malpractice settlements require strict secrecy and the public is never made aware of what happened. Identify the problem and the goal, then consider the choices described in the rest of the chapter for taking action when you have been wronged.

Forgiveness

Many patients, especially if they like their doctors personally but are upset by an error, choose to forgive. Several studies have shown that primary care doctors well liked by their patients—those who spend lots of time, educate patients, use humor, solicit patient opinions, and encourage patients to talk—are far less likely to be sued than those who are not as communicative and caring.

Even if you don't have a strong attachment to the doctor, you may want to put the bad situation behind you, and concentrate on activities that bring contentment rather than stress. You may wish to dissolve the anger that is threatening to consume you. You may simply want to get on with your life. Or you might just feel too sick or too tired to do anything about it.

My six-year-old son had a rare reaction to a drug and his kidneys started to shut down. He was urinating blood and we rushed him to the pediatrician. We were told to bring him 100 miles to the nearest children's hospital. Things began to go wrong in the emergency room. We were there for hours, they did numerous tests, and said they couldn't find anything wrong, but they wanted to admit him for observation. As soon as he was wheeled into the room, he stopped breathing. My husband, an emergency medical technician, started yelling for help. The resident on the floor looked horrified and she froze. I started screaming at her to do something, and the nurses called a "code." People rushed by, they put a breathing tube in, and took him to the pediatric intensive care unit. He was on the ventilator for a week, and in the PICU for two weeks. We really thought that we would lose him. He survived, but with some brain damage.

I think that although there was a series of mistakes made, nothing was done out of vindictiveness. They just screwed up. And they did work hard to get him out of the crisis. However, although we decided not to take any action, I feel a lingering bitterness and I am extremely cautious now with all medical people. I have lost my trust.

An effective way to forgive, as well as preserve your relationship with your doctor, is to schedule an appointment to talk it over with her. If the problem arose from a misunderstanding or erroneous advice from friends, family members, or the curbside lawyer, a face-to-face talk with the doctor may preserve your partnership. Such communication keeps the issues between the two humans involved and may allow for new understanding and growth within the partnership. If the doctor made an error, such a talk allows for an apology or other ways of making amends. Conversely, if there is no conversation and an adversarial relationship develops, the chance for preserving the relationship and allowing change on both sides (maybe the physician needs to improve communication skills or the patient needs to understand the complexities of decision-making) disappears.

Write the doctor

If you are angry at the treatment you received, yet do not want to become embroiled in official complaints or legal conflict, you may choose to educate the doctor about the effects of her actions. If her negligence caused you to become disabled, you might write a letter telling her about how your life has changed—for the worse. One patient who was given a pessimistic prognosis of only six months to live, sends her doctor a Christmas card each year with the notation, "I'm still here!" A patient whose breast cancer diagnosis was delayed by poor care from her gynecologist sends him frequent reminders:

> Dr. Y dismissed the hard, irregularly shaped lump in my breast. "Just a cyst," he reassured me, adding that the mammogram showed nothing to be concerned about. Having heard what I wanted to hear, I went home, relieved. I told myself that this well-respected New York gynecologist, who had performed my hysterectomy a few years earlier, had somehow seen on the mammogram and felt from his examination that this lump was only a benign growth and was sparing me an unnecessary and upsetting surgery. I was grateful.

> A full year later, at my routine checkup, Dr. Y, finding that my lump was still there, did what he should have done in the first place: refer me to a breast surgeon. The biopsy revealed an invasive ductal carcinoma of over three centimeters, large enough to classify me with Stage II breast cancer. The delay could have cost me my life—and it still may.

> I went to see Dr. Y in a state of shock after I'd been diagnosed. I wasn't in any shape to confront him then, and didn't yet understand the magnitude of what he'd failed to do. But he knew, I think. He called me a couple of times, at home. At the time, I was touched by his "concern." It wasn't until several months later, when I joined a support group, and found that just in this small group the majority had similar stories, that I realized kindly Dr. Y was "managing" a potential malpractice situation. One of the women in my group decided to undertake legal action, and won her case—she has since developed metastatic cancer, seven years after her gynecologist failed to refer her for evaluation of the lump in her breast.

> I decided against taking legal action, for myself. But ever since, I have taken every opportunity to send everything pertinent to failure-to-diagnose to this doctor, including my book, with the page marked, my

letter on the subject published in The New York Times, *and anything I've found about litigation in these circumstances. Did you know that failure to diagnose breast cancer is the single most common medical malpractice suit brought against gynecologists? They give workshops for doctors on how to avoid litigation! I did this not only to make him uneasy, but to make him think about what he was doing, and not so cavalierly dismiss lumps in his patients' breasts. Did it work? Who knows...but it has helped me.*

Such actions empower people who have been victimized. They not only feel better, but their actions may actually change a doctor's future actions, preventing other patients from suffering the same mistakes.

State licensing board

Each state has a board that is responsible for licensing and disciplining physicians. While the laws and procedures vary from state to state, generally a physician must be reported to the board by another physician, a patient, or some other person. The complaint—it must be in writing—should be sent to the state board of medical examiners or the equivalent organization in your state. In Washington state, for example, this is the Washington State Medical Quality Assurance Committee, while in New York, it is the State Board of Education. To find out who licenses and disciplines the doctors in your state, call your county or state medical association, listed in the telephone book. If you have trouble finding the agency in the phone book, ask the reference librarian in your local library for help.

I was 37 years old and had severe back pain. I went to a private radiology practice where the doctor both examines the patient and interprets the X rays. During the examination, the radiologist ran his hand down my back while saying, "Gee, it looks fine to me, where does it hurt?" I nearly went through the ceiling from the pain, but he didn't react. He then looked at my X rays and said, "Back looks fine to me." He sent me home. It turns out I had a fractured back and cancerous bone lesions throughout my skeleton. I sent a letter to him, the local medical society, and the state medical board which operates under the aegis of the New York State Education Department. The only response came from the Board of Education, which sent a standard form letter stating, "Thank you for bringing this to our attention." As far as I know, they took no action.

After receiving a complaint, the board decides if a complaint falls within its jurisdiction. Some of the offenses that merit action by licensing boards are:

- Gross negligence (not just making an error, but a gross deviation from the accepted standard of care).

- Repeated negligent acts.

- Professional incompetence.

- Falsifying or failing to adequately maintain medical records.

- Fraudulent claims (most commonly Medicare/Medicaid).

- Mental or physical illness that impairs the ability to practice safely.

- Impairment caused by alcohol or drugs.

- Controlled substance violations (including narcotics).

- Intoxication while taking care of a patient.

- Sexual activity with a patient.

- Unprofessional conduct.

- Conviction of certain crimes not related to patient care.

If the state board determines that action is warranted, a long, and sometimes arduous, process begins. The steps generally followed in most states are: investigation by the board, determination whether action falls under jurisdiction of the board, presentation of charges and evidence, defense, written report sent to appropriate state authority (often the attorney general), administrative action, and a possible series of appeals in state courts. Due process takes a long time.

The only circumstance that may prompt the state to take quick action is if the doctor poses an immediate threat to the public health, safety, or welfare. In these cases, the board has the power to suspend the doctor's license pending a hearing.

If the board finds the doctor guilty of the charges, possible actions that can be taken are: reprimands, probation, fines, censure, revocation or suspension of the doctor's medical license, or limitations put on the doctor's license. If the doctor has a drug or alcohol problem, his license might require participation in a treatment program and continued counseling.

A plastic surgeon in our town has received nineteen complaints in the last five years. Three are still being investigated, action was not taken on six, and ten have resulted in limitations to his license to practice. He has to undergo long-term psychological counseling, be supervised by a com-

mission-approved plastic surgeon, have an approved plastic surgeon
assist during all procedures, not allow nurses to give sedatives, and pay
$2,500 in fines.

Don't be disappointed if your case does not result in action taken against the doctor. According to the Federation of State Medical Boards, only a tiny fraction of the approximately 624,000 physicians in the U.S. had their medical licenses revoked or restricted. The Public Citizen Health Research Group publicizes these low rates, and points out the variability of discipline among the states. For instance, Mississippi disciplined 1.0 percent of its doctors in 1996, while New Hampshire took action against a mere 0.2 percent.[1, 2]

Until recently, doctors who were disciplined in one locality merely moved across state lines to begin a new practice. As noted in Chapter 2, *Finding the Right Doctor*, the U.S. government now maintains a database on all disciplinary actions taken against doctors. Hospitals, HMOs, and other organizations can call this database to check out the background of any physician asking for admitting privileges at their facility.

Peer review

Patient complaints that do not fall under state jurisdiction can be addressed through peer organizations if the offending doctor is a member or employee. Complaints concerning fees, poor judgment, communication problems, or improper behavior are evaluated by national or local organizations such as the following:

- **Medical societies**. Most doctors are members of their county and state medical associations. They frequently also belong to national groups such as the American Medical Association (AMA) or the numerous specialty societies (the American College of Physicians, the American Academy of Pediatrics). To see if your doctor is a member of the AMA, check the *American Medical Association Directory of Physicians in the U.S.*, found in the reference section of your library, hospital library, or medical school library. The AMA is also online at *http://www.ama-assn.org* (go to "Doctor Finder"). Call your state or county medical society to find out if the doctor is a member, and ask how to file a written complaint.

  Usually, an investigation is conducted by a member of the organization's ethics committee, who will interview both the patient and the doctor.

Mediation between the parties may be attempted to settle the dispute. If unresolved, the organization will determine whether the physician is at fault. Action taken may be an official letter, requirement for drug and/or alcohol treatment, removal from the referral list, or expulsion from the organization. Although action by county, state, national, and specialty societies can professionally embarrass a physician and affect the number of referrals, these are not legal proceedings and have no impact on a doctor's license to practice medicine. These actions are secret, so you, a member of the public, have no way to check on your doctor's complaint history with these organizations.

I had a broken back and needed a special brace so that I could protect it while it healed. I went to a physiatrist—a specialist in rehabilitative medicine—to get fitted for the brace. He gave me the wrong type, which not only didn't protect the injury, but aggravated it. When I went for a follow-up MRI, they rolled me into a sitting position and I heard a loud crack and felt excruciating pain. Another fracture. I wrote a letter to the county medical society, and sent the doctor a copy. He admitted he made a mistake and withdrew his bill for his examination, MRI, and brace. I have a friend in physical therapy who sees him occasionally, and he always asks her how I'm doing. I guess he feels remorse.

- **Hospitals**. Hospitals wield considerable power over physicians because they can revoke staff privileges or remove the offending physician from the referral list. If the doctor loses staff privileges, he or she will no longer be able to practice at the hospital, which can seriously affect both income and reputation. Removal from the referral list stops the flow of new patients, also affecting income and reputation.

If you have been ill-treated by a doctor in a hospital, send a certified letter to the hospital administrator explaining the problem, dates, doctor involved, and action that you would like to see taken. Hospitals are especially fearful of suits, so it is often in their financial best interest to take action. Most hospitals review doctors' staff privileges every year, so enough complaints can cause the doctor's privileges to be limited or suspended. If the misconduct is severe, he may be expelled from the hospital staff. Even if the hospital takes no formal action, the letter may serve as a deterrent to the doctor—preventing similar problems for future patients.

- **Medical groups**. Many doctors practice in large groups nowadays, which may help you get action on a complaint. Income for each member depends on the group's good reputation in the community and low malpractice settlements—and one problem physician can dramatically affect both. If you have a problem, write to the group administrator, and copy the letter to each doctor in the group. Peer pressure can sometimes force the doctor to change his or her behavior. In extreme cases of repeated complaints or persistent unethical behavior, the doctor may be forced from the group.

- **Insurance companies or HMOs**. Doctors affiliated with insurance companies or HMOs incur severe displeasure if a patient's complaint suggests the possibility of legal action. Cost is the bottom line. If you have a complaint against a doctor employed by an insurance company or an HMO, send a certified letter to the plan administrator detailing the problem and send a copy to your attorney (make sure you note on the bottom of the letter to the administrator that a copy went to your attorney). The mere suggestion that an attorney may become involved sometimes inspires action.

Malpractice

You can't expect your doctor to be perfect—after all, she's a member of the human race, too. Mistakes are made, sometimes with disastrous results. You also have no legal right to a perfect outcome. Your doctor can do a perfect job and the outcome may not be ideal. However, if you feel that you have been harmed by incompetence or negligence, suing your doctor for malpractice is one option to consider.

An anesthesiologist tells his feelings about the current malpractice climate.

> *I have malpractice insurance because if I harm a patient through negligence, I want him or her to be compensated for any injuries. Most physicians feel this way. Yet, if I have taken care of the patient to the best of my ability and training, being a board certified physician and following appropriate standards of care, and the patient has a bad outcome—that's not malpractice. It is simply a rare, unexpected, or known complication of their illness, treatment, or procedure.*
>
> *The problem with the system is that trial attorneys get a contingency fee (usually one-half to one-third of the settlement) and can walk off with millions of dollars that should go to injured patients for their continuing*

medical expenses and lost incomes. The attorneys usually only take cases when they think they can convince a lay jury that the patient was wronged and the doctor is at fault. For instance, an OB/GYN can do a superb job and a baby can still have severe defects. Even if everything was done correctly and standards of care were followed, the lay jury may find in favor of the patient. This sometimes causes insurance companies to settle cases regardless of whether an error occurred, and the physician has no say in it. To the insurance company it's a matter of saving money, but to the physician it's an admission of guilt.

Consequently, physicians feel compelled to practice defensive medicine. This increases the costs to the patient, the medical system overall, and the medical and malpractice insurance industry. In the end, these increases show up as higher premiums for patients' medical insurance, physicians' malpractice insurance, and higher costs for medications, office visits, professional fees, and hospitalizations.

Medical malpractice occurs when a physician (or other health care professional or hospital) provides negligent medical care to a patient, resulting in financial or physical damage, for which he becomes legally liable to compensate the victim of the wrongful act(s). Despite publicity for large malpractice settlements, malpractice suits are not very common compared to the number of patients actually injured by negligent medical care.

Malpractice claims are not common

In a study of 31,429 hospitalized patients in New York, 1,133 were identified as suffering adverse effects from their medical care. Of these, 280 patients' adverse effects were caused by medical negligence. Surprisingly, only 8 patients filed malpractice claims. The study concluded that "Medical malpractice litigation infrequently compensates patients injured by medical negligence and rarely identifies, and holds providers accountable for, substandard care."[3]

Medical malpractice also occurs when a doctor or other health professional fails to use the skills of an average, prudent, reputable professional in the medical community, resulting in injury, loss, or damage to the patient. Each area of medicine has such "standards of care" that knowledgeable, reasonable physicians are expected to meet or exceed.

Being injured by medical treatment and proving that you are a legal victim of malpractice are two entirely different matters. To win a medical malpractice case based on negligence, you must prove the following:

- A physician-patient relationship exists.

- The standard of medical care in the community was violated.

- Actual damages occurred.

- The substandard care caused the damages. This needs to be proved by a preponderance of the evidence, meaning that you must show there is a greater than 50 percent probability that the damages were caused by the substandard care.

Doctors frequently argue that their substandard care did not change the outcome in any significant way. In other words, if your father died of a heart attack after waiting five hours on a gurney in the hallway of the emergency room, the hospital's lawyer might successfully argue that he would have died anyway due to the severity of the heart attack. However, if a surgeon removed the patient's healthy leg rather than the one with gangrene, as recently happened in Florida, it is considerably harder to argue that no adverse affects to the patient resulted.

To establish the community standard of care and then to prove that it was violated requires the testimony of experts—doctors. Historically, doctors shy away from testifying against their colleagues. One such doctor was quoted in M.D.: Doctors Talk About Themselves:

> I testified against a physician in another city. The patient had gone to him in early pregnancy and said she felt a lump in her breast. The physician had basically said, that's nice dear, and written it down but had done nothing else.
>
> She kept reporting it until finally, in her thirty-sixth week of pregnancy, he said, "Okay, if you insist, we'll get a surgeon to look at it." It was malignant, and by then, it had metastasized. She was delivered immediately, put on chemotherapy and died a year later. They could get no doctor in that city to testify against him, so they came to see me. As far as I'm concerned, the case was clear-cut negligence that warranted compensation to the family and the child who would never know his mother. It was eventually settled for a good amount of money.
>
> ...If the same case had happened in my city, would I have testified against the doctor? It's easy to say yes, of course, but I have to be realistic. There's that old fraternal spirit that still exists...

But I also have to admit to financial considerations. Many of the cases that come to my office are referrals. So I can see some referring doctors saying, "That son of a bitch testified! We won't send any patients there again!"[4]

If you decide to pursue a malpractice suit, the following are some suggested steps to take to improve your chances of success:

- Get your medical records before filing. There is no way to evaluate the merits of your claim unless you have a complete record of all your medical care. If you encounter difficulties getting your records, refer to the Public Health Citizen's *Medical Records: Getting Yours* (listed in *Suggested Reading* at the back of this book).

- Obtain a second opinion. Just because you had a bad outcome doesn't mean that it fits into the legal definition of malpractice. Before wasting time or money, ask another doctor (who is totally independent from the one you are thinking of suing) for an honest evaluation of the treatment you received and how it compares to the community standard of care.

- Hire a good lawyer. Don't hire your uncle's friend or the fellow who drew up your will—you need a lawyer who specializes in medical malpractice. Medical malpractice is legally complex and requires specialized training. Also, a good malpractice lawyer will have knowledge of and access to the medical experts who will provide crucial testimony in court. Malpractice lawyers typically work on a contingency—they usually take one-third of the settlement. If no money is awarded, no fee is owed. However, any costs accrued by the lawyer—copying medical records, payment to expert doctors, court reporters for taking depositions—are passed on to you. These costs can run into thousands of dollars.

- Find out if your state has a screening panel composed of doctors and lawyers who will advise you, your lawyer, and your doctor whether they think there is a legal basis for filing the suit. In some cases, if you choose to pursue a suit against the advice of the panel and lose, the state can levy penalties against you and your attorney.

- If you win the suit, you may collect damages. If you lose, your doctor may be able to counter-sue if your action was taken without a reasonable basis.

- Ask the lawyer to give you a timeline on what will occur and when. Only after you have reviewed the amount of stress, time, money, and risks involved will you have the knowledge necessary to decide whether to file a suit.

When to take action

Whatever action you take, it must be timely. For a medical malpractice claim, for instance, the statute of limitations (the time you have in which to file a legal claim with the court) varies from state to state. It can be as small as one year from the time the injury occurred or was discovered (this also varies) or should have been discovered (by a reasonable and prudent person). These statutes are strictly enforced, and there is no recourse if you file even one day beyond the statute of limitations.

For all other complaint procedures short of malpractice, timeliness is still important though not as legally restrictive. You will be much more likely to get a response that will be helpful to you if you make your concerns known as soon as possible after the event.

Several years ago in Dayton, there was an OB/GYN nicknamed the "Love Doctor" who surgically rearranged women patients' genitals. He never bothered to get permission; he just added it to his authorized surgeries for episiotomies, hysterectomies, etc. A significant number of these women experienced a variety of problems, but he never told them what he had done.

The newsmagazine show "West 57th Street" did an entire segment on his "love surgery" and the complications some women had reported. Naturally, quite a few women sued. When the trials started, part of the legal defense was that the statute of limitations had run out against these women. The court ruled, however, that the time for the statute of limitations did not begin to toll until the show aired.

Reporting criminal activity

If you suspect the actions of a health care worker are against the law, speak up. Examples of reportable offenses are:

- Fraud.
- Misrepresentation of professional qualifications.
- False advertising.

- Practicing without a license.

- Failure to report child abuse.

- Falsification of records.

- Using or selling illegal substances.

Contact your local district attorney or county prosecutor to report criminal activities.

Filing your complaint

Whenever you file a written complaint—whether to the state licensing board, the local medical society, or the prosecuting attorney—give specific and concise information. Leave out inflammatory or emotional remarks. Your goal should be to provide the facts in as clear and professional a manner as possible. Your attorney will file the appropriate paperwork in the case of malpractice.

Facts that should be included are:

- Name of doctor, nurse, dentist, and/or hospital.

- Type of misconduct.

- Dates, times, and places problem occurred.

- Names of persons who have additional information (witnesses, other patients who encountered similar problems with the same doctor). Include written statements from these people, if possible.

- All documentation, such as copies of hospital records, insurance forms, etc.

- Information from other doctors (for instance, if you needed treatment for the injury caused by the first doctor, if you got a second opinion on your current situation, if a doctor witnessed the improper act, etc.).

You take some risks by complaining or taking legal action. Medical societies might ignore you. If you end up in court, the defense attorney may try to confuse or humiliate you. But if you are persistent and convincing, the result can be gratifying. You may be compensated for your injury, help lift an incompetent doctor's license, or be responsible for protecting fellow patients. You might restore your peace of mind. And possibly, justice might triumph.

*The incidents that gave rise to litigation were of a serious nature
and had, in many cases, profound effects on the lives of the patients
involved and their families...Strong emotions were aroused and
both patients and families were often still distressed years after the
original incident. They were disturbed by the absence of explanations, a lack of honesty, the reluctance to apologize, or being treated
like a neurotic...In most cases, these secondary problems contributed to a decision to take legal action.*

*Four main themes emerged from the analysis of reasons for litiga-
tion: standards of care—both patients and families wanted to
prevent similar incidents in the future; explanation—to know how
it happened and why; compensation—for financial losses, pain and
suffering, or to provide care in the future for an injured person; and
accountability—considering that an individual or organization
should be held responsible.[5]*

—Charles Vincent
The Lancet (June 25, 1994)

CHAPTER 12

Clinical Trials

The doctor-patient relationship is commonly portrayed in popular television shows and movies as if the doctor is a tour guide leading a traveler down a well-mapped road to a predictable destination. In truth, often doctor and patient are walking together in the darkness with neither the route nor the destination visible; their open eyes enabling them to make out only shadows.

—Jody Heymann, M.D.
Equal Partners

CLINICAL TRIALS ARE STUDIES designed to objectively determine whether a treatment provides real benefits for patients. Some trials test new drugs, drug dosages, drug side effects, or combinations of drugs. Others test various ways to give a treatment, lifestyles that prevent disease, effect of diet on the progression of disease, the effectiveness of new surgical techniques, or if belonging to support groups affects disease progression.

To help you determine whether a clinical trial might provide the best treatment for your condition, this chapter explains what clinical trials are, who pays for them, ethical issues involved, types of trials, questions to ask about clinical trials, and pros and cons of participating in one. Several patients and doctors share their perceptions on the benefits and possible problems of participating in a controlled clinical trial.

What are clinical trials?

Clinical trials are scientific studies of new methods for treating illness or injuries in human beings. The purpose of all trials is to improve existing treatment. A trial can involve a totally new approach that is thought to be promising or a variation upon current treatments. New methods of early detection and illness prevention are also evaluated in clinical trials. In essence, clinical trials reliably establish the benefits of new therapies, allowing less effective or more harmful therapies to be discarded.

I've been a pediatric oncologist for thirty years. When I started prac-
ticing, very few children survived. Now, for some cancers, there is a 90
percent cure rate. It's unprecedented. And it has occurred because parents
were willing to enroll their children in clinical trials.

Who participates in clinical trials?

Despite the thousands of clinical trials ongoing in the U.S. and abroad,
many patients have never heard of them or been asked to participate. When
would the choice arise? Frequently, doctors invite patients with life-threatening conditions (e.g., cancer) or chronic conditions (e.g., multiple sclerosis)
to join clinical trials. Your doctor might be very interested in research and
offer a clinical trial in his discussion of treatment options. Or you yourself
might take the lead in uncovering the newest research in your quest for the
best science has to offer. Persons with a family history of genetically inher-
ited disease often enter prevention trials in an attempt to postpone or
prevent developing the disease. Occasionally sponsors advertise in the newspaper to get patients to sign up. Sometimes, healthy people join a study
simply to contribute to scientific knowledge.

I am in two nationwide clinical trials now, both of which are con-
ducted by the Women's Health Initiative, George Washington University
Hospital. The first is a ten-year hormone replacement trial, in which half
the women take estrogen and half take a placebo. The second is a
calcium/vitamin D study on osteoporosis. I gave an extensive medical and
family history, and had a thorough physical, including a mammogram. I
go back semi-annually for a recheck. My next visit in May will include
blood work, blood pressure check, weight check, and gynecological exam.
I was asked to join by the researcher and agreed because I wanted to con-
tribute to medical knowledge.

The standard treatment for a given illness sometimes diverges considerably
from innovative state-of-the-art medical care. If standard care is not working
for you, or if your doctor knows of no promising treatments, you might
want to consider a clinical trial. Participation in a clinical trial may involve
some risks, but it also provides an opportunity to receive a treatment on the
cutting edge of research. Steve Dunn describes his search for options on his
web site at *http://www.cancerguide.org*:

I was diagnosed with advanced kidney cancer in late 1989, at the age of 32. Only a month after surgery, it was discovered that my cancer had spread to both lungs and nine bones in my spine. At this point the situation was desperate with no standard treatment, and dismal long term statistics. Early on, some incidents with my doctors, and some help from a friend convinced me that if I wanted the best treatment, it was up to me to find it. I bumbled and stumbled my way through researching my options and through the system, but ultimately I was able to make a good choice of a promising experimental therapy, high dose Interleukin-2 combined with Interferon. To paraphrase Stephen Jay Gould, I found the right information, asked the right questions, and enrolled in the right trial, and it saved my life.

Ethical issues

There are many examples in which patients' rights have been sacrificed upon the altar of science. The infamous Tuskegee Study of Untreated Syphilis in the Negro Male is perhaps the best known. The U.S. Public Health Service, starting in 1932, signed up more than 400 low-income black men in a Macon County, Alabama, study that provided "free treatment" for "bad blood." Despite claims that all participants (many of whom were illiterate) voluntarily consented to participate, it's clear that many did not understand the risks they were accepting or the alternatives in treating their disease. They were not told they had a disease that caused physical deterioration, insanity, and death. They were simply observed, for years, during which time they exposed untold numbers of other people to the disease. The study was officially discontinued in 1972, after most of the participants had died. When the public learned of this experiment, the outrage triggered new rules governing patient consent and regulation of clinical trials.

Despite rules to protect patients, including hospital internal review boards and federal regulations concerning signed consent forms and record-keeping requirements, occasional abuses continue.

Several ethical issues have to be addressed in order to protect patients enrolled in clinical trials. The following sections explain the various components of an ethical clinical trial.

Experimentation without informed consent

In the fall of 1991, hundreds of children on the Standing Rock Sioux Reservation brought home from school a form requesting permission for the children to receive two hepatitis A shots at school, one month apart. The shots were free, and participants received gifts. The form came from the "Hepatitis A Vaccine Prevention Program." It did not tell the parents that their children would be participating in an experimental research program for a vaccine—from a British pharmaceutical company—not approved by the FDA. The tribe felt misled, and relations with the health director (who had approved the study) grew strained. The trial was jointly sponsored by the Centers for Disease Control and the Indian Health Service. The vaccine was eventually determined to be safe.[1]

Informed consent

The opening line of the Nuremberg Code of 1946 is, "The voluntary consent of the human subject is absolutely essential." To give your voluntary consent, you must be fully informed of all potential benefits and risks. The U.S. Guidelines on Human Experimentation require:[2]

- A fair explanation of the procedures to be followed and their purposes, including identification of any procedures that are experimental.

- A description of any attendant discomforts and risks reasonably to be expected.

- A description of any benefits reasonably to be expected.

- A disclosure of any appropriate alternative procedures that might be advantageous for the subject.

- An offer to answer any inquiries concerning the procedures.

- An instruction that the person is free to withdraw his consent and to discontinue participation in the project or activity at any time without prejudice.

- That you do not waive, or appear to waive, any of your legal rights, or release the institution or its agents from liability for negligence.

A truly informed medical decision weighs the relative merits of a therapy after full disclosure of benefits, risks, and alternatives. During the discussions between the doctor(s) and patient, all questions should be answered in language that is clearly understood. There should be no pressure to enroll in the study.

> We had many discussions with the staff prior to signing the informed consent to participate in the clinical trial. We asked innumerable questions, all of which were answered in a frank and honest manner. We researched the previous studies, read the current medical literature, talked it over with physician friends, then made a final list of questions which took the oncologist over an hour to answer. He even pulled out medical texts to back up his answers. We ended up feeling that the trial presented the best chance for a cure, and we also felt good about contributing to knowledge that would help other patients later.

Evan Handler, a 24-year-old actor diagnosed with acute mylogenous leukemia, describes in *Time on Fire* how he was told about a proposed clinical trial at his first meeting with the oncologist:

> He dropped a heavy packet of pages on the meal table next to my breakfast. He took a deep breath, and while he scanned the room with his eyes, and touched and studied the cards and gifts left with me over the weekend, he said, "You'll be part of a randomized study. A computer has already selected a new, experimental treatment protocol for you. Half the patients on the study get the new protocol, the other half get the standard protocol. If you agree to be part of the study, you'll have to sign the informed-consent form I just gave you. If you don't sign it, then you'll automatically get the standard protocol." He took a pen from his shirt pocket, laid it on top of the pages he'd thrown down, and he stood still and looked at me for the first time.
>
> I was sure he was going to say more, but it turned out that he was done, so there was a very long pause. Finally, he said, "Feel free to read it if you want."
>
> ...He sighed deeply and, staring at the ceiling, he said, "We can't get started until you sign it, though."[3]

The above example is an abuse of the informed consent process. Patients, especially those making decisions after having just received a shattering diagnosis of a life-threatening disease, need time to read the information, discuss it with family members and the family physician, formulate questions, have those questions answered, then have time to think over the options.

You should be given the protocol—a lengthy, detailed document that includes the scientific objectives of the trial, a scholarly review of the scientific literature, and an exact treatment plan for patients. In reality, this document is not routinely handed out. Ask for it if it is not provided. You should also be given an informed consent document—listing possible benefits as well as side effects—to take home for thorough review before you sign. Don't be put off by the long list of potential side effects. More important is how common each side effect is versus the potential benefit from the treatment.

Most informed consent forms contain language similar to the following: "The study above has been described to me and I have read all of the information provided. I have had all of my questions answered, and understand that all future questions that I have about this research will be answered by the investigators listed above. I agree to participate in the study."

Doctor-patient issues

Many doctors are uncomfortable dealing with the issue of controversies in treatment, and some are reluctant to include patients in a frank discussion about the unknowns. Some doctors fear that admitting uncertainty undermines their authority. Others simply don't wish to dampen hope in the ultimate success of the proffered treatment plan. It is difficult to reassure patients if there is no clear best treatment for their illness.

Blending the roles of personal physician and research scientist can also be problematic. Some physicians feel that the rigid requirements of clinical trials hamper their ability to determine what is best for their patients. In some cases, physicians are accused of being unfeeling or lacking in compassion if they recommend enrollment in a clinical trial. On the other hand, if a doctor doesn't offer participation in clinical trials, a patient might feel that he isn't getting the best medicine has to offer. In an effort to understand physicians' views on these issues, researchers conducted a questionnaire survey assessing physicians' reasons for not entering patients in a randomized clinical trial for breast cancer. The following reasons were given:[4]

- Concern that the doctor-patient relationship would be affected by a randomized clinical trial (73 percent).

- Difficulty with informed consent (38 percent).

- Dislike of open discussions involving uncertainty (22 percent).

- Perceived conflict between the roles of scientist and clinician (18 percent).

- Practical difficulties in following procedures (9 percent).

- Feelings of personal responsibility if the treatments were not found to be equal (8 percent).

These complicated dynamics can be resolved only by genuine conversation. The doctor needs to present the trial, give the reasons for its design, and thoroughly discuss its similarities and deviations from standard treatment. Then all of your questions must be answered. Any requested documentation, such as previous studies or the entire study document, must be made available.

Valid scientific hypothesis

A new therapy should always have the potential to be less toxic and/or more effective than the standard treatment. A specific question (a hypothesis) should be posed that the trial will answer. The investigators who design the trial, and all scientific reviewers, should agree that the answer to the question being posed is unknown and that the study is designed to make a reliable answer likely. Through laboratory and animal studies, scientists should be able to honestly state that the experimental arm of the proposed trial is not known to be better or worse than the standard.

The trial must have clearly defined objectives and endpoints based on a rational hypothesis. During the informed consent process, ask what the objectives and endpoints are by saying something like, "What is the study hypothesis, when will the study end, and under what conditions will the study be terminated?"

One doctor explains why she refused to refer patients to a particular study for ethical reasons.

> There was a study at a university where I worked that I did not approve of. They were signing people up to use a new, more expensive drug to treat uncomplicated first urinary tract infections. I thought the

drug company was just trying to collect data to use in their advertising for this new, expensive drug when we already had a cheap, effective treatment. I didn't want to be involved.

Plans to modify the experiment

The ethical and legal codes governing medical practice also apply to clinical trials. All clinical trials must be approved by the institutional review board or ethics committee of the hospital in which the treatment is given. These boards, whose purpose is to protect citizens, are made up of scientists, doctors, and sometimes clergy or citizens from the community. In addition, most research is federally funded and regulated, with rules to protect patients.

Large research groups also have review boards that meet at prearranged dates for the duration of the trial to ensure that the risks of all parts of the trial are acceptable relative to the benefits. If one portion ("arm") of the trial is causing unexpected or unacceptable side effects, or appears to be less effective, that portion will be terminated, and the patients enrolled will be given the better treatment. Conversely, if one arm proves to be better than the standard, the trial is terminated and all patients are put on the superior treatment. Your informed consent document should contain language similar to the following: "You will be notified if significant new findings become known that may affect your willingness to continue in the study."

My daughter was enrolled in a trial which attempted to lessen neurotoxicity of leukemia treatment by replacing cranial radiation with higher doses of chemotherapy injected into the cerebrospinal fluid. A few years into the trial, the committee met and discovered a twofold increase in mortality on the experimental arm. That arm was terminated, and the children who had not received cranial radiation were recalled to get it.

What is standard treatment?

Standard treatment is the most effective known treatment for a specific condition or disease. As results from ongoing and completed clinical trials are analyzed, knowledge is accumulated and standard treatments evolve. For decades, women with breast cancer underwent a radical mastectomy, which removed not only the breast, but the muscle underneath as well. In the

1980s, several randomized clinical trials comparing lumpectomy and radiation to radical mastectomy discovered that women with Stage I or II breast cancer do just as well with breast-conserving surgery and radiation. In 1990, the National Institutes of Health endorsed breast-conserving surgery as the preferred treatment for patients with Stage I or II breast cancer. The standard treatment had changed based on the results from clinical trials.

Some clinical trials divide patients into two or more groups (called arms). In these trials, one arm of the trial is the standard treatment, and the other arms are the experimental portions—which scientists hope will prove more effective or less toxic than the standard treatments. In others, the arms compare different standard treatments to resolve any controversies over which one is better.

An example of a trial with two arms is the following study.

Chilly clinical trial improves outcomes for the brain injured

A University of Pittsburgh research team reported its findings from a small clinical trial involving brain injured patients. Eighty-two patients who were in comas from falls, traffic accidents, assaults, and other incidents received standard treatment for their brain injury. Half of the patients were also cooled to a body temperature of 32 to 33 C. degrees for 24 hours. The patients who were unresponsive to pain did not benefit from the cooling, but patients who still responded to pain while in the coma showed much improvement. Six months after being injured, 73 percent of the patients who had been cooled were able to live independently, while only 35 percent of those who received just standard treatment were able to do so.[5]

Types of clinical trials

There are many different kinds of clinical trials, ranging from evaluations of ways to prevent, diagnose, or treat illnesses to the effect of psychological interventions such as visualization or support groups on the progression of disease. Most clinical trials are divided into three phases.

Phase I trials

Phase I trials last only a few days to a few weeks. These studies are the first to take place on humans after results in the laboratory on cells and animals prove promising. The purpose of a Phase I study is to determine safe dosage levels or the best method of delivering the treatment to the patient.

Phase I clinical trials usually involve small numbers of patients (typically 20 to 80 volunteers). Patients with life-threatening diseases sometimes enroll in Phase I studies if no effective treatments are available. In other cases, such as testing new drugs for common ailments, healthy volunteers are recruited.

If the study is evaluating a drug, each patient in the first small group receives a low dose of the drug, and those in the next group each receive a slightly higher dose. Each individual patient receives only one dose. Because treatments in Phase I trials have been tested only in laboratories and on animals, the effects on humans are unknown and can be dangerous.

On average, very few patients with life-threatening illnesses are cured by Phase I trials, but occasionally, patients have dramatic responses. The patients who do not directly benefit from the Phase I treatment are contributing to cures in the future.

Phase II trials

After the maximum dosage or best method of administration is established in a Phase I trial, a Phase II trial is designed to find out whether the new treatment actually stops or slows the progression of disease in humans. For cancer patients, enrollment is limited to small numbers of patients with "measurable" disease, e.g., a tumor with clear margins whose shrinkage is able to be accurately recorded. When a tumor gets smaller, and stays smaller for a month, the patient is considered to have "responded" to the study. If at least 20 percent of the participants in a Phase II study respond to the treatment, the treatment is classified as active against that specific tumor type. Each Phase II study uses patients with the same type of cancer, but there can be several Phase II trials at the same time using the treatment against several different cancers. In addition to monitoring for effectiveness against tumors, Phase II trials record and assess side effects.

> My brother was diagnosed with pancreatic cancer on his fifty-fourth birthday. In this country today, pancreatic cancer is usually a death sentence. In addition to providing emotional support, I have tried to help by searching the Internet for information on drugs and other treatment options. The Johns Hopkins Pancreatic Cancer Chat Room has a lot of information about conventional, experimental, and alternative treatments. This is where I learned about 9-NC, a drug made from the bark of

a tree grown in China. The FDA approved Phase II clinical trials for 9-NC, but it is only available at a facility in Houston. Several families with loved ones using 9-NC shared their experiences in the Chat Room, so we had some idea as to their progress, symptoms, etc. I gave all of this information to my brother and sister-in-law, who discussed it with their oncologists. His doctors felt that this treatment was worth considering because my brother was unlikely to be able to continue conventional treatment much longer. When my brother went to Houston to be evaluated, he was told that two-thirds of the patients in the experiment have either stabilized or improved. We are so grateful that he was accepted in the study and we have this additional source of hope!

If the results from a Phase II study look promising, a duplicate study is initiated to confirm the results. These duplicate studies are a good bet for patients who have not responded to standard therapies and are looking for additional options, or for those needing initial therapy if no effective treatment is known.

Phase III trials

Phase III clinical trials usually compare the standard treatment with promising treatments from Phase II studies for a specific disease or condition. In these studies there is usually one control group—those who are receiving the standard treatment—and one or more experimental groups. Phase III studies enroll large numbers of patients, from hundreds to thousands. The purpose of these large studies is to analyze in a statistically meaningful way whether the new treatment causes more cures, improves quality of life, lengthens remissions, or causes fewer short- and long-term side effects than the standard treatment. Follow-up should be sufficiently long to allow observation of delayed effects. The goal of a Phase III study is to show a tangible benefit to the patient. Studies can range from testing a new chemotherapy drug to comparing the effectiveness of horse chestnut extract with compression stockings for persons with varicose veins.[6]

My son was asked to participate in a Phase III study on a new epilepsy drug. He had tried every other drug on the market, none of which totally prevented his seizures, and all of which had side effects. The doctor pressured us to join the study, and my husband and I were initially willing. But then my son just didn't want to make the many trips to the doctor (120 miles away) that would have been required. He had already been in a three-year study for his leukemia, and the hospital was not a place where he wanted to spend more time. So we tried to get the drug without enrolling in the study. We were finally able to get it after much negotiating, and it dramatically reduced the seizures, but more importantly, did not cause drowsiness or inattentiveness.

Supportive care studies

Supportive care studies try to find better ways to handle side effects of treatment such as nausea, vomiting, or pain. Supportive studies that use drugs to treat these side effects are structured in Phases I, II, and III. Other studies look at the effect of adjuvant therapies—support groups, hypnosis, visualization—on treatment side effects.

> *Way back in 1967-1970, I worked as a supervisor at Children's Hospital in Los Angeles on the adolescent ward. (I am an R.N.) We began a very active project on our terminal patients utilizing test groups. One group received only the medical treatments, i.e., chemotherapy, transplants, drug intervention. The other group received all the same except we also practiced visualization techniques two days a week. We had two R.N.s, a social worker, a therapist, and a psychiatrist on the team. The visualization group lived longer, had higher incidence of remission and/or plateau rates, and generally felt better during their illness.*

Prevention and early detection studies

Prevention studies enroll people who are at high risk of developing a disease because several close relatives have the same disease. These studies usually compare a group of people who receive no special treatment with those who change diet, lifestyle, or take a specific drug to lessen the chances of developing the illness. Prevention studies last for many years, sometimes decades.

An example of a prevention trial using dietary modification is the National Cancer Institute's Polyp Prevention Trial.

Dietary modification trial

The design of the trial is as follows:

Study design: Randomized multi-center, four-year trial.

Sample size: 2,000 males/females.

Eligibility: Older than 35 years, one or more adenomatous polyps

Hypothesis: To determine whether a low-fat, high-fiber diet, as compared with the U.S. customary diet, will reduce the recurrence rate of adenomatous polyps.

Dietary goals: 20 percent of total calories as fat; 18 grams dietary fiber per 1,000 calories.[7]

Early detection studies also use persons at high risk for developing a particular disease. These studies assess various methods of early detection such as periodic X rays, examinations, or blood tests.

I'm in a study to see if diet can help prevent or delay a recurrence of breast cancer. There are three arms: in the first arm, the participants eat seven fruits and vegetables a day and less than 20 percent fat; in the second, participants eat five fruits and vegetables a day and less than 30 percent fat; and in the third arm, there are no diet changes at all. At the beginning of the study, they did blood work and took various measurements of our bodies. Over the eight-year study we will attend cooking classes, have a nutritionist on call to answer any questions, and have periodic checkups.

Every clinical trial has specific eligibility requirements—necessary for scientific accuracy—that limit enrollment. Examples of such restrictions are age, type and extent of disease, amount and type of previous treatment, and other medical conditions. Often patients have some organ (liver, heart, lung, kidney) dysfunction or previous treatment that disqualifies them from participation in a clinical trial.

What is randomization?

An unbiased Phase III study often requires a process called randomization—when a computer randomly assigns a patient to one of the arms of the study. The patient will not know which of the arms (one standard care, two experimental) he will receive until the computer assigns one. One group of patients (the control group) always receives the standard treatment to provide a basis for comparison to the experimental arms. Because neither the physician nor the patient chooses the treatment option, a comparable mix of patients is assured.

> We had a hard time deciding whether to go with the standard treatment or to participate in the study. The "B" arm of the study seemed, on intuition, to be too harsh for her because she was so weak at the time. We finally did opt for the study, hoping we wouldn't be randomized to "B." We chose the study basically so the computer could choose and we wouldn't ever have to think "we should have gone with the study." As it turned out, we were randomized to the standard arm, so we got what we hoped for while still participating in the study.

At the time the clinical trial is designed, there is no conclusive evidence to indicate which arm will prove superior. It is not possible to predict if the patient will benefit from participating in the study. However, there may be significant differences between the arms in length of treatment, toxicity of treatment, and amount of time spent in the hospital. Patients may have a legitimate preference for one arm over the other, and may be able to get the treatment off protocol or in a Phase II trial rather than a Phase III trial.

Costs of clinical trials

In the current climate of cost consciousness, who pays for treatment of patients enrolled in clinical trials is a contentious issue. In the past, insurers paid for patient care costs such as hospitalization, diagnostic tests, physician's fees, and supplies. Experimental drugs for patients enrolled in trials were usually paid for by the National Institutes of Health or pharmaceutical companies. Currently, many insurance plans and HMOs are using more restrictive guidelines and payment schedules, and funding for patients participating in clinical trials is becoming increasingly difficult to obtain. These new policies serve as a deterrent to patients, limit the number of people who enroll in trials, and slow advancement toward more effective treatments. In fact, attempts are being made to roll back federal funding and regulation of the trials themselves.

> I received some very disquieting news today when talking with one of the bone marrow transplant (BMT) doctors at a famous cancer institute. They just received a policy statement from a large insurance provider

stating that it will no longer pay for BMTs for chronic lymphocytic leukemia (CLL). This is a change because it has paid for CLL BMTs in the past.

It strikes me that we again have an insurance company playing doctor. Medical treatment belongs in the hands of the doctors, not in the bottom line of some untrained bureaucrat playing God.

In studies sponsored by pharmaceutical companies, some or all of the costs to the patient, such as the drugs, doctor visits, tests, and travel, may be covered. Treatment at the National Institutes of Health in Bethesda, Maryland, is free. In some clinical trials, costs of research-related injuries are also paid. Before enrolling in a clinical trial, it is important to have in writing what costs will be covered by your insurance as well as the sponsoring company. It is also wise to clarify who will pay for medical care needed if treatment-related injuries occur.

Locating and researching clinical trials

Your disease or condition determines how and where to find information on clinical trials. Usually, a combination of networking—with patients and researchers—as well as searching the scientific literature uncovers all available choices. The following are steps to take to locate and research trials.

- Ask your specialist if she knows of any trials for your disease or condition.

- Ask your family doctor the same question.

- If there is an organization that advocates for your illness, e.g., the American Parkinson Disease Association or the American Heart Association, call and ask them for any information on clinical trials. Appendix C contains lists of organizations for specific diseases.

- If you personally know or know of any physicians who specialize in your condition or disease, call them, briefly describe your situation, and ask if they know of any ongoing or planned trials. National organizations for illnesses often have scientific advisory panels composed of specialists in your condition.

- The Pharmaceutical Research and Manufacturers of America publishes a brochure called "New Medicines in Development" that describes ongoing research into specific diseases. To get a copy, call (202) 835-3450 or write to PhRMA at 1100 15th St. NW, Suite 900, Washington, DC 20005.

- Call nearby medical schools or teaching hospitals and ask to be put on their mailing list. Their newsletters often contain information about clinical trials available at the institution.

- If you have access to the Internet (or have a friend or family member who does), read Steve Dunn's article, "Finding Clinical Trials on the Net" at *http://www.cancerguide.org/clinical_trials.html*.

- For those of you with cancer, the National Cancer Institute (NCI) has created a computer database about cancer and clinical trials called Physician's Data Query (PDQ). PDQ is updated frequently, and will provide both you and your doctor with information on state-of-the-art treatment for your disease, as well as list all trials being offered in the U.S. You will also find the names of the doctors running the trials as well as the hospitals treating patients on the trials. PDQ information can be obtained by calling the Cancer Information Service at 1-800-4-CANCER or on the Internet at *http://cancernet.nci.nih.gov/*. You can also get PDQ statements on your fax machine. Call (301) 402-5874 and request, by pressing a number, the codes for cancer types. Call back, enter the correct code, and you will receive the information by fax. Other than your long distance charge, there is no fee.

- Since much of the research in the U.S. is funded by the federal government, those of you with Internet access could start your research by checking the National Institutes of Health site at *http://cancernet.nci.nih.gov/trials/*. This site contains lists of all the clinical trials funded by the federal government.

- CenterWatch—a private company that collects information on clinical trials—can provide a variety of information about clinical trials sponsored with private and corporate (non-NIH) money. They can be contacted at (617) 247-2327, on the Internet at *http://www.centerwatch.com*, or by email at *Cntrwatch@aol.com*.

- The National Cancer Institute has a wealth of information at their CancerNet web site: *http://www.icic.nci.nih.gov/*.

- Beware of being steered to a trial by just one doctor. Read the trial document yourself, and consider getting a second opinion prior to signing up. Researchers are often eager to enroll patients in their trials and may be biased.

Shortly after my MM (multiple myeloma) became more aggressive and I was re-hospitalized with another vertebral fracture, a local oncologist who also was associated with Memorial Sloan Kettering was called in on my case. She tried to enroll me in a trial of VAD (a type of combination chemotherapy) with a bone marrow transplant to follow. She said it had a very good response rate and that it would probably heal my bone lesions and that this was discussed in the informed consent. She said that I had an 85 percent chance of a cure (I learned later through research that this type of transplant in MM patients has mortality rates approaching 50 percent). She started ordering the tests I would need to go through the chemotherapy before I said yes or had read the informed consent. She kept talking about the informed consent and the journal articles that would back up her claims, but she never produced any of them. Ultimately I put my foot down and said no, and she said, "This is your best bet." She then spent an hour and a half telling my husband how sick I was and that I really needed to receive this treatment. That was five years ago, and I have treated my disease quite successfully with a combination of chemotherapy, herbs, exercise, good nutrition, and acupuncture.

Questions to ask

Prior to asking the following questions, have your doctor describe all studies available for your illness or condition, not only at the institution where you are treated, but anywhere in the country. Get copies of both the entire protocol and the abbreviated patient version for all of these studies and read as much as you can. You might also want to ask friends with medical or science backgrounds to interpret and discuss the information. Discuss any questions you have with the doctor offering the trial as well as your family doctor. To fully understand any clinical trial, the following are suggested questions to ask your doctor or the person(s) who designed the trial:

- What is the purpose of the study?
- Who is sponsoring the study? Who reviews it? How often is it reviewed? Who monitors patient safety?
- What tests and treatments will be done during the study?

- Why is it thought that the treatment being studied is potentially better than standard treatment?

- What is the prior data on this therapy so far? Has it been tested in humans or only on animals? If humans, has it been tested in humans with my disease? What were the results?

- What are the possible benefits?

- What are the possible disadvantages?

- What are all of the potential short-term and long-term side effects of the study? Which side effects are frequent and which are rare? Compare the side effects of the study with those from standard care.

- How will the study affect my daily life?

- How long will the study last? Is this longer or shorter than standard treatment?

- Will participation in the study mean that I will have to change physicians?

- Will the study require more hospitalization than standard treatment?

- What will be my costs for participating in the study?

- Does the study include long-term follow-up care?

- What happens if I am harmed as a result of the study? Who pays for any care that I might need?

- Have insurers been reimbursing for care under this protocol?

- What will be my out-of-pocket costs for the study versus standard treatment?

Pros and cons of clinical trials

After completing your research and having all of your questions answered, it may be helpful to consider the following lists of pros and cons prior to making a decision.

Pros

- Patients receive either the state-of-the-art investigational therapy or the best standard therapy available.

- It can provide an opportunity to benefit from a new therapy before it is generally available.

- Information gained from clinical trials may benefit future patients with your illness or condition.
- Patients enrolled in clinical trials may be monitored more frequently than those receiving the standard treatment.
- Doctors participating in clinical trials tend to be up to date on the latest medical advances.
- Review boards of scientists oversee the operation of the clinical trial.
- Participation in a clinical trial returns some control to patients and sometimes helps them feel that they did everything medically possible for their illness.
- Some clinical trials provide treatment and follow-up care free of charge.

Cons

- The dose of a drug in the early stages of a Phase I trial may be too low to be of therapeutic value.
- Many patients in Phase I and Phase II studies do not benefit from the treatment.
- The experimental arm of a Phase III trial may not provide treatment as effective as the standard or it may generate unexpected side effects or risks.
- Not all patients in a Phase III study receive the new treatment.
- In some studies, patients in one arm receive a placebo.
- Some clinical trials require more hospitalizations, treatments, or clinic visits than standard treatment.
- Insurance may not cover the patient costs or drugs used in the study.

In science, some experiments succeed, while others fail. If you are in the market for a more effective or less toxic treatment, a trial might provide you with the very newest treatment, or it might prove ineffective. In either case, it will give you hope for a better future, satisfaction that you did everything you could to find the best treatments, and knowledge that you helped the patients of the future. Even if you decide not to enroll in a trial, you will learn a great deal about your condition by exploring the newest research options available.

When I was struggling with the decision of whether to join the study, I asked the oncologist how I would ever know if I had made the right decision. He said, "You will never know, and you should never second-guess yourself, no matter how the study turns out. Statistics are about large groups of people, not you. You might relapse no matter what arm you are on, or you might be cured on an arm where most of the other patients relapse. Statistics for you will be either 100 percent or 0 percent, because you will either live or die. I can't tell you which will be the better treatment, that is why we are conducting the study. But no matter what, we will be doing absolutely the best we can."

CHAPTER 13

Researching the Medical Literature

An education isn't how much you have committed to memory, or even how much you know. It's being able to differentiate between what you do know and what you don't.

—Anatole France

NEWLY PUBLISHED MEDICAL TEXTBOOKS are typically two or more years behind the latest medical information and research findings. More than three thousand medical journals, written by and for doctors and scientists, present the most recent innovations. Busy clinicians cannot possibly keep up with this volume of new information. You, however, can access and learn the very newest information about one narrow slice of medicine—your diagnosis. This chapter will introduce you to basic methods to conduct a search for useful information and how to use that knowledge, in partnership with your doctor, to make sound medical decisions.

Should you research?

It used to be that patients took their doctor's advice without a second thought. More and more, people are getting involved in researching their own condition and being more active in the decision-making process. The following are some reasons for researching your condition.

- **Save your life or parts of your body.** No doctor, no matter how dedicated, can keep up on all the newest research in his or her field. With almost a half million technical papers published yearly, it is impossible to read all of the latest scientific findings. You even have an advantage over your doctor—you have only one disease to learn about, and you may also be motivated to devote a large chunk of time to the effort. Patients with rare disorders or diseases for which there is a lot of current research may uncover options that their doctors simply don't know about. If you are insured by an HMO, you have particular reason to put in the effort to learn of the newest treatments. Some HMOs require that their physicians tell you only about treatments for which the HMO will pay.

The OB/GYN who had delivered both of my children mentioned in a routine exam that I had fibroid tumors. I had no symptoms, but he told me that I would need a hysterectomy. The years passed and the tumors grew quite large, but I still had no symptoms. At a yearly exam, he told me that I would need a hysterectomy soon. I still did not understand why. This doctor mentioned in passing a new, less invasive tumor-removal procedure than a hysterectomy, an "electrolysis" using laparoscopy. I searched bookstores, libraries, and the Internet and found some information on fibroids, but none on alternatives to hysterectomy.

I did not want a hysterectomy and I was not convinced that I needed one. And I was not sure that the new "electrolysis" procedure was even a valid option. I decided to get the opinion of a woman doctor. This new doctor had not heard of the new procedure. She felt I needed a hysterectomy, and she said: "I never think about my womb during the day. I wouldn't miss it, neither would you." By this time, I was developing quite heavy menstrual bleeding and becoming convinced that I did need to do "something" about the fibroids. About this time, a woman friend mailed me a clipping of an article about the new electrolysis procedure, which had been printed in the newspaper of a large city.

Still unhappy with my options, I went to a third doctor, again a woman. This woman listened to me and respected my feelings. We discussed the tumors in scientific detail (I'm a chemist) as well as my emotional response to the idea of a hysterectomy. I love this doctor! We ended up deciding to remove the tumors, but not by a hysterectomy. We discussed the article from the newspaper and she agreed to try the electrolysis procedure, as it used techniques with which she was already proficient. During our discussions, we agreed that once the surgery was in progress, if she couldn't remove the fibroids by electrolysis, she would do a myomectomy, wherein she would open as for a C-section and remove the fibroids only: not the uterus. As it turned out, a myomectomy was what she ended up doing. It's been a year and a half since the procedure and I am thrilled with the results.

- **Take back some control.** Ill people typically feel that their lives have spun out of control, that they are powerless to affect their fate. However, researching your medical condition can help reverse this process. You will have a goal on which to focus, and can work diligently to help regain your health. Often, entire families join in the effort to learn of the best options for care. Active participation, rather than passive acceptance, has even been shown clinically to enhance your chances for a longer and healthier life.

I know that some people aren't interested in ingesting gobs of polysyllabic medical jargon, especially when they're in those first horrendous days after diagnosis, but for me information has always been the key to avoiding depression and helplessness when facing a scary medical situation. I remember being enormously frustrated after my first child, Nate, was born with an arrhythmia, near death, and I was trapped in the hospital after a rough C-section with a patronizing doctor and no access to a library! I can only imagine how much different the experience and my interactions with doctors would have been had I been able to have my laptop and modem with me there eight years ago, researching away like I did during all of Joseph's hospitalizations this past year!

- **Enhance the quality of your life**. Often in the heat of the moment, decisions are made to save a life without much weight given to the quality of that life. Researching your condition enables you to understand all of the possible short- and long-term side effects from your menu of options. Only you can evaluate all of the information in light of your values and goals and make the best decision for your unique situation.

I wish I had been more aggressive in finding out the effect of removing many lymph nodes for "staging" as part of my cancer surgery; I don't have lymphedema, but I am concerned that I might one day have it. I don't know if I would have done anything differently, but I feel like I focused too much on "save my life" and "hurry along" and not enough on quality-of-life issues.

- **Make informed decisions**. A thorough review of the literature will give you knowledge of the disease itself as well as all treatment options and any treatment controversies. It will allow you to separate fact from opinion. You will have the basis for asking pertinent and probing questions. After your research, you can discuss your situation with your doctor as a knowledgeable colleague rather than a passive recipient of decisions.

I am embarrassed to admit this now that I have learned better, but I used to think that my doctor was the ultimate authority. I just wasn't raised to think that doctors are fallible or that they should be questioned. I simply went and told them what was wrong, they told me what to do about it, and I did it. No questions asked. I reacted, at first, the same way when I heard my daughter's Wilms' diagnosis. When we got to the children's hospital, the doctor said this is the way it is and this is what we are going to do about it. I just did what I was told. It was only after I met another Wilms' mom and we compared notes that were very different from each other (her daughter was the same age, the same diagnosis, treated at the same time, but at a different facility) that I began to question. I was ignorant enough to think that any treatment was similar, say, to treatment for strep throat. You are diagnosed, there is a set procedure to follow to get rid of it, and everyone is on the same wavelength and in agreement that it is just what is done. Although I have learned better and now research things for myself, I don't think I am alone in my initial type of attitude/response.

- **Reassure self and family that the treatment decision is the best choice**. Unless you have a life-threatening emergency, there is always time to do basic research and get thorough answers to all of your questions. Most people need time to reassure themselves and their families that the recommendations are reasonable and not based on profit (cheaper for the HMO to do nothing than provide a bone marrow transplant), personal opinion (your doctor has been doing it that way for years and isn't interested in innovative options), or difference in philosophy (your doctor wants to stop treatment while you want aggressive care).

While there are numerous reasons for fully understanding your condition and your options for treating it, there are also good reasons why you might want to restrict your research to particular areas, get a friend or family member to help, or not research at all. Following are possible reasons for not researching your condition or evaluating only selected topics.

- **Research is time-consuming**. Especially if your condition is not life-threatening, you might prefer to accept the recommendation of a doctor you trust and reap the benefits of spending your time doing something you enjoy.

  One Easter Sunday morning, I fell and hit my knees on the cement. After the injury healed on the outside, it still hurt on the inside. My internist sent me for X rays and told me it was arthritis. He sent me to a sports physical therapy center where I used machines to work on my knees. They also used heat and light therapies. I started attending water exercise classes three days a week. My doctor gave me different pills to try, but the knees kept hurting. When he gave me dolobid, the pain was gone. I never felt the need to do any research because he was trying different therapies until we found something that I could live with. After he retired, I did ask my new doctor if there was a different drug available that would be as effective, but not as risky for my liver. He suggested that I cut the dose in half to see if it would control the pain as well, and it does.

- **Fear and intimidation**. Wading through technical literature can be intimidating, and for some people the jargon creates additional fear of the illness. However, most people armed with determination and a good medical dictionary rapidly become adept at tracking down information and interpreting it correctly. As with any new language, at first scientific terms may seem strange, but they soon become second nature. In addition, many books and articles are written in lay language—you can start with these.

   I feared taking the time to do the research—I wanted to move on as quickly as possible. It's hard to be confronted with a life-threatening disease and proceed in a leisurely way. It's hard to fight against the impulse to take action, any action. You can also be intimidated by family members or doctors who want you to do what you are told. It's difficult sometimes to buck the expectation of being a "good patient."

- **Dealing with statistics**. Reading dismal statistics can plunge you into despair, whereas discovering positive statistics can give you hope. You need to make sure that you correctly interpret whatever statistics you encounter. Are they based on a small number of patients (small sample size), persons representing your exact condition (age, sex, level of disease), and the most current data? Any of these can skew the numbers so that they are not applicable to your particular situation. If you have access to the Internet, read Stephen Jay Gould's "The Median Isn't the Message" (*http://www.cancerguide.org/median_not_msg.html*) to help you interpret statistics. And above all else, remember that you are not a number—if you are among the 10 percent who are cured, then the statistical chance for survival for you was 100 percent.

   It's terribly difficult reading the cold, hard facts. You are described as a speck, a disease, a clinical morbidity.

- **Confronting ambiguity**. Many patients just want to know "what's going to happen" and have terrible difficulty accepting that the doctor often can't tell them with certainty what is best. Reading scientific papers brings this point home clearly: many experts disagree—sometimes vehemently. You will need to get past the sometimes frightening thought that the experts might know what is best for large groups of patients, but not for one person—you. You are the only person who can take facts and filter them through your personal philosophy, values, and family situation to choose the best path for you.

- **Misunderstanding**. You run a risk when researching your own condition that you might be blinded by your own emotion or misunderstand the facts due to lack of a frame of reference. It's very important to verify all medical information with multiple sources, then take any questions or confusions to your doctor for discussion. Ideally, your doctor should have a wealth of experience treating patients with your condition and a lifetime of learning how to interpret scientific information. Talk it over with her.

  I am very much in support of utilizing well-documented research to guide my treatment decisions. My husband and I spent considerable amounts of time reading journals and gathering statistical data when I was diagnosed. But we also spent a great deal of time soliciting opinions from all the doctors he works with, and ever worked with, because a clinician's experience and assessment based on having seen hundreds of patients is invaluable. A doctor may have seen this outcome, this pattern, this complication in many of his patients before. On the other hand, I have brought studies to the attention of my doctors which they have not yet seen—so we shouldn't assume that their clinical experience is sufficient, either! I think we should make use of clinical experiences/expertise as well as clinical studies, always knowing that neither of them is likely to be 100 percent accurate.

- **Realizing that there are no better options**. Often what prods patients to explore the literature is the hope for a better option to provide relief with the least impact on quality of life. If the research clearly supports embarking on a difficult treatment, it may be a hard thing to face. On the other hand, establishing that the treatment recommended is the best that medicine has to offer can go a long way toward increasing your comfort level.

  I think that knowing there are no better options is a plus. I wanted to do enough research to convince myself that what was being recommended was the best option. If I had found otherwise, my spirits would have dropped like a stone: that would have meant I had to do a lot more directing my own care—changing doctors, more research, probably travel farther, etc. Instead, I learned what was proposed by my doctor was a state-of-the-art treatment, and I felt reassured.

Setting goals

The first step before actual research is to learn about your own condition. From your doctor or specialist you should obtain a diagnosis (or list of symptoms if no diagnosis has been made), a copy of your pathology report (if any), results of all tests, and copies of your entire medical record. You are legally and ethically entitled to all of these documents, but you may have to pay photocopying costs.

> *I've long been an advocate of patient access to medical records, and have always obtained copies of all my treatment records (as well as records for my family members). And I've routinely provided copies of these records to health care providers as appropriate. I might add in this respect that some of the most enthusiastic recipients of copies have been anesthesiologists to whom I have given copies of previous anesthesia reports. They have all told me that they find these reports invaluable and wish all patients would provide them for review.*

If you encounter difficulties getting copies of any medical records, ask anyone you know who is a doctor (Ph.D., dentist, naturopath, chiropractor) to request your records. Usually, the hospital or doctor's office will send them free of charge to another doctor. If you still can't get them, read *Medical Records: Getting Yours*, listed in the *Suggested Reading* at the end of the book.

Some suggested initial research goals are:

* **Find out the standard of care for your illness or condition**. Often, there is an accepted method of treating each illness that competent medical professionals use. To learn if such a standard exists for your situation, call and ask the appropriate academy (listed in Appendix B, *American Boards of Medical Specialties*). For example, if you have kidney stones, call the American Board of Urology and ask to be sent a copy of the treatment guidelines for kidney stones (this information was also published in the *Journal of Urology*, November 1997). For cancer, the standards of care are listed in the PDQ (Physician's Data Query) database at *http://pdqsearch@icicc.nci.nih.gov/*.

- **Find out if there are any controversies in treatment**. Medical journals, and sometimes the popular press, print articles outlining any controversies of treatment. Recent review articles in technical journals are your best bet for an overview of the standard of care for specific conditions. Remember, however, that review articles typically summarize information available two or more years prior to their publication.

  The first place I went after my daughter was diagnosed with cancer was the public library. I soon realized that the books were out of date almost as soon as they were published. I recommend going to a university medical library.

- **Find out the top doctors and treatment centers for your specific illness**. If you require a specialized treatment or surgery, it would not be in your best interest to go to a center that had never done this procedure, or that had a low success rate or an extremely high infection rate. Organizations listed in Appendix C, *Sources of Information on Specific Medical Conditions*, can help you find expert specialists. Also, a company called Best Doctors Worldwide helps patients locate the top physicians, hospitals, and treatment plans available. They can be contacted by phone at 1-800-675-1199, or read about their opinions in the reference book *Best Doctors in America*.

- **Locate disease associations**. Many national associations provide not only factual information, but great emotional support as well. Some groups match persons in similar circumstances who then communicate through letters, phone calls, or email.

- **Find where you can get emotional support from others who have "been there."** Locating people in similar circumstances either through local groups or online communities can provide tremendous reassurance and help. An added benefit is that you may actually get well faster and stay healthy longer if you feel supported. Numerous studies clearly show that emotional support translates into longer and higher quality lives. David Speigel's book *Living Beyond Limits* explores these issues. How to locate these organizations is discussed later in this chapter.

- **Investigate complementary therapies**. Complementary therapies can be used to supplement and enhance Western treatments and deal with underlying conditions (such as poor diet or stress) that contribute to illness. Michael Lerner's book *Choices in Healing* gives a balanced presentation of many complementary therapies.

Getting started

Now that you have identified your goals and are ready to dive into the literature, where do you start?

Buy a good medical dictionary

Whether you are starting from scratch or have a working knowledge of medicine, it's always helpful to own a good quality medical dictionary. Try to look at several before you make a choice. A few have excellent illustrations, others use clear language, and some use very small print and exclusively medical terminology. Five useful ones are *The Bantam Medical Dictionary*, *Dorland's Illustrated Medical Dictionary*, *The HarperCollins Illustrated Medical Dictionary*, *Mosby's Medical Dictionary*, and *Taber's Cyclopedic Medical Dictionary*. Investing in a good dictionary is money well spent as you will return to it again and again. If you need more in-depth information than the dictionary provides, consult *Principles of Anatomy and Physiology*, eighth edition, by G. J. Totora, New York: HarperCollins, 1996.

Read the Merck Manual

Whatever your diagnosis, *The Merck Manual of Diagnosis and Therapy* will explain it thoroughly, albeit in technical language. This comprehensive volume of most medical disorders can be found in libraries and on the Internet at *http://www.merck.com*. It explores causes, symptoms, tests, diagnosis, treatment, and prognosis. The manual's index is thorough, so you will have no difficulty pinpointing the pages that cover your illness or condition. Merck recently published a lay version called *The Merck Manual of Medical Information: Home Edition*. It contains virtually all of the information from the technical version in easy-to-understand, everyday language. The overview you obtain from the Merck manual will help you to formulate questions that further research can answer.

Locate helpful organizations

Finding support organizations and others in similar situations can yield valuable knowledge as well as provide emotional support. Patient groups can be led by professionals (such as a social worker leading an emotional support group that meets at a hospital), can have professionals as resources (such as an M.D. who answers medical questions on an online mailing list), or can be made up entirely of patients who have been there (as in a local, peer-led support group). Patient groups can be primarily for emotional support (face-to-face meetings where patients come to terms with a diagnosis or treatments) or primarily for factual resources (a national patient association that disseminates information about a disease) or, most often, a mixture of emotional and factual resources. Patient support can be conducted in person, over the phone, through newsletters, at conferences, or over the Internet.

Suggested first steps to find a helpful organization are:

- Look through Appendix C at the end of this book.

- Find local support groups by asking your doctor, nurse, or hospital for recommendations. Check the list of support organizations in your local newspaper. If there is no group, or one that does not meet your needs, consider starting one.

- Refer to the *Self-Help Sourcebook: Finding and Forming Mutual Self-Help Groups*, published by the American Self-Help Clearinghouse, Northwest Covenant Medical Center, 25 Pocono Road, Denville, NJ 07834, (973) 625-7101. This resource contains the names, addresses, phone and fax numbers, and a short description of hundreds of self-help groups.

- Consult the *Encyclopedia of Associations* (Detroit: Gale Research) available at the reference desk in your local library. This three-volume set lists more than 23,000 national and international organizations.

- If none of the above list your illness, contact the National Organization for Rare Disorders (NORD), P.O. Box 8923, New Fairfield, CT 06812, 1-800-999-6673 or (203) 746-6518 (in Connecticut). NORD is a federation of thousands of individuals and professionals and more than 140 not-for-profit health organizations—each focusing on one or more rare diseases.

- Call the National Information Center for Orphan Drugs and Rare Diseases at 1-800-300-7469.

Support groups and organizations can provide practical and technical information, emotional support, connection with others with a similar condition, or political advocacy. Often, such groups publish newsletters and journals that discuss current medical studies, contain book reviews, organize pen pal services, and contain articles on the illness or related issues. If you find one or more appropriate organizations, write, call, fax, or email to ask them to send you all available information about your illness and related support organizations. In particular, ask if they have compiled a resource guide.

One morning when I was in my early twenties, I was watching Good Morning America while I got ready for work. They were reporting the death of Flo Hyman—women's volleyball silver medalist. The address for the National Marfan Foundation flashed up on the screen. It stopped me in my tracks. I scribbled it down and immediately contacted them. I went to the next annual meeting, and it was just incredible. I was in a room full of tall, skinny people who all looked just like me. Up until then I had never met a single living soul with Marfan syndrome.

I went around the room armed with a notebook, open ears, and an open mind. I asked them what medications (beta blockers) they were taking, if any, for mitral valve prolapse (a common heart problem for persons with Marfan) and to keep their blood pressure down. I also asked how they handled their scoliosis (curvature of the spine), and what routine testing they had done. If they lived in my area, I also asked for the names of their cardiologists and orthopedic surgeons, since it's reassuring to find doctors who treat patients with the same condition.

They had clinics there staffed by doctors who were the national experts in treating Marfan. I signed up for each one. It was an important piece of my research to see what each specialist had to say. It was the first time in my life that I received specific suggestions on what to avoid (contact sports) and what exercise was appropriate. Prior to this, I had merely been told, "Don't exert yourself, just do whatever's comfortable." As a result, I did hardly any physical activity so I was out of shape which was not good for my heart, either. I am also able to use the literature they provide to help negotiate with my doctors on frequency and types of testing I need.

I go to the annual meetings whenever possible and find them to be a wealth of technical and emotional support. For instance, I met a woman who recently had an aortic graft (which I may need at some point), and though she looked thin and fragile (an often typical look for a Marfan patient, whether you've had surgery or not), her attitude and emotional and physical energy were amazing. She told me that she had never felt better, that she was finally able to do everyday activities like walking up a flight of stairs without getting short of breath. She had only positive things to say, which really reassured me and encouraged me to view the outcome of the surgery as positive.

Support groups and discussion groups can also be found online. Refer to the section "Using the Internet" later in this chapter to learn how to find these groups.

Ask your family and friends to help

Friends and family members generally pitch in to help if asked. Some of the situations that make it difficult or impossible to research your condition by yourself are: when you are in the hospital, when you are stunned after receiving a diagnosis of a life-threatening or life-altering illness, or when you are too sick to muster the energy for reading. You may be surprised at the speed with which friends and family swing into action when they have a goal. Just ask—they may care desperately, but just not know what to do that truly helps.

> When my daughter was diagnosed with leukemia, I knew that I needed lots of information—fast—and I wasn't in a position to get it. So I talked a nurse into photocopying 12 copies of the proposed protocol and I sent it to my brother (a science professor), my sister (getting a graduate degree at Harvard), and ten friends who were doctors or married to doctors. I asked them all to send me abstracts from Medline searches on state-of-the-art treatment for childhood acute lymphoblastic leukemia. I asked the doctors to go to their chiefs of pediatric oncology with the long list I provided describing the medical particulars of my daughter's case, and ask them what they would do if she was their daughter.

> All ten chiefs said that the proposed protocol was developed by a cooperative group representing the best minds in pediatric oncology. They differed, however, on whether to use cranial radiation or increased chemotherapy. The numbers of opinions helped me to clarify the options. The pages and pages of abstracts supplied me with the newest research on the topic. After reviewing the abstracts, I would call my "troops" and ask them to find, copy, and send me specific journal articles to read. After a month of focused study (I was stuck in the hospital and couldn't sleep anyway) I knew quite a bit about the newest and most effective treatments for childhood leukemia. And I never set foot in a library.

Finding the experts

Information-seeking patients often go directly to the foremost experts in the field to hear the newest findings. You may get a chilly reception, but more often than not, the researcher will answer your questions or direct you to the most recent publications in your area of interest. Prepare well before you make contact to ensure your best chances of getting what you need. Write up a brief, clear description of your diagnosis or condition, and a short list of specific questions. Being respectful and concise will increase your chances of getting helpful information.

In some cases, patients even negotiate to send their records to the expert for a second opinion over the telephone, or they make arrangements to carry their records for an appointment in person. This is most common for rare, so-called orphan diseases, for which there are merely a few knowledgeable researchers and clinicians experienced in treating the disease. For any telephone conference or question-and-answer session, be prepared to pay for the physician's time. The following dialogue gives one possible approach:

Caller: Hello, Dr. Smith, thank you for taking my call. My name is Mr. Jones, and I was recently diagnosed with Marfan syndrome. Is this a convenient time for me to ask a few specific questions about your research?

Dr. Smith: Yes, but I have only about ten minutes before I am due in a meeting.

Caller: Thank you, I will be brief. I recently read your article in X journal on grafting aortic aneurysms. I have an aneurysm on the ascending aorta that is three centimeters in diameter. Are there current guidelines available or would you give your recommendations on the appropriate time to consider surgery?

Dr. Smith: I can't give you advice on your particular situation, but I'd be glad to tell you about existing opinions. As you probably know, there is a controversy concerning…[lengthy explanation follows].

Caller: Thank you for that helpful explanation. I know you also have a clinical practice. My doctor is recommending a yearly cardiac catheterization, but I have read that MRIs are just as effective and less likely to have side effects. I have a metal rod in my spine to correct my scoliosis. What do you recommend for your patients in this situation?

Dr. Smith: In my opinion…[lengthy explanation follows].

Caller: That is good information to hear. I especially appreciate the references to the current literature. I have just one more question. Do you have a printed list of yearly diagnostic tests that you recommend to your patients?

The caller was able to get useful information by being knowledgeable, concise, and polite. The expert responded favorably and provided some helpful suggestions. The following are several ways to locate experts.

- **Get abstracts from Medline or a similar computer database on your illness or condition**. Abstracts are available from the Internet, local library, or hospital library. You may need to go to a hospital or medical school library to pick out the full text of the articles you wish to read: The best are recent review articles (they discuss all of the current literature on a topic so you get an excellent overview) or the latest, most pertinent articles. If you are unable to visit a specialized library, call your regional library's interlibrary loan service and arrange to have the article sent to you. Professional journal articles list the institutions of the authors. Call information for the city involved (Cambridge, Massachusetts, for Harvard; Memphis, Tennessee, for St. Jude's) to get the telephone number for the university or hospital of the lead researchers. Then prepare your questions, and call the researcher.

> *When my son was diagnosed with histiocytosis, the fellow gave us research papers on the newest findings. I looked in the back of the papers and read which hospitals the authors worked at. I called information for the number of the hospital, and called and asked to speak to Dr. So & So. I almost always had to leave a message. Every doctor I ever called returned the call. I had all of my questions answered—and on their dime! I discovered that since it was an orphan disease, there was not much published, and the doctors did not have a very good network for sharing information. I was frequently showing my son's doctors new research information. So much so that it became embarrassing after a while. But our primary specialist, Dr. C., was always so open to new information and just a joy to work with.*

- **Look on the masthead of the literature from any disease-specific organizations you have contacted**. Often, the group lists a scientific advisory panel containing experts in the field. You can get their telephone numbers from the organization or by looking them up in the *American Medical Association (AMA) Directory of Physicians in the U.S.* at your local library.

- **Locate computer support groups dealing with your illness, and ask for names of experts**. To find these groups, refer to the section in this chapter called "How to find emotional support." It's perfectly acceptable to ask these groups for names of the foremost experts. If you put

"Medical" on the subject line of your email to the group, doctors that monitor the group are more likely to respond. The following is a response to a question about pancreatic cancer posed to a large Internet discussion group:

> *David, I don't know that much about your friend's particular situation. The best suggestion that I have is putting this information on the Johns Hopkins Chat Room at http://www.path.jhu.edu/pancreas then select "chat room." You can ask for private email responses, but chances are that others will post underneath your message. Tell your friend good luck, and congratulations for beating the doctors' prognosis!*

Using public libraries

Your local library is connected to a huge number of printed and electronic resources. Even if your library doesn't have the book or journal you want in their collection, most likely they can get it for you. Here are the basics for tapping into the vast wealth of material in the library system.

Finding a book

All of the books available in your local library will be listed in a card catalog or on a computer. If you do not know how to use these, ask the reference librarian to help you. You will be able to find out from the catalog or computer if the book is available in your local library or any of the branches in the system. If it is in the library, you can get it from the shelf. If you can't find it, tell the reference librarian and she will double-check, then put a trace on it. You will be notified when it is found.

If the book is in at another branch, you can either drive there to pick it up or put in a request to have it sent to your local library. Most library systems have a van that shuttles books between libraries, so it often takes only a few days to arrive. Some libraries give you the option of getting a phone call or a postcard to notify you when the book is available.

If the book has been checked out by someone else, ask the reference librarian to put it on reserve for you. When the book is returned, you will be notified to come pick it up. Libraries usually hold books for only a week, so it needs to be picked up promptly. If there are special circumstances, call and ask them to extend the hold. Unless another patron has a reservation on the book, they will continue to hold it until you can pick it up.

When I had severe back pain, with numbness down my leg, and my
doctor told me to keep up my normal levels of activity, I felt that I needed
to start reading. I went to the local library and got out seven books on
back pain. Two were very good—sort of walked you through the different
options from A to Z. Four were not as thorough or well written, but basically gave the same advice. So I was starting to think that what they outlined was the generally accepted treatment. One book, though, was off the
wall. It said that the pain was all in your head and the power of positive
thinking would cure it. That taught me to always read a range of material. I read enough so that I realized my doctor wasn't giving me good
advice, and I got a second opinion.

If the book you want is not in the collections of any of the libraries in the
system, ask the reference librarian to arrange an interlibrary loan. This
means that the library will borrow it from another library system for you.
You can even obtain medical texts from university or medical school libraries. Your local library will receive the book in the mail, and will call you or
send you a card to tell you of its arrival.

If the book is not available through interlibrary loan, you can ask the library
to purchase it for their collection. They will usually do this only if it has
been recently published, they have money budgeted for new purchases, and
they feel it will be useful to others.

Finding a magazine or journal article

Libraries usually have a computerized magazine/journal index that you can
search by topic. If, for instance, you want to find articles about diabetes in
lay magazines, enter "diabetes" on the subject line, and see what is available.
There should be clear directions posted on how to proceed.

If you are looking for a specific magazine, go to the area where the library
displays magazines (usually in alphabetical order). Often, the previous year's
monthly issues are stacked below the current issue. For an older issue of a
popular lay magazine, ask the reference librarian for its location. It may be
in the stacks (a sometimes nonpublic area of the library), on microfilm or
fiche, or in electronic form on a computer.

Public libraries sometimes stock well-known medical journals such as *The
Journal of the American Medical Association* and *The New England Journal of
Medicine*, although you will probably have to visit a specialized library to

find other medical journals. If the library has an Internet connection, you can go to *http://www.nlm.nih.gov* and find more than twenty-four medical journals online.

If you cannot locate a specific journal article in any of your local libraries, ask the reference librarian to arrange an interlibrary loan. He will check to see whether the journal is available from any of their sources. Usually, rather than sending you the journal through interlibrary loan, the library that owns the journal will make a copy of the requested article and send it to you in the mail. This may be a free or a fee service.

Never hesitate to consult the reference librarian if you have any questions or problems. They are typically very friendly people who genuinely like to help people find what they need.

Using a medical library

You can find technical information at medical school or hospital libraries. Large hospitals often have resource rooms, which contain nontechnical information, and libraries, which contain medical texts and journals. Medical school libraries usually have the largest and most comprehensive collections. To find the nearest medical library open to the public, call the National Network of Libraries of Medicine at 1-800-338-7657.

If the hospital library is closed to the public, you may still be able to use it. Just walk in, tell the librarian about your diagnosis, and ask to use the library. In the following story, a mother tells of how she worked around the rules:

> *When my daughter was critically ill, I really needed information to stay sane. I just walked into the hospital library and started searching for journals that contained articles I wanted to copy. I knew what articles I needed from relatives who had sent me lists of abstracts that they pulled off Medline. The librarian looked at me curiously, so I told her I had a sick child and needed information on which to base treatment decisions. I pulled out a stack of blank paper from my satchel, and said with a smile, "See, I didn't want to inconvenience you so I brought my own paper." She told me to go ahead. When taking magazines off the shelf, I always used the colored cardboard markers so that I wouldn't misfile a magazine when I returned it. I put my paper in their photocopy machine and used it to copy two stacks of articles—one for me and one for the doctor.*

Another patient turned to her doctor for help:

> Since my doctor's office is right next to the hospital library, I asked her if she could get me in. She talked to them, I was allowed in, and the librarian helped me quite a bit. Sweet-talking them helps.

Most medical libraries subscribe to computer services such as Medline or Grateful Med, which provide summaries of medical articles. Know the topics that you want to research, and ask the librarian to help you use the computer service. The machine will print out a list of abstracts (a paragraph summarizing the information contained in the article) dealing with the requested topic. After reviewing the list, choose the articles that you would like to read, and ask the librarian to help you locate the correct issue of each journal. Rather than feeding dimes (or quarters) into their copy machine, ask if they have a card that can be purchased at a discount for quantity copying.

If the library does not have Medline or a similar computer database, ask the librarian to show you how to use the Index Medicus, a print index to the world's biomedical literature. It is published monthly by the National Library of Medicine and indexes articles from more than three thousand journals.

Using a university library

If you live closer to a university library than a medical library, call the librarian to ask if they subscribe to Medline or other medical databases. Ask if the public is allowed to use it, and, if so, whether an appointment is required. Steve Dunn, in his Internet site *http://cancerguide.org/sdunn_story.html*, describes giving a recent journal article to his doctor:

> I found out that not only could my doctors give me references, but I could give them references, too. When I first showed Dr. Todd the Rosenberg paper, she practically grabbed it out of my hand, wanting to make a copy right then.

You may also be able to search the collections of your local public library, medical libraries, or university libraries using your home computer. Call the library and ask how to access the collection by computer.

Purchasing a book

If you prefer to buy books rather than borrow them from the library, you can do so at your local bookstore, or through an online or mail order bookstore. To save time, call ahead to see if they have the book in stock. If they don't, ask them if they can order it. They will check their computer, and tell you if it is available, the cost, and the estimated time of arrival. If you plan to pick it up at the bookstore, ask them to call you when it arrives.

Using the Internet

An astonishing amount of information is available at more than 12,000 medical sites on the Internet. What used to take hours or days of research is now available at your fingertips in the comfort of your own home. You can roam through libraries all over the world, as well as download information in minutes from huge databases like Medline or Healthstar. You can reach out for support from others in similar circumstances. One mother of a sick child welcomed a new parent to her online group by saying, "A group like ours provides something that no one else can—true empathy, because we have either walked in your shoes, or perhaps we're still wearing them."

While this wealth of information helps immensely when researching a medical condition, there is a down side. The huge number of people using the Internet has spawned chat rooms, bulletin boards, discussion lists, and thousands of FAQs (frequently asked questions) that may or may not contain accurate information. The Food and Drug Administration is scrambling to develop guidelines to help Internet users identify bogus medical sites. Currently, the best ways to evaluate health and medical information on the Internet are common sense (if it seems too good to be true, beware) and consultation with your doctor. The California Medical Association has a good site full of practical ways to verify online information at *http:// www.CMAnet.org*.

How to find technical information

Do not feel threatened by the abundance of information available. Amateurs can conduct thorough searches by simply learning a few entry points (often from a friendly librarian), then experimenting. If you join an Internet discussion group, you might even get some pointers from the legion of gifted medical researchers who help beginners. If you are ill, or have limited time to make decisions, you could hire a professional to gather the information for you (consult Appendix E, *Medical Information Search Companies*).

The Internet is like a spider web: large, intricate, and, in a way, beautiful. You can enter at one point and circle around and around until you are lost, or you can take notes and methodically explore a small corner at a time. You may even find all the information you need from just one or two technical databases.

What follows is a brief description of a few basic places to begin your search. Because the Internet is constantly changing, some of the following addresses may quickly become out of date. If you cannot locate one of the resources, you can ask a librarian to help you conduct a search for it.

Medline

The richest source of medical information on the Internet is Medline. This database, compiled and maintained by the National Library of Medicine (NLM), is a collection of medical journal citations and abstracts covering virtually every aspect of medicine. It contains more than nine million records from more than 3,800 biomedical journals. According to the NLM, Medline is searched more than 20,000 times a day.

There are many ways to search Medline. You can purchase software such as Grateful Med to make searching the NLM databases easier, or you can use programs that give free access to the database. Grateful Med allows access to Medline, Aidsline, and Healthstar, and is available from National Technical Information Service (NTIS), 5285 Port Royal Road, Springfield, VA 22161, and on the Internet at *http://www.ntis.gov/*.

One of the best (to date) of the free methods for searching Medline is the NLM's PubMed at *http://www.nlm.nih.gov*. As with any other online database, you find your way to information by entering search terms or choosing menu items, and narrowing or widening your search, depending on what you find. For example, at the time this book was written, searches on PubMed took place as follows, but the precise user interface and steps used to search will probably change over time.

When you go to the PubMed site, you will see an empty box next to the "search" button. Enter a topic in the box, such as "lyme disease" and click on "search." The program tells you how many citations (or "hits") are available for that topic. Lyme disease resulted in 3,972 hits. As you can see, in some cases you will need to narrow the search or you will waste valuable time scrolling through endless lists of journal abstracts. To narrow the search, simply add another search term. Type a comma after "lyme disease" and put in the second item. For example, you might want to learn about diagnosis of lyme disease, so type in "lyme disease, diagnosis" and click on "search."

PubMed allows you to control the limits on publication dates. You can choose to view abstracts from the last 30 days, 60 days, 90 days, 180 days, 1 year, 2 years, 5 years, or 10 years. If you have a chronic condition, and you check Medline once a month, this feature prevents you from receiving hundreds of old citations that you have already seen. If you have difficulty with any of the above steps, or wish to learn more about options in the program, click on the "help" button on the sidebar to the left. Using PubMed, millions of citations are at your fingertips, and you control what slice of the information pie you would like to view.

If you wish to conduct an advanced search, click on that button on the left sidebar. If you wish PubMed to divide the information into topics, type in one subject, e.g., "rett syndrome," and change the mode setting from "automatic" to "list terms." In this case, after typing in "rett syndrome" and clicking on "search," a window appears that contains a list similar to the one shown below.

rett syndrome	(541)
rett syndrome/blood	(7)
rett syndrome/cerebrospinal fluid	(22)
rett syndrome/chemically induced	(1)
rett syndrome/classification	(4)
rett syndrome/complications	(57)
rett syndrome/diagnosis	(108)
rett syndrome/drug therapy	(12)
rett syndrome/economics	(1)
rett syndrome/enzymology	(6)
rett syndrome/epidemiology	(29)
rett syndrome/etiology	(11)
rett syndrome/genetics	(59)
rett syndrome/history	(1)
rett syndrome/immunology	(2)

rett syndrome/metabolism	(33)
rett syndrome/mortality	(1)
rett syndrome/nursing	(1)
rett syndrome/pathology	(32)
rett syndrome/pathophysiology	(116)
rett syndrome/psychology	(32)
rett syndrome/radiography	(5)
rett syndrome/radionucliotide imaging	(7)
rett syndrome/rehabilitation	(9)
rett syndrome/surgery	(1)
rett syndrome/therapy	(13)
rett syndrome/urine	(2)

You can also experiment with the search field setting in PubMed. The default setting is "all fields." However, you can also search using author name, journal name, text word, title word, and several other methods.

In addition to searching the databases, you can go directly to the journals themselves. Several prestigious medical journals are online, some with full text, others with only abstracts of the articles. *The New England Journal of Medicine* (*http://www.nejm.org*) and *The Journal of the American Medical Association* (*http://www.ama-assn.org/public/journals/jama/*) are both available online. The NLM site (*http://www.nlm.nih.gov*) links to more than twenty-four biomedical journals, some free, some by subscription only.

Other databases

Literally thousands of databases are on the Internet, with more sprouting daily. A few of the major sources of medical information are provided here. Several books that delve into how to find and use information on the Internet are listed in *Suggested Reading* at the end of this book. Beyond that, new vistas will open as you become more adept at exploring the Net.

- **Hardin Meta Directory of Internet Health Sources.** Hardin Meta Directory pages have pointers to the most complete and frequently cited lists for dozens of medical topics. For subjects not yet listed, go directly to the comprehensive index sites that are included. *http://www.lib.uiowa.edu/hardin-www/md.html*.

- **Medical Matrix.** Peer-reviewed, up-to-date clinical medical resources. MedMatrix also gives links to hundreds of sites ranked by medical experts. *http://www.medmatrix.org.*

- **Aidsline.** Contains references to journal articles, theses, technical reports, meetings, books, and audiovisuals on Acquired Immunodeficiency Syndrome (AIDS). Aidsline is available on Grateful Med. Aidsline, Aidstrials, Cancerlit, and five other databases are also available for a flat fee of $14.95 per month at Healthgate (*http://healthgate.com*). This fee covers searching any of eight databases, displaying abstracts, and printing the search results.

- **Aidstrials.** Information on active and closed clinical trials of substances being tested for use against AIDS and related diseases.

- **Cancerlit.** Contains references to published journal articles, meeting abstracts, government reports, monographs, and other sources covering cancer and related topics.

- **Healthfinder.** The federal government's new entry point for a vast collection of health information. *http://www.healthfinder.gov.*

- **Med Help International.** One of the largest consumer health information libraries in the world. When you search their medical library, you will receive all available matches for six sources: their Medical Glossary, articles from their Medical Library, articles from their News Room, messages from the Medical Forums, articles from other Internet sites, and support groups that contain the keyword(s) you entered. *http://med-help.org.*

- **National Organization for Rare Disorders, Inc. (NORD).** A nonprofit group dedicated to helping people with rare orphan diseases (defined as a disease affecting fewer than 200,000 Americans) and assisting the organizations that serve them. Their database contains information on more than 1,050 disorders, written in nontechnical language. For $5, NORD will send you a report on any disease in their database. *http://www.pcnet.com/~orphan/*, email *76703.301@compuserve.com,* or write to NORD, P.O. Box 8923, New Fairfield, CT 06812.

- **OncoLink™.** A text and multimedia service offering a wide variety of cancer-related information, including articles, handbooks, newsletters, writings by patients and their families. *http://cancer.med.upenn.edu/.*

- **Physician's Data Query (PDQ).** A cancer database maintained by the National Cancer Institute that contains up-to-date treatment and clinical trial information. There are two versions: one for patients in nontechnical language (containing far less actual information) and one for professionals (uses technical language and contains statistics). The same information is available by phone at the Cancer Information Line at 1-800-4-CANCER. *http://pdqsearch@icicc.nci.nih.gov/.*

- **Psych Central.** Psychologist John Grohol has assembled a comprehensive online listing of all web sites, newsgroups, mailing lists, and support information for online mental health. *http://www.coil.com/~grohol/.*

- **PharmInfoNet**™. Devoted to delivering useful, up-to-date, and accurate pharmaceutical information to health care providers, pharmacists, and patients. *http://www.pharminfo.com.*

Evaluating the information

How can you determine what information is accurate and what is bunk? The following suggestions will help you evaluate the content and reliability of this wealth of medical information.

- Who is the author? Technical information should come from a known authority who published the results in a peer-reviewed journal.

- Is the site advertising a product or service? If so, is it clear where content ends and the ad begins? Both overt and subtle salesmanship are commonly found on the Internet.

- Are the claims for the treatment or therapy substantiated? If no scientific supporting evidence (e.g., specific peer-reviewed journal articles) is referenced, be leery.

- Are testimonials from individuals used to back up claims? If so, shy away from the results. True science is based on the statistically significant results obtained from large numbers of people undergoing the treatment.

- If a health practitioner is making claims using grandiose language such as "new revelation," "earthshaking," or "miraculous cure," check his credentials. He may be unlicensed, incompetent, or a scam artist.

- Are conspiracy themes promoted? Many sites claim that there is a conspiracy by the pharmaceutical companies to discredit their particular product. View such claims with caution.

A site that contains information on sites pushing fraudulent information is *http://www.quackwatch.com*. As with any information, verify before acting. Take any questions you have to your doctor and discuss the validity of the options you locate.

How to find emotional support

On the Internet, patients discover self-help communities where they share stories and swap information on the newest treatments and most experienced doctors. Large Internet service providers like AOL and CompuServe have forums and medical message centers on a host of medical topics. There are also hundreds of Internet message centers—called "listserv discussion groups" or "mailing lists"—on specific medical topics, where patients and often physicians share experiences and information. Such discussions not only offer emotional support, but can literally make the difference between life and death, as the following story shows.

> *If I had not been able to search the Internet, I would probably be dead. Because of the Internet, I am about to embark on a very unique medical adventure. I have been accepted into a vaccine clinical study at the University of Michigan. I found Dr. S. and the clinical study because Donna, a leiomyosarcoma survivor who lives in Minnesota, posted a note on cancer-L (a discussion list for cancer patients) by way of a neighbor in December '95. I found her note and called her. She gave me the phone number of Tim, another leiomyosarcoma survivor, who gave me information about the vaccine study and Dr. S.'s phone number.*
>
> *I did not want to call Dr. S. without first knowing something about the study. By nature, I am a cautious person. So I put a plea on cancer-L, asking for information about vaccine studies that included sarcoma patients. Joan provided me with the information that led me to the two sites that are or will be involved in vaccine studies. Although both studies are funded by the National Cancer Institute (NCI), neither study is included in a list of NCI or non-NCI funded clinical studies recently sent to me through calling the 1-800-4-CANCER number. A gene study now in progress at the University of Michigan also was not included.*
>
> *I cannot imagine having an extremely rare cancer and living without the Internet. I now have a list of about 65 leiomyosarcoma survivors that I am corresponding with either through the Internet or via snail mail or the telephone. Had I not had Internet access, I would not know one*

person with leiomyosarcoma. Most of the people I have written to have noted that I was the first person they had encountered who shared our common problem.

Another member of a large discussion group greeted a newcomer to the "club that no one wants to join" with the following message:

Most of us are on this List to share what we have learned, ferret out promising treatments that may be unknown to those living away from large treatment centers, and rejoice in the companionship of others who have "been there."

In addition to emotional support, many discussion groups share the newest treatments for specific maladies and news on available clinical trials. Many of these groups have computer-savvy owners who can tell you the location of most medical resources on the Web, as well as members who have spent years learning about and fighting a specific disease or condition. In addition, some physicians who specialize in the disorder monitor the lists and give detailed answers to medical questions, although they don't advise or prescribe.

Thousands of discussion groups (also called mailing lists) are available on the Internet. A few examples of the variety of subjects covered are:

- **Alzheimer's.** For patients, researchers, and caregivers. *Major-domo@wubios.wustl.edu.*
- **BreastCancer.** For patients, families, researchers, and physicians. *Listserv@morgan.ucs.mun.wvnet.*
- **CSF-L.** Open list for persons suffering from chronic fatigue syndrome. *listserv@list.nih.gov.*
- **Diabetic.** For diabetic patients. *Listserv%pccvm.bitnet@cmsa.berkely.edu.*
- **Menopaus.** For persons dealing with menopause. *Listserv@psuhmc.maricopa.edu.*
- **Ped-onc.** For parents of children with cancer. *Listserv@listserv.acor.org.*
- **Sorehand.** For persons who suffer from carpal tunnel syndrome. *Listserv@ubvm.cc.buffalo.edu.*

To locate a particular mailing list on the Internet, check out:

- *http://www.geocities.com/HotSprings/1505/guide.html.*
- *http://www.liszt.com.*
- *http://medinfo.org* for a list of cancer listservs.

To join a mailing list, send an email message to that list's Internet listserv address. Leave the subject line blank, and put "subscribe (name of list) your first name, your last name" in the body of the message. For example, if I wanted to join Sorehand, I would put the following in the message: *subscribe Sorehand Nancy Keene*. After you sign up, you will be sent a detailed welcome message telling you everything you need to know about the group—including how to unsubscribe. Keep this message in a safe place for future reference. In some cases you need to decide whether to get individual emails or a daily digest of all the emails sent to the list in the previous twenty-four hours. Some lists generate hundreds of messages a day, so determine what is the best method for you.

Most members of mailing lists are "lurkers," that is, they read the messages, but don't post (or send) replies to the group. Lurking is perfectly acceptable in discussion group circles. What is not acceptable is making derogatory remarks about other members of the group (called flaming) or posting commercial messages. Most members also appreciate brevity—especially since some people pay for the time they use their Internet connections. Long-windedness can be expensive. It is always a good idea to see if the list has a FAQ—a document covering frequently asked questions and their answers—before asking a question of the group.

If you respond to a post, put that post's heading on your reply's subject line. For instance, for your first post you might put "introduction" on the subject line. All responders will also put "introduction" on the subject line so that you can quickly determine which messages are responses to your original message.

If you have a personal comment to make to an individual, send it to his private email address. Only post replies to the group that have a general interest. This keeps the list traffic down and keeps off-topic discussions to a minimum.

You have little to lose and plenty to gain by participation in an online discussion group. However, a few basic precautions are in order:

• Always verify information. Although most persons sharing information and advice in groups mean well, they may not always have their facts straight. On the other hand, some persons are extraordinarily knowledgeable. You can protect yourself by carefully researching all suggestions.

- Beware of hucksters hawking miracle products (some salespeople on the Internet have become very sophisticated). Any treatments backed up only by testimonials without scientific scrutiny should be avoided.

- Use care in subscribing to numerous lists, especially if you use a service that charges per message. Some groups generate only a few messages a day, while active groups can post hundreds. Start off slowly.

- If you are treated discourteously, either ignore it or respond privately. Ongoing arguments annoy other members of the list, and can be expensive as well. If you subscribe to a group that tends to be argumentative, consider checking out other groups with a more civil tone.

- Don't download files from the list unless you first use an antivirus program. At present, you can't get a computer virus from an email, but you certainly can from a downloaded file.

Professional information searches

This chapter has discussed many issues involved in conducting your own research. Reasons to do the research yourself are plentiful. You will learn more about your illness by conducting the search for information on your own. You may uncover areas of interest that you would like to pursue. It's either free or relatively inexpensive. In addition, if you search yourself, you will acquire a useful skill that may prove helpful in the future.

However, if you need rapid answers to your questions or are unable to do the research yourself, you can hire a specialist to conduct the search. If you choose to use a professional service, investigate it prior to entering into an agreement. Some questions to ask prior to making a decision are:

- How long have you been in business?

- What is the training and background of the searchers?

- What type of searches does your company specialize in?

- What sources do you use? How up to date are they?

- How much does the service cost?

- Exactly what information will I get for this price? All abstracts? How many full-text articles? How much general information? All technical information? All information in lay terms?

- How specific will the information be?

- Do you include information on complementary and alternative therapies?

- What type of guarantee (if any) do you give?

- Can you provide a sample output?

Once you've decided on the company, explain in detail the information you want. Be explicit. Do not say, "I want to know the best treatment for lung cancer." Instead, give specific medical information about yourself ("I'm a 56-year-old female with small cell lung cancer with metastases to the liver, and I need information on any Phase I and Phase II clinical trials using immunotherapy to treat this illness"). The professional searcher will not recommend treatment options. Rather, he will give you the information that may help you to better understand your illness and its treatment options. You must make your own decisions.

Appendix E, *Professional Medical Search Organizations*, contains a list of search organizations.

Making decisions

In virtually all cases, your physician is committed to providing you with the very best medical care available. But there are many unknowns in medicine. Treatment options may be available, and individual responses to treatments vary. Thus, the best choice for you may not be clear.

Doctors, like all humans, are fallible. They may not know every option available, and in some cases, may not be up to speed on the latest research. You, on the other hand, can become extremely knowledgeable in one narrow area of medicine, but this cannot duplicate a medical education and years of experience. Sharing the information that you have researched, and making decisions in partnership with your doctor, provides you with the best of both worlds. An educated patient, armed with the newest studies, and a doctor, with a wealth of clinical experience and broad medical education, can join forces to make decisions better than either could make alone.

> My doctor was wonderful. He explained to me about not reading outdated information and reviewed any reading material I discussed with him in a very informative, comforting way. I always felt like he was completely open with me. In fact, I truly feel in my heart that that man is part of the reason I'm a biomedical librarian now. He knew I was a "reader" and that didn't bother him. He always remembered my interests

and activities. He always asked about them. Always, always, always, he talked with me in a way that made me feel hopeful. That was one of the greatest gifts I've ever gotten.

Deciding how to talk over the results of your research is important. If you've always been somewhat passive and barge in one day with reams of journal articles, demanding an instant response, you may get a frosty reception. If you prepare your doctor ahead of time, it will be time well spent. You could, for instance, say any of the following:

- I've found that information gives me comfort. I'm going to spend some time reviewing the newest research and treatment options. I'd like to come discuss these articles with you to get your viewpoint. Would you like me to fax the articles to your office several days before my next appointment? Or do you have another method that you would prefer?

- I've been doing some research on my condition, and have found some helpful information. I'd like to share this information with you and also get your thoughts on a few questions that it has raised.

- I'm going to do some research on my illness. My goal is to be an informed patient who makes good decisions. I'd like to fax, mail, or drop off some articles so that we can discuss them at our next appointment. Is this okay with you?

One patient remarked that his doctor was turned off by any mention of the Internet because he associated it with misinformation and scams. The patient would put in a cover note that accompanied the articles he dropped off, "This information is from a nonprofit organization that specializes in my illness. I found some information in it that I would like your opinion on." On the other hand, some doctors steer their patients to the Internet, and look forward to discussing the information found. One family practitioner remarked, "The process of gathering information and doing something helps. It's therapeutic."

Attempt to stake out the territory between passivity and aggression. Be assertive, but friendly. Try to project the sense that you and your doctor are on the same team, with the same goal—working together to improve your health. If you respect your doctor by giving him adequate time to read and digest the material, and then have a reasonable discussion, you both benefit.

The steps toward making sound medical decisions are: research, evaluation, discussion with your doctor, weighing the risks versus the benefits of all options, considering your personal values, then deciding. Such a pragmatic approach benefits both patient and doctor. You can feel confident that you have made the best possible decision—based on the newest research—yet tailor-made to your unique circumstances. Remember, always, that knowledge is power.

Being an active participant in my care has really helped me feel in charge and on top of things, and I think it has helped career-wise; I'm now a biomedical librarian, and my information specialty is hematology/oncology. I've always had a little line I draw—I read about my risks and about Hodgkin's, but I know that when I start to feel edgy I can put the book or journal article down and walk away. And that's what I do. It's been my experience that both pediatric and adult cancer survivors/patients vary on how much they want to know. My boyfriend, a brain tumor survivor, is almost the opposite—he knows what they tell him, and is perfectly happy with that. On the other hand, I like being able to come back and talk about current trends in the use of post-splenectomy antibiotic prophylaxis, etc., with my hematologist. To each his/her own!

Ethics Codes and Bills of Rights

AMA Principles of Medical Ethics

1. A physician shall be dedicated to providing competent medical service with compassion and respect for human dignity.

2. A physician shall deal honestly with patients and colleagues, and strive to expose those physicians deficient in character or competence, or who engage in fraud or deception.

3. A physician shall respect the law and recognize a responsibility to seek changes in those requirements which are contrary to the best interests of the patient.

4. A physician shall respect the rights of patients, of colleagues, and of other health professionals, and shall safeguard patient confidences within the constraints of the law.

5. A physician shall continue to study, apply, and advance scientific knowledge, make relevant information available to patients, colleagues, and the public, obtain consultation, and use the talent of other health professionals when indicated.

6. A physician shall, in the provision of appropriate patient care, except in emergencies, be free to choose whom to serve, with whom to associate, and the environment in which to provide medical services.

7. A physician shall recognize a responsibility to participate in activities contributing to an improved community.

Source: *Code of Medical Ethics: Current Opinions With Annotations* Copyright © 1996 American Medical Association.

The Consumer Bill of Rights and Responsibilities

The Advisory Commission on Consumer Protection and Quality in the Health Care Industry was appointed by President Clinton to draft a consumer bill of rights. The draft, released in November 1997 and called "The Consumer Bill of Rights and Responsibilities," is summarized below.

1. **Information disclosure.** Consumers have the right to receive accurate, easily understood information, and some require assistance in making informed health care decisions about their health plans, professionals, and facilities.

2. **Choice of providers and plans.** Consumers have the right to a choice of health care providers that is sufficient to ensure access to appropriate high-quality health care.

3. **Access to emergency services.** Consumers have the right to access emergency health care services when and where the need arises. Health plans should provide payment when a customer presents to an emergency department with acute symptoms of sufficient severity—including severe pain—such that a "prudent layperson" could reasonably expect the absence of medical attention to result in placing that consumer's health in serious jeopardy, serious impairment to bodily functions, or serious dysfunction of any bodily organ or part.

4. **Participation in treatment decisions.** Consumers have the right and responsibility to fully participate in all decisions related to their health care. Consumers who are unable to fully participate in treatment decisions have the right to be represented by parents, guardians, family members, or other conservators.

5. **Respect and nondiscrimination.** Consumers have the right to considerate, respectful care from all members of the health care system at all times and under all circumstances. An environment of mutual respect is essential to maintain a quality health care system. Consumers must not be discriminated against in the delivery of health care services consistent with the benefits covered in their policy or as required by law based on race, ethnicity, national origin, religion, sex, age, mental or physical disability, sexual orientation, genetic information, or source of payment. Consumers who are eligible for coverage under the terms and conditions of a health plan or program as required by law must not be discriminated against in marketing and enrollment practices based on race, ethnicity, national origin, religion, sex, age, mental or physical disability, sexual orientation, genetic information, or source of payment.

6. **Confidentiality of health information.** Consumers have the right to communicate with health care providers in confidence and to have the confidentiality of their individually identifiable health care information protected. Consumers also have the right to review and copy their own medical records and request amendments to their records.

7. **Complaints and appeals.** All consumers have the right to a fair and efficient process for resolving differences with their health plans, health care providers, and the institutions that serve them, including a rigorous system of internal review and an independent system of external review.

8. **Consumer Responsibilities.** In a health care system that protects consumers' rights, it is reasonable to expect and encourage consumers to assume reasonable responsibilities. Greater individual involvement by consumers in their care increases the likelihood of achieving the best outcomes and helps support a quality-improvement, cost-conscious environment. Such responsibilities include:

- Take responsibility for maximizing healthy habits, such as exercising, not smoking, and eating a healthy diet.

- Become involved in specific health care decisions.

- Work collaboratively with health care providers in developing and carrying out agreed-upon treatment plans.

- Disclose relevant information and clearly communicate wants and needs.

- Use the health plan's internal complaint and appeals processes to address concerns that may arise.

- Avoid knowingly spreading disease.

- Recognize the reality of risks and limits of the science of medical care and the human fallibility of the health care professional.

- Be aware of a health care provider's obligation to be reasonably efficient and equitable in providing care to other patients and the community.

- Become knowledgeable about his or her health plan coverage and health plan options (when available), including all covered benefits, limitations and exclusions, rules regarding use of network providers, coverage and referral rules, appropriate processes to secure additional information, and the process to appeal coverage decisions.

- Show respect for other patients and health workers.

- Make a good faith effort to meet financial obligations.

- Abide by administrative and operational procedures of health plans, health care providers, and Government health benefit programs.

- Report wrongdoing and fraud to appropriate resources or legal authorities.

American Hospital Association's Patient's Bill of Rights

Effective health care requires collaboration between patients and physicians and other health care professionals. Open and honest communication, respect for personal and professional values, and sensitivity to differences are integral to optimal patient care. As the setting for the provision of health services, hospitals must provide a foundation for understanding and respecting the rights and responsibilities of patients, their families, physicians, and other caregivers. Hospitals must ensure a health care ethic that respects the role of patients in decision making about treatment choices and other aspects of their care. Hospitals must be sensitive to cultural, racial, linguistic, religious, age, gender, and other differences as well as the needs of persons with disabilities.

The American Hospital Association presents A Patient's Bill of Rights with the expectation that it will contribute to more effective patient care and be supported by the hospital on behalf of the institution, its medical staff, employees, and patients. The American Hospital Association encourages health care institutions to tailor this bill of rights to their patient community by translating and/or simplifying the language of this bill of rights as may be necessary to ensure that patients and their families understand their rights and responsibilities.

These rights can be exercised on the patient's behalf by a designated surrogate or proxy decision maker if the patient lacks decision-making capacity, is legally incompetent, or is a minor.

1. The patient has the right to considerate and respectful care.

2. The patient has the right to and is encouraged to obtain from physicians and other direct caregivers relevant, current, and understandable information concerning diagnosis, treatment, and prognosis. Except in emergencies when the patient lacks decision-making capacity and the need for treatment is urgent, the patient is entitled to the opportunity to discuss and request information related to the specific procedures and/or treatments, the risks involved, the possible length of recuperation, and the medically reasonable alternatives and their accompanying risks and benefits. Patients have the right to know the identity of physicians, nurses, and others involved in their care, as well as when those involved are students, residents, or other trainees. The patient also has the right to know the immediate and long-term financial implications of treatment choices, insofar as they are known.

3. The patient has the right to make decisions about the plan of care prior to and during the course of treatment and to refuse a recommended treatment or plan of care to the extent permitted by law and hospital policy and to be informed of the medical consequences of this action. In case of such refusal, the patient is entitled to other appropriate care and services that the hospital provides or transfer to another hospital. The hospital should notify patients of any policy that might affect patient choice within the institution.

4. The patient has the right to have an advance directive (such as a living will, health care proxy, or durable power of attorney for health care) concerning treatment or designating a surrogate decision maker with the expectation that the hospital will honor the intent of that directive to the extent permitted by law and hospital policy. Health care institutions must advise patients of their rights under state law and hospital policy to make informed medical choices, ask if the patient has an advance directive, and include that information in patient records. The patient has the right to timely information about hospital policy that may limit its ability to implement fully a legally valid advance directive.

5. The patient has the right to every consideration of privacy. Case discussion, consultation, examination, and treatment should be conducted so as to protect each patient's privacy.

6. The patient has the right to expect that all communications and records pertaining to his/her care will be treated as confidential by the hospital, except in cases such as suspected abuse and public health hazards when reporting is permitted or required by law. The patient has the right to expect that the hospital will emphasize the confidentiality of this information when it releases it to any other parties entitled to review information in these records.

7. The patient has the right to review the records pertaining to his/her medical care and to have the information explained or interpreted as necessary, except when restricted by law.

8. The patient has the right to expect that, within its capacity and policies, a hospital will make reasonable response to the request of a patient for appropriate and medically indicated care and services. The hospital must provide evaluation, service, and/or referral as indicated by the urgency of the case. When medically appropriate and legally permissible, or when a patient has so requested, a patient may be transferred to another facility. The institution to which the patient is to be transferred must first have accepted the patient for transfer. The patient must also have the benefit of complete information and explanation concerning the need for, risks, benefits, and alternatives to such a transfer.

9. The patient has the right to ask and be informed of the existence of business relationships among the hospital, educational institutions, other health care providers, or payers that may influence the patient's treatment and care.

10. The patient has the right to consent to or decline to participate in proposed research studies or human experimentation affecting care and treatment or requiring direct patient involvement, and to have those studies fully explained prior to consent. A patient who declines to participate in research or experimentation is entitled to the most effective care that the hospital can otherwise provide.

11. The patient has the right to expect reasonable continuity of care when appropriate and to be informed by physicians and other caregivers of available and realistic patient care options when hospital care is no longer appropriate.

12. The patient has the right to be informed of hospital policies and practices that relate to patient care, treatment, and responsibilities. The patient has the right to be informed of available resources for resolving disputes, grievances, and conflicts, such as ethics committees, patient representatives, or other mechanisms available in the institution. The patient has the right to be informed of the hospital's charges for services and available payment methods.

The collaborative nature of health care requires that patients, or their families/ surrogates, participate in their care. The effectiveness of care and patient satisfaction with the course of treatment depend, in part, on the patient fulfilling certain responsibilities. Patients are responsible for providing information about past illnesses, hospitalizations, medications, and other matters related to health status. To participate effectively in decision making, patients must be encouraged to take responsibility for requesting additional information or clarification about their health status or treatment when they do not fully understand information and instructions. Patients are also responsible for ensuring that the health care institution has a copy of their written advance directive if they have one. Patients are responsible for informing their physicians and other caregivers if they anticipate problems in following prescribed treatment.

Patients should also be aware of the hospital's obligation to be reasonably efficient and equitable in providing care to other patients and the community. The hospital's rules and regulations are designed to help the hospital meet this obligation. Patients and their families are responsible for making reasonable accommodations to the needs of the hospital, other patients, medical staff, and hospital employees. Patients are responsible for providing necessary information for insurance claims and for working with the hospital to make payment arrangements, when necessary.

A person's health depends on much more than health care services. Patients are responsible for recognizing the impact of their life-style on their personal health.

Hospitals have many functions to perform, including the enhancement of health status, health promotion, and the prevention and treatment of injury and disease; the immediate and ongoing care and rehabilitation of patients; the education of health professionals, patients, and the community; and research. All these activities must be conducted with an overriding concern for the values and dignity of patients.

American Board of Medical Specialties

The American Board of Allergy and Immunology, Inc.
510 Walnut Street, Suite 1701
Philadelphia, PA 19106-3699
Tel: (215) 592-9466
Fax: (215) 592-9411
http://www.abai.org

The American Board of Anesthesiology, Inc.
4101 Lake Boone Trail
The Summit, Suite 510
Raleigh, NC 27607-7506
Tel: (919) 881-2570
Fax: (919) 881-2575

The American Board of Colon and Rectal Surgery, Inc.
20600 Eureka Road, Suite 713
Taylor, MI 48180
Tel: (734) 282-9400
Fax: (734) 282-9402
email: *admnabcrs@aol.com*

The American Board of Emergency Medicine, Inc.
3000 Coolidge Road
East Lansing, MI 48823
Tel: (517) 332-4800
Fax: (517) 332-2234
http://www.abem.org

The American Board of Family Practice, Inc.
2228 Young Drive
Lexington, KY 40505-4294
Tel: (606) 269-5626 or 1-888-995-5700
Fax: (606) 335-7509
http://www.abfp.org

The American Board of Internal Medicine, Inc.
510 Walnut Street, Suite 1700
Philadelphia, PA 19106-3699
Tel: (215) 446-3500 or 1-800-441-ABIM
Fax: (215) 446-3470

The American Board of Medical Genetics, Inc.
9650 Rockville Pike
Bethesda, MD 20814-3998
Tel: (301) 571-1825
Fax: (301) 571-1895
http://www.faseb.org/genetics

The American Board of Neurological Surgery, Inc.
6550 Fannin Street, Suite 2139
Houston, TX 77030
Tel: (713) 790-6015
Fax: (713) 794-0207

The American Board of Nuclear Medicine, Inc.
900 Veteran Avenue, Room 13-152
Los Angeles, CA 90024-1786
Tel: (310) 825-6787
Fax: (310) 825-9433

The American Board of Obstetrics and Gynecology, Inc.
2915 Vine Street
Dallas, TX 75204-1069
Tel: (214) 871-1619
Fax: (214) 871-1943
http://www.abog.org

The American Board of Ophthalmology, Inc.
111 Presidential Boulevard, Suite 241
Bala Cynwyd, PA 19004
Tel: (610) 664-1175
Fax: (610) 664-6503
http://www.abop.org

The American Board of Orthopaedic Surgery, Inc.
400 Silver Cedar Court
Chapel Hill, NC 27514
Tel: (919) 929-7103
Fax: (919) 942-8988

The American Board of Otolaryngology, Inc.
2211 Norfolk Street, Suite 800
Houston, TX 77098-4044
Tel: (713) 528-6200
Fax: (713) 528-1171
http://www.aboto.org

The American Board of Pathology, Inc.
P.O. Box 25915
Tampa, FL 33622
Tel: (813) 286-2444
Fax: (813) 289-5279
http://www.abpath.org

The American Board of Pediatrics, Inc.
111 Silver Cedar Court
Chapel Hill, NC 27514-1651
Tel: (919) 929-0461
Fax: (919) 929-9255
http://www.abp.org

The American Board of Physical Medicine and Rehabilitation, Inc.
Norwest Center
21 First Street SW, Suite 674
Rochester, MN 55902
Tel: (507) 282-1776
Fax: (507) 282-9242

The American Board of Plastic Surgery, Inc.
Seven Penn Center
1635 Market Street, Suite 400
Philadelphia, PA 19103-2204
Tel: (215) 587-9322
Fax: (215) 587-9622

The American Board of Preventive Medicine, Inc.
9950 West Lawrence Avenue, Suite 106
Schiller Park, IL 60176
Tel: (847) 671-1750
Fax: (847) 671-1751
http://www.abprevmed.org

The American Board of Psychiatry and Neurology, Inc.
500 Lake Cook Road, Suite 335
Deerfield, IL 60015
Tel: (847) 945-7900
Fax: (847) 945-1146
http://www.abpn.com

The American Board of Radiology, Inc.
5255 East Williams Circle, Suite 3200
Tucson, AZ 85711
Tel: (520) 790-2900
Fax: (520) 790-3200
http://www.theabr.org

The American Board of Surgery, Inc.
1617 John F. Kennedy Boulevard, Suite 860
Philadelphia, PA 19103
Tel: (215) 568-4000
Fax: (215) 563-5718
http://www.absurgery.org

The American Board of Thoracic Surgery, Inc.
One Rotary Center, Suite 803
Evanston, IL 60201
Tel: (847) 475-1520
Fax: (847) 475-6240

The American Board of Urology, Inc.
2216 Ivy Road, Suite 210
Charlottesville, VA 22903
Tel: (804) 979-0059
Fax: (804) 979-0266

Sources of Information on Medical Conditions

This appendix lists dozens of organizations that provide information and emotional support for persons with specific medical conditions. Thousands of such groups exist, however. To locate a group not listed, contact one of the following clearinghouses of information.

The American Self-Help Clearinghouse
Northwest Covenant Medical Center
25 Pocono Road
Denville, NJ 07834
1-800-367-6274 or (973) 625-7101

National Self-Help Clearinghouse
25 West Forty-third Street, Room 620
New York, NY 10036
(212) 642-2944

National Organization for Rare Disorders (NORD)
P.O. Box 8923
New Fairfield, CT 06812
1-800-999-6673
email: *orphan@nord-rdb.com*
http://www.pcnet.com/~orphan/

HealthTouch
http://www.healthtouch.com

AIDS

National CDC HIV/AIDS Hotline
1-800-342-AIDS (24 hours) or
(202) 245-6867 from Alaska or Hawaii; call collect.

Gay Men's Health Crisis
129 West Twentieth Street
New York, NY 10011
(212) 807-6655 (hotline)

HIV Information Exchange and Support Group
610 Greenwood
Glenview, IL 60025
(847) 724-3832

Addison's disease

National Adrenal Disease Foundation
505 Northern Boulevard, Suite 200
Great Neck, NY 11021
(516) 487-4992
email: *nadf@aol.com*
http://medhelp.netusa.net/www.nadf.htm

Alcoholism

Alcoholics Anonymous
P.O. Box 459
Grand Central Station
New York, NY 10163
(212) 870-3400
http://www.aa.org

Anemia

Aplastic Anemia Foundation
P.O. Box 613
Annapolis, MD 21404
1-800-747-2820
email: *aafacenter@aol.com*
http://www.aplastic.org

Franconi's Anemia Research Fund
1902 Jefferson Street, Suite 2
Eugene, OR 97405
1-800-828-4891 or (541) 687-4658
http://www.rio.com/fafund

Allergies

Asthma and Allergy Foundation of America
1125 Fifteenth Street NW, Suite 502
Washington, DC 60611
1-800-727-8462

Alzheimer's disease

Alzheimer's Association
919 North Michigan Avenue, Suite 1000
Chicago, IL 60611
1-800-272-3900
http://www.alz.org

Alzheimer's Disease Education and Referral Center
P.O. Box 8250
Silver Springs, MD 20907
1-800-438-4380
http://www.alzheimers.org

Arthritis

Arthritis Foundation
1314 Spring Road
Atlanta, GA 30309
1-800-283-7800 or (404) 972-9036

Canadian Arthritis Society
393 University Avenue, Suite 1700
Toronto, Ontario M5G 1E6
Canada
(416) 979-7228

Spondylitis Association of America
P.O. Box 5872
Sherman Oaks, CA 91413
1-800-777-8189
http://www.spondylitis.org

Asthma

American Lung Association
1740 Broadway
New York, NY 10019-4374
1-800-732-9339
http://www.alaw.org

National Foundation for Asthma, Inc.
P.O. Box 30069
Tucson, AZ 85751
(520) 323-6046

Ataxia

National Ataxia Foundation
2600 Fernbrook Lane, Suite 119
Plymouth, MN 55447
(612) 553-0020
http://www.ataxia.org

Autism

Autism Society of America
7910 Woodmont Avenue, Suite 650
Bethesda, MD 20814
(301) 657-0881

Blindness

American Foundation for the Blind
11 Penn Plaza, Suite 300
New York, NY 10001
1-800-AF-BLIND (1-800-232-5463)
http://www.afb.org

Blind Children's Center
4120 Marathon Street
Los Angeles, CA 90029
1-800-222-3566
http://www.blindsctr.org/bcc

Blood disorders

Aplastic Anemia Foundation
P.O. Box 613
Annapolis, MD 21404
1-800-747-2820

Cooley's Anemia Foundation (Thalassemia)
129-09 Twenty-sixth Avenue, Suite 203
Flushing, NY 11354
1-800-522-7222
http://www.thalassemia.org

National Association for Sickle Cell Disease
200 Corporate Point, Suite 495
Culver City, CA 90230
1-800-421-8453 or (301) 215-3722

National Hemophilia Foundation
116 West Thirty-second Street, Eleventh Floor
New York, NY 10001
1-800-42-HANDI (1-800-424-2634)
http://www.hemophilia.org

Cancer

American Brain Tumor Association
2720 River Road, Suite 146
Des Plaines, IL 60018
1-800-886-2282 or (847) 827-9910
email: *info@abta.org*
http://www.abta.org

American Cancer Society
1599 Clifton Road NE
Atlanta, GA 30329
1-800-227-2345 or (404) 320-3333
http://www.cancer.org

Cancer Information Service of the National Cancer Institute
1-800-4-CANCER

Cure for Lymphoma Foundation
215 Lexington Avenue
New York, NY 10016
(212) 213-9595
http://www.cfl.org

International Myeloma Foundation
2129 Stanley Hills Drive
Los Angeles, CA 90046
1-800-452-2873
http://www.myeloma.org

Leukemia Society of America
600 Third Avenue
New York, NY 10016
1-800-955-4572
http://www.leukemia.org

National Brain Tumor Foundation
785 Market Street, Suite 1600
San Francisco, CA 94103
1-800-943-CURE (1-800-934-2873)
email: *nbtf@braintumor.org*
http://www.braintumor.org

National Alliance of Breast Cancer Organizations (NABCO)
9 East Thirty-seventh Street, Tenth Floor
New York, NY 10016
1-800-719-9154 or (212) 719-0154
email: *nabcoinfo@aol.com*
http://www.nabco.org

Skin Cancer Foundation
245 Fifth Avenue, Suite 1403
New York, NY 10016
1-800-SKIN490 or (212) 725-5176
email: *info@skincancer.org*

Y-ME Breast Cancer Organization
212 West Van Buren, Fourth Floor
Chicago, IL 60607
1-800-221-2141 (24-hour hotline)
1-800-986-9505 (Spanish)
http://www.yme.org

Carpal tunnel syndrome

American Carpal Tunnel Syndrome Association
P.O. Box 6730
Saginaw, MI 48608

Cerebral palsy

United Cerebral Palsy Association
1660 L Street NW, Suite 700
Washington, DC 20036
1-800-872-5827
http://www.ucpa.org

Chronic fatigue syndrome

Chronic Fatigue and Immune Dysfunction Syndrome Association
P.O. Box 220398
Charlotte, NC 28222-0398
1-800-442-3437

Coma

Coma Recovery Association
100 East Old Country Road, Suite 9
Mineola, NY 11501
(516) 746-7714

Cystic fibrosis

Cystic Fibrosis Foundation
6931 Arlington Road
Bethesda, MD 20814
1-800-FIGHTCF (1-800-344-4823)
http://www.cff.org

Deafness

National Institute on Deafness and Other Communication Disorders
Information Clearinghouse
1 Communication Avenue
Bethesda, MD 20892
1-800-241-1044
http://www.nih.gov/nidcd

Depression

National Depressive and Manic Depressive Association
730 North Franklin, Suite 501
Chicago, IL 60610
1-800-82-NDMDA (1-800-826-3632)
http://www.ndmda.org

Diabetes

National Diabetes Association
P.O. Box 25757
1660 Duke Street
Alexandria, VA 22314
1-800-ADA-DISC (1-800-232-3472)

National Diabetes Information Clearinghouse
1 Information Way
Bethesda, MD 20892
(301) 654-3327
http://www.niddk.nih.gov

Drug abuse

Narcotics Anonymous
P.O. Box 9999
Van Nuys, CA 91409
(818) 773-9999
http://www.wsoinc.com

Eating disorders

The American Anorexia/Bulimia Association
165 West Forty-sixth Street, #1108
New York, NY 10036
(212) 575-6200
http://members.aol.com/amanbu/

Overeaters Anonymous
P.O. Box 44020
Rio Rancho, NM 87174
(505) 891-2664
http://www.overeatersanonymous.org

Endometriosis

Endometriosis Association
8585 North Seventy-sixth Place
Milwaukee, WI 53223
1-800-992-3636

Epilepsy

Epilepsy Foundation of America
4351 Garden City Drive
Landover, MD 20785
1-800-EFA-1000 (1-800-332-1000) or (301) 459-3700

Eye diseases

National Eye Institute
Building 31, Room 6A 32
31 Centre MSC 2510
Bethesda, MD 20892
(301) 496-5248

Fibromyalgia

Fibromyalgia Network
P.O. Box 31750
Tucson, AZ 85715
1-800-853-2929
http://www.fmnetnews.com

Genetic disorders

March of Dimes Birth Defects Foundation
1275 Mamaroneck Avenue
White Plains, NY 10605
1-888-MODIMES (1-888-663-4637) or (914) 428-7100
http://www.modimes.org

Headaches

American Council for Headache Education
1-800-255-ACHE (1-800-255-2243)
http://www.achenet.org

National Headache Foundation
5252 North Western Avenue
Chicago, IL 60625
1-800-843-2256
http://www.headaches.org

Heart disease

American Heart Association
7320 Greenville Avenue
Dallas, TX 75231
1-800-AHA-USA1 (1-800-242-8721)
http://www.amhrt.org/index.html

The Coronary Club, Inc.
9500 Euclid Avenue
Cleveland, OH 44195
1-800-478-4255 or (216) 444-3690
http://www.heartline/news.org

Hemophilia

National Hemophilia Foundation
116 West Thirty-second Street, Eleventh Floor
New York, NY 10001
1-800-424-2634
http://www.hemophilia.org

Hereditary hemochromatosis

Iron Overload Diseases Association
433 Westwind Drive, Dept. L
North Palm Beach, FL 33408
(561) 653-7543
http://www.ironoverload.org

Impotence

Impotence Institute of America/Impotence Anonymous
119 South Ruth Street
Maysville, TN 37803
(615) 983-6092

Incontinence

The Simon Foundation for Continence
P.O. Box 835
Wilmette, IL 60091
1-800-237-4666

Infertility

Resolve, Inc.
1310 Broadway
Somerville, MA 02144
Business office: (617) 623-1156
National HelpLine: (617) 623-0744
Fax: (617) 623-0252
http://www.resolve.org

Intestinal problems

Crohn's and Colitis Foundation of America
386 Park Avenue South
New York, NY 10017
1-800-932-2423

Intestinal Disease Foundation
1323 Forbes Avenue, Suite 200
Pittsburgh, PA 15219
(412) 261-5888

Kidney disease

American Association of Kidney Patients
100 South Ashley Drive, Suite 280
Tampa, Fl 33602
1-800-749-2257
http://www.aakp.org

Kidney Transplant/Dialysis Association
(617) 267-3747

National Kidney Foundation
30 East Thirty-third Street, Suite 1100
New York, NY 10016
1-800-622-9010 or (212) 889-2210
http://www.kidney.org

Polycystic Kidney Research Foundation
4901 Main Street, Suite 200
Kansas City, MO 64112
1-800-753-2873
http://www.kumc.edu/pkrf/

Leprosy

American Leprosy Missions
1 Alm Way
Greenville, SC 29601
1-800-537-7679
http://www.leprosy.org

Liver problems

American Liver Foundation
1425 Pompton Avenue, Suite 1-3
Cedar Grove, NJ 07009
1-800-223-0179

Lung disease

American Lung Association
1740 Broadway
New York, NY 10019
1-800-LUNG-USA (1-800-586-4872)
(212) 315-8700 or (212) 245-8000

Lupus

American Lupus Society
3914 Del Amo Boulevard, Suite 922
Torrance, CA 90503
1-800-331-1802

Lupus Foundation of America
4 Research Place, Suite 180
Rockville, MD 20850
1-800-558-0121

Lyme disease

American Lyme Disease Foundation
293 Route 100
Somers, NY 10549
1-800-876-5963
http://www.aldf.com

Lymphedema

National Lymphedema Network
2211 Post Street, Suite 404
San Francisco, CA 94115
1-800-541-3259
http://www.hooked.net/users/lymphnet

Marfan syndrome

National Marfan Foundation
382 Main Street
Port Washington, NY 11050
1-800-862-7326
http://www.marfan.org/factsheet.html

Multiple sclerosis

National Multiple Sclerosis Society
733 Third Avenue
New York, NY 10017
1-800-FIGHT-MS (1-800-344-4867) or (212) 986-3240
http://www.nmss.org

Muscular dystrophy

Muscular Dystrophy Association
3300 East Sunrise Drive
Tucson, AZ 85718
1-800-572-1717 or (602) 529-2000

Osteoporosis

National Osteoporosis Foundation
1150 Seventeenth Street NW, Suite 500
Washington, DC 20036
1-800-223-9994 or (202) 223-2226
http://www.nof.org

Parkinson's disease

American Parkinson's Disease Association
1250 Hylan Boulevard
Staten Island, NY 10305
1-800-223-2732 or (718) 981-8001
http://www.apdaparkinson.com

Premenstrual syndrome

PMS Access
P.O. Box 9326
Madison, WI 53715
1-800-222-4PMS (1-800-222-4767)

Prostate problems

American Prostate Society
1340 Charwood Road, Suite F
Hanover, MD 21076
1-800-308-1106

Psoriasis

National Psoriasis Foundation
6600 Southwest Ninety-second Avenue, Suite 300
Portland, OR 97223
1-800-723-9166
http://www.psoriasis.org

Sexually transmitted diseases

American Social Health Association
P.O. Box 13827
Research Triangle Park, NC 27009
1-800-230-6039
http://www.sunsite.unc.edu/asha

Spinal bifida

Spinal Bifida Association of America
4590 MacArthur Boulevard NW, Suite 250
Washington, DC 20007
1-800-621-3141

Stroke

Courage Stroke Network
7272 Greenville Avenue
Dallas, TX 75231
1-800-553-6321

National Institute of Neurological Disorders and Stroke
31 Centre Drive
Building 31, Room 8A-16
Bethesda, MD 20892
(301) 496-5751

American Stroke Foundation, Inc.
898 Park Avenue
New York, NY 10021
1-800-759-7592 or (212) 734-3461

Sources of Information on General Medical Topics

Newsletters

Harvard Health Letter
P.O. Box 380
Boston, MA 02117
http://www.countway.med.harvard.edu/publications/
Health_Publications/.index.html

Harvard Women's Health Watch
Harvard Medical School Health Publications Group
164 Longwood Avenue
Boston, MA 02115

Health After 50
Johns Hopkins Medical Center
P.O. Box 420179
Palm Coast, FL 32142

Mayo Clinic Health Letter
P.O. Box 53899
Boulder, CO 80322
1-800-678-5747, extension 45
http://www.ivi.com/ivistore/common/htm/letter.htm

University of California at Berkeley Wellness Letter
P.O. Box 420148
Palm Coast, FL 32142
(904) 446-4675
http://www.enews.com/magazines/ucbwl

Organizations

Child abuse

National Clearinghouse on Child Abuse and Neglect Information
P.O. Box 1182
Washington, DC 20013
1-800-FYI-3366 (1-800-394-3366) or (703) 385-7565

Childbirth

American Society for Psychoprophylaxis in Obstetrics (Lamaze Method)
1200 Nineteenth Street NW, Suite 3
Washington, DC 20036
1-800-368-4404

Cesareans: Support, Education, and Concern
22 Forest Road
Framingham, MA 01701
(508) 877-8266

Informed Home Birth: Informed Birth and Parenting
P.O. Box 3675
Ann Arbor, MI 48106
(313) 662-6857

International Childbirth Education Association
P.O. Box 20048
Minneapolis, MN 55420
1-800-624-4934

Children and teens

Association for the Care of Children's Health
19 Mantua Road
Mount Royal, NY 08061
(609) 224-1742

Child Find
1-800-I AM LOST (1-800-426-5678)

National Academy for Child Development
P.O. Box 380
Huntsville, UT 84317
Tel: (801) 621-8606
Fax: (801) 621-8389
email: *nacdinfo@nacd.org*
http://www.nacd.org/

National Center Hotline for Missing and Exploited Children
1-800-843-5678

Consumer groups

Center for Medical Consumers and Health Care Information
237 Thompson Street
New York, NY 10012
(212) 674-7105

People's Medical Society
462 Walnut Street
Allentown, PA 18102
(610) 770-1670

Public Citizen Health Research Group
1600 Twentieth Street NW
Washington, DC 20009
(202) 588-1000

Drug information

Food and Drug Administration
Office of Consumer Affairs
5600 Fishers Lane, HFE-50
Rockville, MD 20857
(301) 847-4420

Elder health issues

American Association of Retired Persons (AARP)
601 E Street NW
Washington, DC 20049
1-800-424-3410

National Citizen's Coalition for Nursing Home Reform
1424 Sixteenth Street NW, Suite 202
Washington, DC 20036
(202) 332-2275

Older Women's League
666 Eleventh Street NW, Suite 700
Washington, DC 20001
(202) 738-6686

Family planning

Planned Parenthood Federation of America
810 Seventh Avenue
New York, NY 10019
1-800-829-7732 or (212) 541-7800

Hospice

Children's Hospice International
2202 Mount Vernon Avenue, Suite 3C
Alexandria, VA 22301
1-800-24CHILD (1-800-242-4453)
http://www.chionline.org

National Hospice Organization
1901 North Moore Street, Suite 901
Arlington, VA 22209
1-800-658-8898 or (703) 243-5900
http://www.nho.org

National Institute for Jewish Hospice
P.O. Box 48025
Los Angeles, CA 90048
1-800-446-4448

Hospital accreditation

Joint Commission on Accreditation of Healthcare Organizations
One Renaissance Boulevard
Oak Brook Terrace, IL 60181
(630) 916-5600

Insurance problems

Patient Advocacy Foundation
739 Thimble Shoals Boulevard, Suite 704
Newport News, Virginia 23606
Tel: 1-800-532-5274
Fax: (757) 873-8999
http://www.patientadvocate.org

Patient Advocacy Coalition
3801 East Florida Avenue, Suite 400
Denver, CO 80210
(303) 512-0544

Learning disabilities

Learning Disabilities Association
4156 Library Road
Pittsburgh, PA 15234-1349
Tel: (412) 341-1515
Fax: (412) 344-0224
email: *ldanatl@usaor.net*
http://www.ldanatl.org/

Living wills and health care proxies

Choice in Dying
200 Varick Street
New York, NY 10014
1-800-989-WILL

Medicare/Medicaid information

Health Care Financing Administration, Office of Public Affairs
U.S. Department of Health and Human Services
Hubert H. Humphrey Building, Room 435-H
200 Independence Avenue SW
Washington, DC 20001
1-800-638-6833 (Medicare hot line)

Mental health

National Mental Health Association
1021 Prince Street
Alexandria, VA 22934
1-800-969-6642
http://www.nmha.org

Organ donations

The Living Bank
P.O. Box 6725
Houston, TX 77265
1-800-528-2971
http://www.livingbank.org

Women's health

National Women's Health Network Information Clearinghouse
(202) 628-7814

Office of Research on Women's Health
National Institutes of Health
(301) 402-1770

Medical Information Search Companies

The Health Resource, Inc.
564 Locust Avenue
Conway, AR 72032
Tel: 1-800-949-0090 or (501) 329-5272
Fax: (501) 329-9489
email: *moreinfo@thehealthresource.com*
http://www.thehealthresource.com

Institute for Health & Healing Information Service
2040 Webster Street
San Francisco, CA 94115
(415) 923-3680 (recording)
(415) 923-3681 (direct line)
Fax: (415) 673-2629

MEDcetera, Inc.
4515 Merrie Lane
Bellaire, TX 77401
1-800-748-6866 or (713) 666-6891
email: *pgeyer@netropolis.net*

Medical Information Foundation
2420 Sand Hill Road, Suite 101
Menlo Park, CA 94025
Tel: 1-800-999-1999 or (515) 326-6000
Fax: (415) 326-6700

Michigan Information Transfer Source
The University of Michigan
106 Hatcher Graduate Library
Ann Arbor, MI 48109
Tel: (313) 763-5060
Fax: (313) 763-6803
email: *pkmakin@umich.edu*
http://www.lib.umich.edu/libhome/services/mits/index.html

Personal Health Care Advocates
8000 Tower Crescent Drive, Suite 1350
Vienna, VA 22182
Tel: (703) 760-7838
Fax: (703) 760-7899

Schine On-Line Services
39 Brinton Avenue
Providence, RI 02906
Tel: 1-800-346-3287 or (401) 751-0120
Fax: (401) 751-7955
email: *schine@findcure.com*
http://www.findcure.com

Notes

Chapter 1: Taking Charge of Your Medical Care

1. Eric Cassell, M.D., *The Healer's Art: A New Approach to the Doctor-Patient Relationship* (New York: Lippincott, 1976), 62.

2. Lewis Thomas, "Leech, Leech, Etcetera," in *The Youngest Science: Notes of a Medicine Watcher* (New York: Viking Press, 1983), 59-60.

3. Max Lerner, *Wrestling with the Angel: A Memoir of My Triumph Over Illness* (New York: W. W. Norton, 1990), 139.

4. Patch Adams, M.D., *Gesundheit!* (Rochester, Vermont: Healing Arts Press, 1993), 33.

5. Perri Klass, M.D., *A Not Entirely Benign Procedure: Four Years as a Medical Student* (New York: Signet, 1987), 48.

6. C. A. Gatsonis et al., "Variations in the Utilization of Coronary Angiography for Elderly Patients with an Acute Myocardial Infarction," *Medical Care* 33, no. 6 (June 1995): 625-642.

7. Peter Berczeller, M.D., *Doctors and Patients: What We Feel About You* (New York: Macmillan, 1994), 17.

8. Sherwin B. Nuland, M.D., *How We Die: Reflections on Life's Final Chapter* (New York: Alfred A. Knopf, 1994), 248.

9. Cynthia Carver, M.D., *Patient Beware: Dealing with Doctors and Other Medical Dilemmas* (Scarborough, Ontario: Prentice Hall Canada, Inc., 1984), 8.

10. John Pekkanen, *M.D.: Doctors Talk About Themselves* (New York: Delacourt, 1988), 55.

11. A. G. Lawthers et al., "Physicians' Perception of the Risk of Being Sued," *Journal of Health, Politics, Policy and Law* 17, no. 3 (Fall 1992): 463-82.

12. P. H. Hughes et al., "Prevalence of Substance Abuse Among U.S. Physicians," *Journal of the American Medical Association* 267, no. 17 (6 May 1992): 2333-9.

13. "Physician, Cherish Thyself. The Hazards of Self Prescribing," *Journal of the American Medical Association* 267, no. 17 (6 May 1992): 2373-4.

14. T. A. Brennan et al., "Incidence of Adverse Effects and Negligence in Hospitalized Patients: Results of the Harvard Medical Practice Study I," *New England Journal of Medicine* 324, no. 6 (7 February 1991): 370-76.

15. Richard A. Knox, "Doctor's Orders Killed Cancer Patient: Dana-Farber Admits Drug Overdose Caused Death of Globe Columnist, Damage to Second Woman," *Boston Globe*, 23 March 1995.

16. E. L. Allan et al., "Dispensing Errors and Counseling in Community Practice," *American Pharmacist* NS35, no. 12 (December 1995): 25-33.

Chapter 2: Finding the Right Doctor

1. James E. Payne, M.D., *Me Too: A Doctor Survives Prostate Cancer* (Waco, Texas: WRS Publishing, 1995), 72.

2. J. M. Read and R. M. Ratzan, "Yellow Professionalism: Advertising by Physicians in the Yellow Pages," *New England Journal of Medicine* 316, no. 21 (21 May 1987): 1315-19.

3. Pekkanen, *M.D.: Doctors Talk About Themselves*, 138-139.

4. Payne, *Me Too*, 16.

5. Edward Rosenbaum, M.D., *A Taste of My Own Medicine: When the Doctor Is the Patient* (New York: Random House, 1988), 161.

Chapter 3: Getting What You Need from Managed Care

1. The National Committee for Quality Assurance, "The State of Managed Care Quality," *http://www.ncqa.org/news/report.htm*.

2. James W. Saxton, "The Physician's Legal Duty as the Patient's Advocate," *Medical Practice Communicator* 4, no. 6 (1997): 1, 7.

3. J. Kassirer, "Managed Care and the Morality of the Marketplace," *New England Journal of Medicine* 333, no. 1 (July 1995): 50.

4. Alan J. Steinberg, M.D., *The Insider's Guide to HMOs: How to Navigate the Managed-Care System and Get the Health Care You Deserve* (New York: Penguin Books, 1997), 52-54.

5. John R. Hayes, "Knowledge is Money," *Forbes*, 13 February 1995, 188.

6. The National Committee for Quality Assurance, "The State of Managed Care Quality," *http://www.ncqa.org/news/report.htm*.

7. Ellen Joan Pollock, "Managed Care's Focus on Psychiatric Drugs Alarms Many Doctors," *Wall Street Journal*, 1 December 1995.

8. Laura Johannes, "Some HMOs Now Put Doctors on a Budget for Prescription Drugs," *Wall Street Journal*, 22 May 1997.

9. Steinberg, *The Insider's Guide to HMOs*, 33-34.

10. Steinberg, *The Insider's Guide to HMOs*, 133.

11. Howard Gleckman, "My Dad's Harrowing Trip Through a Medicare HMO," *Business Week*, 4 August 1997, 34.

12. Susan Brink, "The Cancer Wars at HMOs," *US News and World Report*, 5 February 1996.

Chapter 4: Communication

1. Lerner, *Wrestling with the Angel*, 33.

2. Jody Heymann, *Equal Partners: A Physician's Call for a New Spirit of Medicine* (Boston: Little, Brown and Company, 1995), 48.

3. E. L. Idler and S. Kasl, "Health Perceptions and Survival: Do Global Evaluations of Health Status Predict Mortality?" *Journal of Gerontology* 46, no. 2 (March 1991): 55-65.

4. D. Roter, M. Lipkin Jr., and A. Korsgaard, "Sex Differences in Patients' and Physicians' Communication During Primary Care Medical Visits," *Medical Care* 29, no. 11 (November 1991): 1083-93.

5. Berczeller, *Doctors and Patients*, 106.

6. Rosenbaum, *A Taste of My Own Medicine*, 131.

7. Klass, *A Not Entirely Benign Procedure*, 73.

8. Norman Cousins, *Anatomy of An Illness as Perceived by the Patient: Reflections on Healing and Regeneration* (New York: W. W. Norton, 1979).

9. Payne, *Me Too*, 2.

10. H. B. Beckman and R. M. Frankel, "The Effect of Physician Behavior on the Collection of Data," *Annals of Internal Medicine* 101, no. 5 (November 1984): 692-96.

11. W. Levinson et al., "Physician-Patient Communication: The Relationship with Malpractice Claims Among Primary Care Physicians and Surgeons," *Journal of the American Medical Association* 277, no. 7 (1997): 553-59.

12. Austin Flint, *Medical Ethics and Etiquette: The Code of Ethics Adopted by the American Medical Association* (New York: D. Appleton and Company, 1883), 34.

13. S. Greenfield, S. H. Kaplan, and J. E. Ware Jr., "Expanding Patient Involvement in Care: Effects on Patient Outcomes," *Annals of Internal Medicine* 102, no. 4 (April 1985): 520-28.

Chapter 5: Physician Rights and Responsibilities

1. "American College of Physicians Ethics Manual, Third Edition," *Annals of Internal Medicine* 117, no. 11 (1 December 1992): 948.

2. A. Greenspan et al., "Incidence of Unwarranted Implantation of Permanent Cardiac Pacemakers in a Large Medical Population," *New England Journal of Medicine* 318, no. 3 (January 1988): 158-162.

3. Arthur Frank, *At the Will of the Body: Reflections on Illness* (Boston: Houghton Mifflin, 1991), 27.

4. Levinson, "Physician-Patient Communication," 553-59.

5. Diane Komp, M.D., *A Child Shall Lead Them: Lessons About Hope from Children with Cancer* (San Francisco: HarperCollins, 1993), 132.

6. R. B. Burns et al., "As Mammography Use Increases, Are Some Providers Omitting Clinical Breast Examination?" *Archives of Internal Medicine* 156, no. 7 (8 April 1996): 741-44.

7. "Ethical Considerations in the Allocation of Organs and Other Scarce Medical Resources Among Patients," *Archives of Internal Medicine* 155 (1995): 2013-17.

8. D. A. Taira et al., "The Relationship Between Patient Income and Physician Discussion of Health Risk Behaviors," *Journal of the American Medical Association* 278, no. 17 (5 November 1997): 1412-17.

9. Gleckman, "My Dad's Harrowing Trip," 34.

10. Edith Gittings Reid, *The Great Physician* (London: Oxford University Press, 1931), 46.

11. Barbara Webster, *All of a Piece: A Life with Multiple Sclerosis* (Baltimore: The Johns Hopkins University Press, 1989), 124.

12. "American College of Physicians Ethics Manual, Third Edition," 950.

13. Reynolds Price, *A Whole New Life* (New York: Atheneum, 1994), 13.

14. Heymann, *Equal Partners*, 134.

15. Oath of Geneva, *http://www.sequel.net/~twilight/oath7.htm.*

16. "American College of Physicians Ethics Manual, Third Edition," 948.

17. Reid, *The Great Physician*, 154.

18. Cousins, *Anatomy of An Illness*.

Chapter 6: Patient Rights and Responsibilities

1. Levinson, "Physician-Patient Communication," 553-59.

2. Advisory Commission on Consumer Protection and Quality in the Health Care Industry, "Consumer Bill of Rights and Responsibilities" (1997), 20-21.

3. "Consumer Bill of Rights and Responsibilities," 53-56.

4. Rosenbaum, *A Taste of My Own Medicine*, 37.

5. Webster, *All of a Piece*, 126.

6. S. Greenfield and S. H. Kaplan, "Patients' Participation in Medical Care: Effects on Blood Sugar Control and Quality of Life in Diabetes," *Journal of General Internal Medicine* 3, no. 5 (September 1988): 448-57.

7. S. H. Kaplan, S. Greenfield, and J. E. Ware Jr., "Assessing the Effects of Physician-Patient Interactions on the Outcomes of Chronic Disease," *Medical Care* 27, no. 3 Supplemental (March 1989): S110-S127.

8. Sandra Boodman, "Medicine's Dirty Little Secret: Hospitals Promote Hand Washing to Stem Spread of Infection," *Washington Post,* 30 September 1997, Health, 12.

9. J. M. Teno et al., "Preferences for Cardiopulmonary Resuscitation: Physician-Patient Agreement and Hospital Resource Use," *Journal of General Internal Medicine* 10 (April 1995): 179-186.

10. R. L. Kravitz et al., "Recall of Recommendations and Adherence to Advice Among Patients with Chronic Medical Conditions," *Archives of Internal Medicine* 153, no. 16 (23 August 1993): 1869-78.

11. N. Col et al., "The Role of Medication Noncompliance and Adverse Drug Reactions in Hospitalization of the Elderly," *Archives of Internal Medicine* 150 (April 1990): 841-45.

12. Joseph E. Harding, "Second Opinion," in *A Piece of My Mind: A Collection of Essays from JAMA,* edited by Bruce B. Dan and Roxanne K. Young (New York: Random House, 1990), 96-97.

13. Webster, *All of a Piece,* 123.

14. J. M. McGinnis and W. H. Foege, "Actual Causes of Death in the U.S.," *Journal of the American Medical Association* 270 (1993): 2207-12.

Chapter 7: Problem Solving

1. Francesca Thompson, *Going for the Cure* (New York: St. Martin's Press, 1989), 221.

Chapter 8: Getting a Second Opinion

1. "AMA Principles of Medical Ethics," *Code of Medical Ethics: Current Opinions With Annotations* (AMA, 1996).

2. S. G. Martin et al., "Impact of Mandatory Second Opinion Program on Medicaid Surgery Rates," *Medical Care* 20, no. 1 (January 1982): 21-45.

3. J. I. Epstein et al., "Clinical and Cost Impact of Second-Opinion Pathology Review of Prostate Biopsies Prior to Radical Prostatectomy," *American Journal of Surgical Pathology* 20, no. 7 (July 1996): 851-57.

4. Heymann, *Equal Partners,* 75.

Chapter 9: Changing Doctors

1. Brennan, "Incidence of Adverse Effects," 370-76.

Chapter 10: Questions to Ask About Tests, Drugs, and Surgery

1. Cousins, *Anatomy of An Illness.*

2. Rosenbaum, *A Taste of My Own Medicine*, 100.

3. P. W. Marcello et al., "Routine Preoperative Studies: Which Studies in Which Patients?" *Surgical Clinics of North America* 76, no. 1 (February 1996): 11-23.

4. R. G. Wiencek et. al., "Usefulness of Selective Preoperative Chest X-ray Films. A Prospective Study," *American Surgery* (July 1987): 396-98.

5. R. A. Wood and R. A. Hoekelman, "Value of the Chest X-ray as a Screening Test for Elective Surgery in Children," *Pediatrics* 67, no. 4 (April 1981): 447-52.

6. D. Klingman et al., "Measuring Defensive Medicine Using Clinical Scenarios," *Journal of Health, Politics, Policy and Law* 21, no. 2 (Summer 1996): 185-217.

7. Pekkanen, *M.D.: Doctors Talk About Themselves*, 164.

8. Lawthers, "Physicians' Perceptions on the Risk of Being Sued," 463-82.

9. E. A. Boohaker et al., "Patient Notification and Follow-up of Abnormal Test Results. A Physician Survey," *Archives of Internal Medicine* 156, no. 3 (12 February 1996): 327-31.

10. Sandra Boodman, "Now That Two Popular Weight Loss Drugs Are Off the Market, What's Left for Dieters?" *Washington Post*, 16 Sept 1997, Health, 11-15.

11. Brennan, "Incidence of Adverse Effects," 370-76.

12. E. L. Allan et al., "Dispensing Errors and Counseling in Community Practice," *American Pharmacist* NS35, no. 12 (December 1995): 25-33.

13. D. Einstadter et al., "Variation in the Rate of Cervical Spine Surgery in Washington State," *Medical Care* 31, no. 8 (August 1993): 711-18.

14. A. Lee-Feldstein, H. Anton-Culver, and P. J. Feldstein, "Treatment Differences and Other Prognostic Factors Related to Breast Cancer Survival. Delivery Systems and Outcomes," *Journal of the American Medical Association* 271, no. 15 (20 April 1994): 1163-68.

15. Thomas Scully and Celia Scully, *Playing God: The New World of Medical Choices* (New York: Simon & Schuster, 1988), 75.

Chapter 11: Taking Action if You Have Been Wronged

1. *The Washington Post*, 1 April 1997, Health, 8.

2. Public Citizen, *http://www.citizen.org.*

3. A. R. Localio, "Relation Between Malpractice Claims and Adverse Effects Due to Negligence: Results of the Harvard Medical Practice Study III," *New England Journal of Medicine* 324, no. 6 (7 February 1991): 245-51.

4. Pekkanen, *M.D.: Doctors Talk About Themselves*, 182-183.

5. Charles Vincent, Magi Young, and Angela Phillips, "Why Do People Sue Doctors? A Study of Patients and Relatives Taking Legal Action," *Lancet* 343 (25 June 1994): 1612.

Chapter 12: Clinical Trials

1. Bill Sloat and Keith Epstein, "Using Our Kids as Guinea Pigs," *Cleveland Plain Dealer*, 16 December 1996.

2. Federal Register, 39, 105, 30 May 1974, 18917.

3. Evan Handler, *Time on Fire: My Comedy of Terrors* (Boston: Little, Brown and Company, 1996), 21.

4. "Physicians' Reasons for Not Entering Eligible Patients in a Randomized Clinical Trial of Surgery for Breast Cancer," *New England Journal of Medicine* 310 (1984): 1363-67.

5. D. W. Marion et al., "Treatment of Traumatic Brain Injury with Moderate Hypothermia," *New England Journal of Medicine* 336, no. 8 (20 February 1997): 540-46.

6. C. Diehm et al., "Comparison of Leg Compression Stocking and Oral Horse Chestnut Seed Extract in Patients with Chronic Venous Insufficiency," *Lancet* 347 (1996): 292-94.

7. R. T. Chlebowski and M. Grosvenor, "The Scope of Nutrition Intervention Trials with Cancer-Related Endpoints," *Cancer* 74, no. 9 (1 November 1994): 2734-38.

Suggested Reading

Patient-physician relationships

Barasch, Marc Ian. *The Healing Path: A Soul Approach to Illness*. New York: Penguin Books, 1995.

Callahan, Daniel. *The Troubled Dream of Life: In Search of a Peaceful Death*. New York: Simon & Schuster, 1993.

Cassell, Eric, M.D. *The Healer's Art: A New Approach to the Doctor-Patient Relationship*. Philadelphia: J. B. Lippincott Company, 1976.

Dan, Bruce, M.D., and Roxanne Young. *A Piece of My Mind*. Boston: Feeling Fine, 1988.

Hilfiker, David, M.D. *Healing the Wounds: A Physician Looks at His Work*. New York: Pantheon Books, 1985.

Inlander, Charles B., ed. *People's Medical Society Health Desk Reference: Information Your Doctor Can't or Won't Tell You*. New York: Hyperion, 1996.

Katz, Jay. *The Silent World of Doctor and Patient*. New York: The Free Press, 1984.

Kleinman, Arthur, M.D. *The Illness Narratives: Suffering, Healing and the Human Condition*. New York: Basic Books, 1988.

Pekkanen, John. *M.D.: Doctors Talk About Themselves*. New York: Delacorte Press, 1988.

Podell, Richard, M.D., and William Proctor. *When Your Doctor Doesn't Know Best*. New York: Simon & Schuster, 1995.

Preston, Thomas, M.D. *The Clay Pedestal: A Renowned Cardiologist Reexamines the Doctor-Patient Relationship*. New York: Charles Scribner's Sons, 1986.

Rosenfeld, Isadore, M.D. *Second Opinion: Your Medical Alternatives*. New York: Simon & Schuster, 1981.

Vergehese, Abraham. *My Own Country: A Doctor's Story*. New York: Vintage Books, 1995.

Illness narratives written by doctors

Heymann, Jody, M.D. *Equal Partners: A Physician's Call for a New Spirit of Medicine*. New York: Little, Brown and Company, 1995.

Payne, James, M.D. *Me Too: A Doctor Survives Prostate Cancer.* Waco, Texas: WRS Publishing, 1995.

Rosenbaum, Edward, M.D. *A Taste of My Own Medicine.* New York: Random House, 1988.

Illness narratives written by patients

Broyard, Anatole. *Intoxicated by My Illness: And Other Writings on Life and Death.* New York: Fawcett, 1992.

Cousins, Norman. *Anatomy of an Illness as Perceived by the Patient: Reflections on Healing and Regeneration.* New York: W. W. Norton & Company, 1979.

Dubus, Andre. *Broken Vessels.* Boston: David R. Godine, 1991.

Frank, Arthur W. *At the Will of the Body: Reflections on Illness.* Boston: Houghton Mifflin Company, 1991.

Handler, Evan. *Time on Fire: My Comedy of Terrors.* New York: Little, Brown and Company, 1996.

Lerner, Max. *Wrestling with the Angel: A Memoir of My Triumph Over Illness.* New York: W. W. Norton & Company, 1990.

Mayer, Musa. *Examining Myself: One Woman's Story of Breast Cancer Treatment and Recovery.* Boston: Faber and Faber, 1993.

Price, Reynolds. *A Whole New Life.* New York: Atheneum, 1994.

Thompson, Francesca, M.D. *Going for the Cure.* New York: St. Martin's Press, 1989.

Webster, Barbara D. *All of a Piece: A Life with Multiple Sclerosis.* Baltimore: The Johns Hopkins University Press, 1989.

Medical ethics

Annas, George J. *The Rights of Patients: The Basic ACLU Guide to Patient Rights,* revised edition. Ottawa, New Jersey: Humana Press, 1992.

Caplan, Arthur. *Due Consideration: Controversy in the Age of Medical Miracles.* New York: Wiley, 1997.

Caplan, Arthur. *Moral Matters: Ethical Issues in Medicine and the Life Sciences.* New York: Wiley, 1995.

Dubler, Nancy, and David Nimmons. *Ethics on Call: Taking Charge of Life-and-Death Choices In Today's Health Care System.* New York: Vintage, 1993.

Hilfiker, David, M.D. *Healing the Wounds: A Physician Looks at His Work.* New York: Pantheon Books, 1985.

Hilton, Bruce. *First Do No Harm: Wrestling with the New Medicine's Life and Death Dilemmas.* Nashville: Abingdon Press, 1991.

Macklin, Ruth. *Enemies of Patients.* Oxford: Oxford University Press, 1993.

Scully, Thomas, M.D., and Celia Scully. *Playing God: The New World of Medical Choices*. New York: Simon & Schuster, 1987.

Coping with hospitalization

Blau, Sheldon, M.D., and Elaine Fantle Shimberg. *How to Get Out of the Hospital Alive—A Guide to Patient Power*. New York: Macmillan General Reference, 1997.

Inlander, Charles. *Take this Book to the Hospital with You*. St. Martin's Mass Market Paper, 1997.

Keene, Nancy, and Rachel Prentice. *Your Child in the Hospital*. Sebastopol, California: O'Reilly & Associates, 1997.

McCann, Karen Keating. *Take Charge of Your Hospital Stay*. New York: Insight Books, 1994.

Scheller, Mary Dale. *Building Partnerships in Hospital Care*. Palo Alto, California: Bull Publishing Company, 1990.

Medical self-help books

Berkow, Robert, and Mark H. Beers, eds. *The Merck Manual of Medical Information: Home Edition*. Whitehouse Station, New Jersey: Merck & Company, 1997.

Cox, Kathryn, ed. *The Good Housekeeping Illustrated Guide to Women's Health*. New York: Hearst Books, 1994.

Goldberg, Ken, M.D. *How Men Can Live as Long as Women*. The Male Health Center, 1993. Call (214) 490-6253.

Hoffman, Eileen, M.D. *Our Health, Our Lives: A Revolutionary Approach to Total Health Care for Women*. New York: Pocket Books, 1996.

Inlander, Charles, and Paula Brisco. *The Consumer's Guide to Medical Lingo*. Allentown, Pennsylvania: People's Medical Society, 1992.

Public Citizen. *Medical Records; Getting Yours*. 1995. $10. To order this book, you can send a check payable to Public Citizen at 1600 20th Street NW, Washington, DC 20009. Please be sure to include $4.00 shipping and handling. Or call (202) 588-1000 and ask for the publications office.

Weisse, Allen B., M.D. *The Man's Guide to Good Health*. Yonkers, New York: Consumer Reports Books, 1991. Call 1-800-500-9760.

Finding the best doctor or hospital

Arnot, Robert, M.D. *The Best Medicine: How to Choose the Top Doctors, the Top Hospitals, and the Top Treatments*. Reading, Massachusetts: Addison-Wesley, 1992.

Boyden, K., ed. *Medical and Health Information Directory: A Guide to Associations, Agencies, Companies, Institutions, Research Centers, Hospitals, Clinics, Treatment Centers, Educational Programs, Publications, Audiovisuals, DataBanks, Libraries, and Information Services in Clinical Medicine*, 4th edition, 3 volumes. Detroit: Gale, 1993.

Ernst, F. W., M.D. *Now They Lay Me Down to Sleep... What You Don't Know About Anesthesia and Surgery May Harm You*. Dothan, Alabama: E & P Publishers, 1997.

Naifeh, Steven, and Gregory Smith. *The Best Doctors in America: 1996-97*. 3rd edition. Aiken, South Carolina: Woodward/White, 1997.

Smith, Gregory, and Steven Naifeh. *Making Miracles Happen*. New York: Little, Brown and Company, 1997.

Avoiding questionable doctors

Public Citizen. *Physicians Disciplined for Sex-Related Offenses*. Washington, DC: Public Citizen, 1997.

Public Citizen. *13,012 Questionable Doctors*. Washington, DC: Public Citizen, 1996.

Research

Baldwin, Fred, and Suzanne McInerney. *Infomedicine*. New York: Little, Brown and Company, 1996.

Barrett, Daniel. *NetResearch: Finding Information Online*. Sebastopol, California: O'Reilly & Associates, 1997.

Ferguson, Tom, M.D. *Health Online: How to Find Health Information, Support Groups and Self-Help Communities in Cyberspace*. New York: Addison Wesley, 1996.

Freed, Melvyn, and Karen Graves. *The Patient's Desk Reference: Where to Find Answers to Medical Questions*. New York: Macmillan, 1994.

Hogarth, Michael, M.D., and David Hutchison. *An Internet Guide for the Health Professional*. Sacramento, California: New Wind Publishing, 1996.

Millenson, Michael L. *Demanding Medical Excellence: Doctors and Accountability in the Information Age*. Chicago: University of Chicago Press, 1997.

Naythons, Matthew, and A. Catsimatides. *The Internet: Health, Fitness & Medicine Yellow Pages*. New York: Osborne McGraw-Hill, 1995.

Rees, Alan M., ed. *The Consumer Health Information Sourcebook*. Phoenix: Oryx Press, 1994.

Slack, Warner V. *Cybermedicine: How Computing Empowers Doctors and Patients for Better Health Care*. San Francisco: Jossey-Bass, 1997.

Managed care

American Association of Retired Persons (AARP). *Managed Care: An AARP Guide*. 1-800-424-3410.

Anders, George. *Health Against Wealth: HMOs and the Breakdown of Medical Trust*. New York: Houghton Mifflin, 1996.

Connolly, John J. *How to Find the Best Doctors, Hospitals, and HMOs for You and Your Family*. New York: Castle Connolly Medical, 1995.

Steinberg, Alan. *The Insider's Guide to HMOs: How to Navigate the Managed-care System and Get the Health Care You Deserve*. New York: Penguin, 1997.

Alternative and complementary therapies

Cousins, Norman. *Head First: The Biology of Hope and the Healing Power of the Human Spirit*. New York: Penguin Books, 1989.

Golman, Daniel, and Joel Gurin. *Mind/Body Medicine*. Yonkers, New York: Consumer Report Books, 1993.

Lerner, Michael. *Choices in Healing: Integrating the Best of Conventional and Complementary Approaches to Healing*. Cambridge, Massachusetts: The MIT Press, 1994.

Moyers, Bill. *Healing and the Mind*. New York: Doubleday, 1993.

Tyler, Varro. *The Honest Herbal: A Sensible Guide to the Use of Herbs and Related Remedies*. Binghamton, New York: Haworth Press, 1993.

Weil, Andrew, M.D. *Spontaneous Healing: How to Discover and Enhance Your Body's Natural Ability to Maintain and Heal Itself*. New York: Alfred A. Knopf, 1995.

Index

A

abandonment by physician, 126-127
ABMS Directory of Board-Certified
    Medical Specialists, 34
Adams, Dr. Patch
    advance directive, 136
    doctor's detachment, 3-4
advocate
    during appointments, 164-165
    during tests, 211
    right to have, 141-142
    when in hospital, 65
AMA (American Medical Association)
    Council of Ethical and Judicial Af-
        fairs, 118
    Directory of Physicians, 34, 239
    Principles of Medical Ethics, 301
American Board of Medical Special-
    ties, 275, 307-310
American College of Physician's Ethics
    Manual, obligations be-
    tween patient and doc-
    tor, 109-110
American Hospital Association's Pa-
    tient's Bill of Rights, 303-
    306
American Medical Association. *See*
    AMA
appreciation, showing, 100-102
attorneys
    HMO appeals, 72
    malpractice claims, 244-245
authorization for care from HMO, 63-
    64

B

Berczeller, Dr. Peter
    expecting obedience from pa-
        tients, 9
    withholding information from pa-
        tients, 81
Best Doctors Worldwide, 276
bills
    pay promptly, 108
    paying, 151-152
    problems with, 161-162
    talking about problems, 89-90
Bills of Rights and Ethic Codes, 301-
    306
blood pressure, high, 219, 221
blood products, refusal of, 135-136
board certification, 30-33
books
    finding in library, 283-287
    medical dictionary, 277
    purchasing, 287
boredom, of doctor, 10

C

CancerGuide, 264
CancerNet, 264
capitation, 38, 51-54
Carver, Dr. Cynthia
    examination by student doctors,
        10-11
Cassell, Dr. Eric
    healing medicine, 2
Center for the Study of Service, 61
CenterWatch, 264

compliance with treatment plan, 106, 148-149
conditions, sources of information on, 311-330
confidentiality
    doctor's responsibility to maintain, 125-126
    patient's right to, 138-139
conflict resolution, 162-173. *See also* problems, solving
Consumer Bill of Rights and Responsibilities, 301-303
Consumer Federation of America, 72
Cousins, Norman
    partnership with doctor, 129
credentials of doctor, 29-36
criminal activity, report, 245-246
curiosity, intellectual, 9

D

decision making
    based on research, 271-272, 297-298
    informed consent required, 116-118
    mutual, 94-100
    See also communication
defensive medicine, 12-13, 208
diagnosis
    based on test results, 215
    second opinion if uncertain, 178-179
dictionary, medical, 277
disagreements between doctors and patients, 157-158, 170-171
disclosure, 118
    hospitals, disclosure by, 134
    right to facts, 133-134
    time provided for full disclosure, 133
diseases, sources of information on, 311-324

Doctor Finder, 239
doctors
    changing, 191-204. *See also* changing doctors
    communicating with, 88-94
    credentials, 29-36
    decisions influenced, 5-14
    finding right, 19-41. *See also* finding right doctor
    historical view, 2-5
    impaired, 13-14
        taking action against, 238
    payment systems, 36-39
    practice, types of, 24-25
    relationships, types of, 25-26, 76-79
    responsibilities, 109-127, 301
        AMA Principles of Medical Ethics, 301
        confidentiality, 125-126
        hope, promote, 122-123
        informed consent, 116-118
        limits, know,124-125
        new information, current with, 120
        no abandonment, 126-127
        reasonable care and skill, 109-110
        respect and kindness, 110-111
        risky behaviors, discuss, 119-120
        service, 109
        time, providing adequate, 114-116
        treat person, not body, 121
        waiting time reasonable, 113-114
    rights, 103-108
        compliance with treatment, 106
        conversation, limited social, 107
        courtesy from patient, 104

finding right doctor (*continued*)
  specialists, 23-24
  training, 30
forgiveness, after medical errors, 234-235
formularies, 48, 59
Frank, Arthur
  uncaring physician, 112

G
gag orders, 58
gatekeepers, 47, 66
Gould, Stephen Jay
  making sense of statistics, 86-87
  "The Median Isn't the Message," 87
grievances
  after injury, 234-241
  managed care, 68
  See also problems, solving
group practice, 25

H
Handler, Evan
  clinical trial explanation, 253
healers, 127-128
health
  behaviors that affect, 119
  patient responsibility for, 18, 153-155
health maintenance organization
  (HMO), 68-71. *See also*
  managed care
healthy lifestyle, 18
  patient responsibility for, 153-155
Heymann, Dr. Jody
  getting second opinions, 178, 187
  trusting physicians, 77
hope, 122-123
hospitalization
  advocate, right to, 65
  limitations on stays, 48
  mistakes, 224
  problems during, 171-172

hospital records
  confidentiality of, 138-139
  getting copies, 139-140
humor, helps communication, 93-94
hypertension, side effects of medication for, 219, 221

I, J
illness
  compliance with treatment plan, 148-149
  information about, obtaining, 132-133
  participation in treatment decisions, 134-135
  prevention of, 7-8
  responsibility to learn about, 146-147
  right to refuse treatment for, 135-137
impaired doctors, 13-14, 233-249
independent practice association
  (IPA), 51-52. *See also*
  managed care
Index Medicus, 286
information searches, professional, 296-297, 331-332
informed consent, 116-118
  for clinical trials, 252-253
informed decision making, 271-272
injury, by doctor, 233-249
insurance
  requiring second opinion, 176
  See also managed care
interlibrary loan, 285
Internet
  evaluating information, 292-293
  locating technical information, 287-292
  MEDLINE, 288-290
  other medical databases, 290-292
  PubMed, 288-290
  support groups, 282

interruptions
  how to stop, 91
  prevention, 91
intervention, levels of, 8
interviewing potential doctors, 39-41

K

Klass, Dr. Perri
  abnormal pregnancies, 4
Komp, Dr. Diane
  questions, overwhelmed by, 115

L

language
  blaming language by doctors, 85
  jargon, 82
  statistics, making sense of, 86-88
  See also communication
lawyers. See attorneys
Lerner, Max
  roles of patient and doctor, 3
letter to doctor
  after error, 236-237
  to leave doctor's practice, 203
  to solve problems, 165-166
  when filing complaint, 246
libraries
  finding an article, 284
  finding a book, 283
  interlibrary loans, 285
  medical, 285-286
  public, 283-285
  university, 286-287
  See also researching medical literature
limitations on drug use, HMO, 48, 59
limitations on hospital stays, 48
listserv discussion group, 293-296
living will, 136

M

malpractice
  claims not common, 242
  definition, 242-243

malpractice suits
  communication prevents, 112-113
  how to file, 244-245
  physician perceptions, 13
  statute of limitations, 245
managed care
  appeals, 68-71
  arbitration, 63
  authorization, 63-64
  complaints about doctor, 241
  definition, 46-50
  denial of services, 69
  emergency room policies, 60
  formularies, 48, 59
  gag orders, 58
  gatekeepers, 47, 66
  grievances, 53-54
  limitations on hospital stays, 48
  payment methods
    capitation, 38, 51-54
    fee-for-service, 36-37, 50-51
    salary and bonuses, 37-38
  plan, picking a, 56-61
  point-of-service option, 59, 63
  preventing problems, 62-65
  problems
    solving, 68-73
    types of, 66-68
  restrict access to clinical trials, 262
  types of plan
    fee-for-service, 50-51
    health maintenance organization (HMO), 68-71
    independent practice association (IPA), 51-52
    preferred provider organization (PPO), 52-53
    utilization management committee, 49
"The Median Isn't the Message," 87
medical charts
  confidentiality of, 138-139
  copies of, 139-140
  understanding, 84

prognosis, based on test results, 217
protocol, for clinical trial, 254
Public Citizen Health Research Group,
    35-36
PubMed, 288

Q

questions
    about clinical trials, 265-266
    about medications, 219-222
    about surgery, 228-231
    about tests and procedures, 209-
        217
    deciding on HMO, 56-61
    interviewing potential doctor, 39-
        41
    keep asking, 99
    when giving doctor your history,
        92

R

rare disorders, national organization
    for, 278
recommendations for doctors, 28
records, medical
    confidentiality, 138-139
    copies of, 139-140
    falsifying, 238
relationship with doctor
    types of, 25-27
        adversarial, 77
        collegial, 78
        paternal, 76
researching medical literature, 269-
    299
    finding experts, 280-283
    getting research help, 280
    Internet resources, 287
        emotional support, 293-296
        evaluation, 292-293

technical information, 287-
    292
libraries, using
    medical libraries, 286
    public libraries, 283-285
    university libraries, 286
making decisions, 297-299
professional information search-
    es, 296-297, 331-332
reasons not to research, 272-274
    ambiguity, confronting, 273-
        274
    fear, 273
    misunderstanding informa-
        tion, 274
    options, lack of better, 274-
        275
    statistics, 273
    time-consuming, 272-273
reasons to research, 269-272
    improve quality of life, 271
    make informed decisions,
        271-272
    reassurance, 272
    save life or limb, 269
    take back control, 270
resources
    Internet, 287-296
    libraries, 283-286
setting research goals
    complementary therapies,
        276
    controversies, 276
    doctors, top, 276
    emotional support, 276
    organizations, 276
    standard of care, 275
residents
    definition, 30
    doing procedures, 11
    right to refuse treatment from,
        135

responsibilities. *See* doctors, responsibilities; ethics; patient responsibilities

rights. *See* doctors, rights; ethics; patient rights

risks
 of clinical trials, 266-267
 of medications, 218
 of surgery, 226

Rosenbaum, Dr. Edward
 communication with doctors, 83
 need for advocate in hospital, 141
 selecting doctor, 44

S

salaries, of doctors, 37-38

Scully, Dr. Thomas
 treatment options, learning about, 231-232

searches, professional, 296-297, 331-332

second opinions, 175-189
 information gained, using, 187-190
 obtaining, 184-187
 when you need one, 175-184
  choosing treatment for life-threatening condition, 180-181
  diagnosis uncertain, 178-179
  doctor recommends, 176
  insurance company requires, 176
  surgery or major procedure recommended, 177-178
  symptoms persist, 179
  uncomfortable with treatment, 182

selecting doctor, 19-41. *See also* finding right doctor

Self-help clearinghouse, 278

specialists, 23-24
 American Board of Medical Specialties, 275, 307-310
 credentials and training, 29-33

performing procedures, 210
 superspecialists, 24

staff, befriending, 89

state medical licensing board, 35, 237-239

statistics, 86-88
 interpretation, 86-87
 probabilities, 87
 researching, 273

Steinberg, Dr. Alan
 activist HMO consumers, 65

student doctors, 10-11
 definition, 30
 right to refuse treatment from, 135

support organizations, 276-278
 encyclopedia of, 278
 on the Internet, 293-296

surgeons
 questions to ask prior to surgery, 228-231

surgery
 children's surgeries, 231
 geographical variation, 227
 inpatient or outpatient, 230
 questions to ask, 228-231
 rate of complications, 229
 recuperation time, 230
 risks, 226

T

talking to doctors. *See* communication

testing facility
 certification, 210
 qualifications, 210

test results, 212-214
 diagnosis, 215
 prognosis, 217
 treatment, 215-216

tests
 over-prescribed, 208
 patient demand for, 208
 questions to ask about children's procedures, 212

tests (continued)
questions to ask about tests, 209-212
routine, 206
understanding results of, 214-217
diagnosis, 215
prognosis, 217
treatment, 215-216
waiting for results, 212-214
Thomas, Dr. Lewis
loss of healing touch, 2-3
training credentials, 29-33
transfusions, refusal of, 135-136
treatment
based on test results, 216-217
communication about, 146
compliance with, 148-149
controversies of, 254
end-of-life decisions on, 136
patient participation, 134-135
right to refuse, 135-137
second opinions, 175-184
standard, 256-257
treatment guidelines, 97, 216
trust, loss of, 196-197
Tuskegee study of untreated syphilis, 251

U
U.S. Guidelines on Human Experimentation, 252-253
U.S. Pharmacopoeia Drug Information for the Consumer, 222
utilization management committee, 49

V
value system, match between doctor and patient, 8

W
waiting
excessive, 161
reason to change doctors, 194-195
to see doctor, 137
Webster, Barbara
doctor has different perspective, 153
treat the person, not the body, 121
unrealistic expectations, 144
will, living, 136

About the Author

Nancy Keene is one of the original developers of the O'Reilly Patient-Centered Guides series. She has been involved with the medical world for over two decades— both as a caregiver and a patient. Nancy's first book was *Childhood Leukemia: A Guide for Families, Friends, & Caregivers*, which was a blend of technical information and stories from over forty parents, children with cancer, and their siblings. Her second book was *Your Child in the Hospital: A Practical Guide for Parents*.

Nancy has long been interested in working with the medical profession to achieve results, rather than working against it. She organized the first ever parent/oncology staff panel at the hospital where her daughter was treated for leukemia to improve communication and to provide adequate pain relief for children undergoing repeated painful procedures. The *Journal of the American Medical Association* recently published her essay "He Lifted His Eyes," about a doctor who soothed her daughter's fears prior to surgery. Nancy spends considerable time talking with parents of children newly diagnosed with cancer, and is a tireless defender of children's medical rights.

Colophon

Patient-Centered Guides are about the experience of illness. They contain personal stories as well as a mixture of practical and medical information.

The pictures on the covers of our Guides reflect the personal side of the medical experience.

The cover of *Working with Your Doctor: Getting the Healthcare You Deserve* was designed by Edie Freedman using Photoshop 4.0 and QuarkXpress 3.32. The fonts on the cover are Onyx and Berkeley. Cover photo © 1998 Comstock, Inc.

The interior design is by Nancy Priest and Edie Freedman using Berkeley and Franklin Gothic fonts. The text was implemented in FrameMaker 5.5 by Mike Sierra. Composition was by Claire Cloutier LeBlanc, Sebastian Banker, and Will Plummer. The book was copyedited by Lunaea Hougland and proofread by Phyllis Lindsay. Sheryl Avruch and Melanie Wang provided quality assurance. The index was written by Nancy Keene.

Patient-Centered Guides™

Questions Answered
Experiences Shared

We are committed to empowering individuals to evolve into informed consumers armed with the latest information and heartfelt support for their journey.

When your life is turned upside down, your need for information is great. You have to make critical medical decisions, often with what seems little to go on. Plus you have to break the news to family, quiet your own fears, cope with symptoms or treatment side effects, figure out how you're going to pay for things, and sometimes still get to work or get dinner on the table.

Patient-Centered Guides provide authoritative information for intelligent information seekers who want to become advocates of their own health. They cover the whole impact of illness on your life. In each book, there's a mix of:

- **Medical background for treatment decisions**
  We can give you information that can help you to intelligently work with your doctor to come to a decision. We start from the viewpoint that modern medicine has much to offer and also discuss complementary treatments. Where there are treatment controversies we present differing points of view.

- **Practical information**
  Once you've decided what to do about your illness, you still have to deal with treatments and changes to your life. We cover day-to-day practicalities, such as those you'd hear from a good nurse or a knowledgeable support group.

- **Emotional support**
  It's normal to have strong reactions to a condition that threatens your life or changes how you live. It's normal that the whole family is affected. We cover issues like the shock of diagnosis, living with uncertainty, and communicating with loved ones.

Each book also contains stories from both patients and doctors — medical "frequent fliers" who share, in their own words, the lessons and strategies they have learned when maneuvering through the often complicated maze of medical information that's available.

We provide information online, including updated listings of the resources that appear in this book. This is freely available for you to print out and copy to share with others, as long as you retain the copyright notice on the print-outs.

> *http://www.patientcenters.com*

Patient-Centered Guides

Published by *O'Reilly & Associates, Inc.*
Our products are available at a bookstore near you.
For information: **800-998-9938** • **707-829-0515** • **info@oreilly.com**
101 Morris Street • Sebastopol • CA • 95472-9902

Other Books in the Series

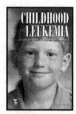 ## Childhood Leukemia
A Guide for Families, Friends, and Caregivers
By Nancy Keene
ISBN 1-56592-191-7, Paperback, 6 x 9", 539 pages, $24⁹⁵

This complete guide offers detailed and precise medical information for parents that includes day-to-day practical advice on how to cope with procedures, hospitalization, family and friends, school, social, emotional, and financial issues, as well as tools to be strong advocates for their child.

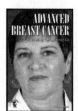 ## Advanced Breast Cancer
Holding Tight, Letting Go, 2nd Edition
By Musa Mayer
ISBN 1-56592-522-X, Paperback, 6 x 9", 520 pages (est.), $19⁹⁵

This updated edition contains new information on medical treatments for metastatic breast cancer. It offers the stories of 40 women and men as they live with metastatic breast cancer, often for many years. The book covers coping with the shock of recurrence, treatment decisions, managing side effects and pain, finding support, family issues, and dealing with emotions.

 ## Your Child in the Hospital
A Practical Guide for Parents
By Nancy Keene & Rachel Prentice
ISBN 1-56592-346-4, Paperback, 5 x 8", 128 pages, $9⁹⁵

This hands-on book provides tips and wisdom that will help make any hospital stay easier. It includes essential information on preparing your child, common procedures, surgery, pain management, feelings and behavior, keeping family life going, the nuts and bolts of hospital records, billing, insurance, and how to seek financial assistance.

 ## Choosing a Wheelchair
A Guide for Optimal Independence
By Gary Karp
ISBN 1-56592-411-8, Paperback, 5¼ x 8", 190 pages, $9⁹⁵

This is the only book of its kind that describes technology, wheelchair options, and the selection process to help identify the chair that can provide optimal independence. The book also includes difficult-to-find information on small, niche manufacturers and their chairs.

Patient-Centered Guides
Published by O'Reilly & Associates, Inc.
Our products are available at a bookstore near you.
For information: 800-998-9938 • 707-829-0515 • info@oreilly.com
101 Morris Street • Sebastopol • CA • 95472-9902

Here at Patient-Centered Guides we're dedicated to providing the most comprehensive practical, medical, and emotional information to readers such as yourself. Please take a moment to fill out the card below so we can learn how to better serve you and others.

We do not sell our mailing list to outside firms.

We'd appreciate hearing from you

Which book did this card come from?

_____

Why did you purchase this book?
❑ I am directly impacted
❑ A family member or friend is directly impacted
❑ I am a health-care practitioner looking for information
  to recommend to patients and their families
❑ Other _____

How did you first find out about the book?
❑ Recommended by a friend/colleague/family member
❑ Recommended by a doctor/nurse
❑ Saw it in a bookstore
❑ Online
❑ Other _____

❑ *Please send me the Patient-Centered Guides catalog.*

What sources do you use to gather your medical information?
❑ Friends/family   ❑ A library
❑ Your doctor   ❑ Your nurse(s)
❑ Television (which shows?)
❑ Newspapers (which newspapers?)
❑ Magazines (which magazines?)
❑ Newsletters (which newsletters?)
❑ The Internet (which newsgroups,
  mailing lists or Web sites?)
❑ Support Groups (which groups?)
❑ Other _____

What other medical conditions are of concern to you, your family, and community?

_____

_____

Name

Company/Organization (Optional)

Address

City   State   Zip/Postal Code   Country

Telephone   Internet or other email address (specify network)

BUSINESS REPLY MAIL

FIRST CLASS MAIL   PERMIT NO. 80   SEBASTOPOL, CA

Postage will be paid by addressee

O'Reilly & Associates, Inc.
101 Morris Street
Sebastopol, CA 95472-9902
Attn: Patient-Centered Guides